New Health Technologies: Managing Access, Value and Sustainability

OECD
BETTER POLICIES FOR BETTER LIVES

Please cite this publication as:
OECD (2017), *New Health Technologies: Managing Access, Value and Sustainability*, OECD Publishing, Paris.
http://dx.doi.org/10.1787/9789264266438-en

ISBN 978-92-64-26642-1 (print)
ISBN 978-92-64-26643-8 (pdf)

Photo credits: © Yannis Jacoby-Koaly pour Pykha.com.

Corrigenda to OECD publications may be found on line at: *www.oecd.org/publishing/corrigenda*.

Foreword

Technology has been a dominant force in health and medicine, contributing to longer and healthier lives for many people. An early milestone is the aseptic technique, devised in the 19th century, which dramatically reduced avoidable deaths. Antibiotics and vaccines remain, to this day, among the most successful health technologies. Since then, medicine has been strongly associated with technological progress, as a visit to any modern clinic, pharmacy or hospital confirms. Some technologies – insulin, for example, or treatment for heart attacks and stroke – have been remarkably valuable. Others, however, have delivered fewer gains.

Adoption of technology is a major driver of health expenditure growth. Policy makers constantly seek to reconcile access to innovative treatments with affordability, while maintaining incentives for innovation. Therapies tailored precisely to an individual's biology, digital innovations, and revolutionary technologies such as 3D bioprinting all present opportunities but also a complex set of technical, ethical, and financial challenges. Drugs tailored to a person's genetics may be expensive and unaffordable. Other new treatments are highly cost-effective, even at high prices, but if the conditions they treat are common, financial sustainability becomes a concern. Use of personal health data creates massive opportunities for health system improvement, research and disease surveillance, but requires the right governance frameworks to realise these benefits while managing risks.

Making the most of this complex landscape requires new policies and approaches. Policy frameworks governing the development and use of health technologies are not designed for the 21st century. Decision makers should modernise these frameworks to make the most of new technologies while also protecting patients and the public, spending resources more wisely, and fostering the "right" type of innovation in the future.

Many biomedical technologies are approved and adopted based on limited evidence of safety and effectiveness. Assessment of their performance under real-world conditions is rare. Many technologies are sometimes used inappropriately for little or no health gain. This compromises safety, is wasteful and undermines value to society. It is also no longer sustainable. Collecting real-world evidence, smarter use of information, education and engagement of providers and patients, and more transparent reporting of outcomes, are some of the policy levers that can encourage appropriate use of health technologies and inform decisions about the scope to be covered by payers. The prices paid for technologies must reflect their real-world health benefits compared to alternatives, and be adjusted based on evidence about their actual impact. Payers must be equipped with the necessary powers to adjust prices and withdraw payment for ineffective technologies. And more debate is needed on ways to deal with the budget impact of highly effective, but very costly treatments.

Developing the "right" type of innovation – safe, effective and affordable, aligned to population health needs – must be actively encouraged. Strong regulation and payment policy play a key role. Efforts to look over the horizon, identify promising trends and foster development of products that benefit health and deliver value for money are also needed, requiring greater collaboration across health systems and countries.

Given the continuing evolution of health technology in new and unexpected directions, managing new health technologies will remain a priority. Faced with budget constraints and the desire to offer patients access to most effective innovations, policy makers should think anew about the health innovation model. Leveraging the power of Big Data to make the current system work better, reviewing technologies that bring only limited health benefits, and thinking through novel approaches to manage areas where the current model does not work, are just a few of the needed solutions.

Acknowledgements

The preparation of this report was co-ordinated by Valérie Paris, who also co-authored several chapters. Chapter 1 was written by Valérie Paris, Luke Slawomirski and Allison Colbert, Chapter 2 by Luke Slawomirski, Allison Colbert and Valérie Paris, Chapter 3 by Valérie Paris and Allison Colbert, Chapter 4 by Valérie Paris, Luke Slawomirski and Allison Colbert, Chapter 5 by Valérie Paris, Allison Colbert, and Nicolas Delaunay, Chapter 6 by Luke Slawomirski and Jillian Oderkirk.

The team would like to acknowledge country delegates and experts, delegates from the European Commission, as well as members of the Business and Industry Advisory Committee to the OECD (BIAC), for their valuable comments on the draft and suggestions at the various stages of the project, in particular during the expert meeting of 22 March 2016 and the OECD Health Committee meeting of 28-29 June 2016.

This report has also benefited from the expertise, material and comments received from Stefano Bonacina (Karolinska Institutet), Michel Grignon (McMaster University), Iñaki Gutiérrez Ibarluzea (Osteba), Ruth Lopert (George Washington University), Andrew Stevens (Birmingham University), and Adrian Towse (Office of Health Economics).

At the OECD, the authors wish to thank Ane Auraaen, Léa Maitre (now at the Barcelona Institute for Global Health ISGlobal, Spain) and Ronni Gamzu (currently at the Tel Aviv Sourasky Medical Center, Israel), who contributed to initial research for various chapters, as well as Francesca Colombo, Mark Pearson, and Stefano Scarpetta from the Directorate of Employment, Labour and Social Affairs who provided thoughtful comments on initial drafts. Thanks also go to Natalie Corry, Duniya Dedeyn, Susannah Nash, and Isabelle Vallard for their administrative support and to Gaëlle Balestat, Lucy Hulett, and Alastair Wood for statistical and design support. The report was edited by Amy Gautam. We also thank Marlène Mohier for her help in preparing the manuscript.

Table of contents

Tables

Figures

Acronyms and abbreviations

3D	Three dimensional
AMI	Acute myocardial infarction
AMR	Antimicrobial resistance
CED	Coverage with evidence development
CMS	US Centers for Medicare & Medicaid Services
CT	Computed tomography
DNA	Deoxyribonucleic acid
DRG	Diagnosis-related group
EHR	Electronic health record
EMA	European Medicines Agency
EMR	Electronic medical record
FDA	US Food and Drug Administration
FFS	Fee-for-service
GDP	Gross domestic product
HCQI	OECD Health Care Quality Indicators
HIV/AIDS	Human immunodeficiency virus/acquired immunodeficiency syndrome
HTA	Health Technology Assessment
ICER	Incremental cost-effectiveness ratio
ICT	Information and communications technology
ICU	Intensive care unit
IHD	Ischaemic heart disease
IVD	In-vitro diagnostic
KCE	Belgian Health Care Knowledge Centre
LBWI	Low-birth-weight infant
LDT	Laboratory-developed test
MEA	Managed entry agreement
mHealth	Mobile health
MRI	Magnetic resonance imaging
NGO	Non-governmental organisation
NGS	Next-generation sequencing
NHS	UK National Health Service
NICE	UK National Institute for Health and Clinical Excellence
PAC	Pulmonary artery catheter
PM	Precision medicine
PMDA	Japanese Pharmaceuticals and Medical Devices Agency
PRIM	Patient-Reported Incident Measure
PROM	Patient-Reported Outcome Measure
QALY	Quality-adjusted life-year

R&D	Research and development
RCT	Randomised controlled trial
RWE	Real-world evidence
UDI	Unique device identification
WHO	World Health Organization

Executive summary

New technologies are entering health care systems at an unprecedented pace: remote sensors, robotics, genomics, stem cells, and artificial intelligence are on the cusp of becoming a normal part of medical care. Medicines can now be combined with nanotechnologies and digital tools. 3D printing is already used to manufacture implants, and bioprinting is expected soon to modify organ transplantation. Precision medicine, which establishes links between individuals' biology and their diseases, promises to increase our understanding of diseases and help better target treatments. Vast amounts of electronic data related to health and wellness are being generated by health systems and by individuals. Collectively, these data hold valuable information that could foster improvement in all health system activities, from clinical care to population health, to research and development.

These new technologies provide immense opportunities but also raise novel challenges for all health stakeholders, including policy makers, regulatory authorities, payers, physicians and patients.

New technologies challenge regulatory pathways in many ways. New types of products often combine technologies (medical devices, diagnostics and medicines) that are typically assessed before market entry by separate entities. The development of precision medicine, especially in cancer, involves new forms of clinical trials, sometimes including very few patients, questioning current standards for market approval. Regulators are pressured to provide rapid access to medicines for severe conditions with no available alternative.

Regulators recognise the need to strengthen regulation of medical devices, which has traditionally been less stringent than that of pharmaceuticals. The burgeoning field of mobile health (mHealth) is also a challenge for policy makers. The sheer volume and variety of new mHealth products, as well as the risks related to security of personal health data, calls for new regulatory models to determine what is safe and useful to patients, providers and the public.

More needs to be done after market entry to ensure sustainable access to innovative therapies while guaranteeing safety and efficient use of resources. Too often, products are only assessed for safety and performance at market entry. Monitoring these aspects as well as clinical utility in real life can manage risks for patients and identify devices that perform better than others.

In the pharmaceutical sector, the proliferation of high-cost medicines calls current pricing models into question. The launch prices of drugs for cancer and rare diseases are increasing, sometimes without commensurate increase in health benefits for patients. Payers increasingly struggle to pay for high-cost medicines targeting very small populations, which are becoming the "new normal" in the pharmaceutical sector. New treatments for hepatitis C, which are very effective and cost-effective, are unaffordable to many who would benefit in almost all OECD countries because of their high budget impact.

Despite much discussion about the potential of Big Data and information systems for public health goals of research, health system improvement and disease surveillance, progress is needed in many countries to set laws and policies that permit and enable use of health and health care data in a secure fashion.

Technology can only generate value in health care systems if the health benefits of these technologies outweigh the costs they impart. This can only be achieved by promoting access to and appropriate use of technologies that are safe, performant, effective and clinically useful.

This report analyses policies affecting the use of pharmaceuticals, medical devices, precision medicine, and digital technology (mainly the use of health data). It recommends policy makers to:

Steer investments in biomedical research and development (R&D) and prepare for upcoming technologies in the health sector

- Further co-ordinate efforts to identify gaps in global biomedical R&D and encourage research through co-operation between countries and stakeholders, with well-designed incentives.
- Engage in co-operative horizon scanning to better prepare for new technologies that have the potential to be disruptive or to raise financing challenges.

Adapt policies to regulate market entry of new technologies

- Ensure that quicker access to promising pharmaceuticals for severe unmet needs does not unduly compromise patient safety. Patients should be adequately informed about the quasi-experimental status of products with incomplete pre-market evidence.
- Strengthen regulation of medical devices to improve safety and performance, especially for those associated with higher patient risk. Improve post-market surveillance, notably through the implementation of a system that enables product identification. Increase efforts to monitor performance of medical devices in routine clinical use by leveraging health data, and share information across countries and regions.
- Adapt regulation to new technology types, including hybrid technologies, by promoting co-ordination between entities that typically manage separately different types of technologies.
- Adopt a regulatory framework for mHealth products, which ensures safety and manages risks to privacy and security, encourages high-value innovation, and prevents ineffective, unsafe and low-value products from flooding the market and crowding out the more beneficial ones.

Use health technology assessment, coverage and pricing policies to encourage value-for-money

- Use new methods to guarantee quicker access to treatments where effectiveness is uncertain or very different across indications, while also seeking to reduce uncertainty about the impact of treatments. Coverage with evidence development schemes, that have been used for pharmaceuticals (e.g. in the Netherlands, Sweden, and the United States) or for medical devices (e.g. in Australia, France, Germany, the Netherlands, Switzerland, the United Kingdom and the United States), can be used, provided that new evidence is produced on time and coverage conditions are revised accordingly.

- Promote a "lifecycle approach" for Health Technology Assessment (HTA) across all types of biomedical technology, whereby coverage and pricing decisions are not set only once at market entry, but regularly re-assessed.
- Develop methods to produce evidence on safety and effectiveness of treatments in real life (so-called "real-world evidence"), especially based on routinely collected data. Use these data to compare effectiveness and cost-effectiveness of treatments and influence care processes, complementing information collected from clinical trials.
- Regularly update provider payment schedules and introduce ad-hoc payments, as necessary, to encourage adoption of value-adding and cost-effective technologies.
- Rebalance negotiating powers of payers and manufacturers in the pharmaceutical sector. This could be achieved through increased transparency and cooperation between payers and international joint procurement initiatives – tested in Europe and Latin America. In the case of oncology, innovative pricing methods could be developed, such as bundled or indication-based payment. Performance-based pricing agreements (used in Italy and England) should be applied parsimoniously to avoid high administration costs and make sure that new evidence generated is made available to the community.
- Re-assess orphan drug legislation to make sure incentives are not diverted from their initial vocation to encourage R&D investments in areas that would not be explored otherwise.

Harness the potential of health data while managing risks appropriately

- Implement sound, fit-for-purpose governance frameworks to make the most of health data, while managing the risks appropriately. While no country has, to date, implemented the ideal information infrastructure and health data governance, potential models for harnessing opportunities include Denmark, Finland, Iceland, Israel, Korea, New Zealand, Norway, Singapore, Sweden and the United Kingdom (England and Scotland).
- Ensure strong data governance and technical and operational readiness to capitalise on the opportunity presented by Electronic Health Record (EHR) systems. A recent OECD survey suggests that Canada, Denmark, Finland, New Zealand, Singapore, Sweden, the United Kingdom (England and Scotland) and the United States are advanced in putting EHR data to work.

Chapter 1

New health technologies: Managing access, value and sustainability

by
Valérie Paris, Luke Slawomirski *and* Allison Colbert

This chapter presents an overview of the analytical report prepared by the OECD Secretariat for the 2017 Health Ministerial on "New Health Technologies: Managing Access, Value and Sustainability". The report discusses the need for an integrated and cyclical approach to managing health technology to mitigate clinical and financial risks and to ensure acceptable value for money. This synthesis chapter considers how health care systems and policy makers should adapt in terms of the development, assessment and uptake of health technologies. Following a brief examination of the past adoption and impact of medical technology, this synthesis chapter focuses on opportunities linked to new and emerging technologies as well as current challenges faced by policy makers. It concludes with a suggested new governance framework to address these challenges.

We thank Mark Pearson and Francesca Colombo for detailed comments on earlier versions of this chapter. We thank all country delegates and experts, as well as BIAC members, for their comments on earlier drafts and suggestions at various stages of the project, in particular during the expert meeting of 22 March 2016.

Introduction

Technology has profoundly affected the way medicine is practised and health care delivered. Thanks in large part to innovations in medical technology, modern health service is virtually unrecognisable from a few decades ago. While technology has delivered undisputable benefits to human health, however, it has done so at considerable cost. As such, the value – the health benefits compared to the costs[1] – of health technology is often called into question. Seen in these terms, not all technology, new or existing, may be worth the expenditure.

The health technology landscape is continually changing, with innovation moving in new directions: artificial intelligence, remote sensors, robotics, 3D printing, "Big Data", genomics, stem cells and more (Box 1.1). Introduction of these new technologies into health care systems sometimes represents disruptive changes in processes, relationships and resourcing. In a context of limited resources as well as rising public expectations for effective and affordable health care, policy makers must think pro-actively about the potential impact of new technology on sustainability, health gains and costs. Changing

Box 1.1. **Health technology – a basic taxonomy**

Health technology and innovation is defined as the application of knowledge to solve practical clinical and health problems, including products, procedures and practice styles that alter the way health care is delivered. Such a definition includes biomedical technology – such as medicines, medical devices and diagnostics (Dx) – as well as enabling technology such as mobile health (mHealth) and "Big Data". The definition also includes innovations in processes and care delivery. Process innovation is addressed in this report when it is a product of, or related to, the development and introduction of other types of technology. For example, single-day surgical procedures were enabled through development of medical equipment that permitted minimally invasive access to internal bodily structures, while digital technology has driven process redesign across all care settings.

Figure 1.1. **Health technology – a basic taxonomy**

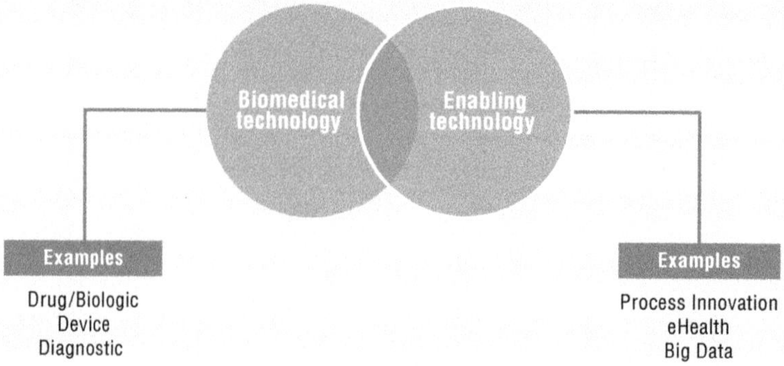

market dynamics for health technology necessitate new regulatory models and incentives. Existing institutions, regulatory pathways and reimbursement systems may no longer be fit for purpose.

This report considers how health care systems and policy makers should adapt in terms of the development, assessment and uptake of health technologies. The ultimate objective of health policy is to improve population health, often under budget constraints. To act towards this objective, policy makers need to:

- encourage development and adoption of technologies that help improve population health,
- ensure equitable access to these technologies, and
- promote the sustainability of health care systems.

This implies that technologies should be delivered at a price that offers value for money and is affordable. These principles guide the discussion and recommendations of this report.

Following a brief examination of past adoption and impact of medical technology, this synthesis chapter focuses on opportunities linked to new and emerging technologies as well as current challenges faced by policy makers. The chapter then suggests a new framework to address these challenges. The overarching theme is the need for an integrated and cyclical approach to managing health technology to mitigate clinical and financial risks and ensure acceptable value.

1. Impact of health technologies on health and health spending: Lessons from the past

The past provides some lessons for the development of policies to harness both emerging and existing technologies to achieve the objectives listed above. Progress in medical science has resulted in major advances in society's understanding of disease and its ability to develop and improve treatments. Numerous examples exist of immense health benefits derived from medical technology. While the costs of these innovations vary, most have delivered a decent return on the resources invested in their development and use (i.e. value). But some innovations have delivered little or no health benefit (but incurred considerable costs) and some were even harmful.[2]

Technology has influenced how health care is delivered in many ways: by expanding the number of treatable conditions and patient types; by substituting for existing interventions or targeting them more accurately; by intensifying the level of treatment for given conditions; and by changing processes of care delivery. The diffusion of health technology in concert with other factors such as income levels, reimbursement systems, medical culture and demographic change – has been a strong driver of the remarkable rise in health care expenditure in OECD countries since the mid-20th century. Depending on the approach used, attempts to estimate the direct impact of health technology on expenditure range from one-fifth to as high as 70% (Chernew and Newhouse, 2012). Given the differences between health care systems and the incentives they provide to actors and stakeholders, no single figure can be applied across all health systems. However, given the rising share of national income spent on health care across OECD countries, any point within the range of estimates is likely to be considerable. As health spending invariably displaces other areas of expenditure that also generate welfare, such as education, housing and infrastructure, the opportunity cost of expenditure driven by the adoption of health technology must be considered.

Based on research focusing on a subset of high-impact illnesses such as cardio-vascular diseases (CVD), cancer and infectious diseases in the United States, the additional cost of introducing technology in the past appears to have delivered acceptable levels of value and can therefore be deemed "worth it". Overall, the resources devoted to the development and application of health technology have yielded satisfactory results, generally measured through longevity gains and survival. However, this research is constrained by: 1) assumptions around attributing the health effect of the technologies examined against other, non-medical factors influencing human health; and 2) the absence of quality data on patient and population health outcomes extending beyond mortality into dimensions such as quality of life and function. Nevertheless, recognition is growing that in more recent decades, the escalating expenditure on technology-enabled therapies may not be matched by commensurate health gains. The cost-benefit function may be trending towards unfavourable territory, suggesting that a more prudent approach to implementation and adoption of technology is required in the future.

The impact of technology on patients, populations and health care systems is highly variable depending on the technology, its application, the disease or patient group, and the context in which it is used. Seen through the lens of value, health technology can be grouped into three types (Chandra and Skinner, 2008, 2012). The first type is technology that is effective in achieving its therapeutic aim and delivers high value. Cheap, "low-tech" technologies that can be broadly applied across populations feature strongly in this group. Costly interventions can also deliver considerable value if they are effective and their target population is clearly defined. Well-defined indication is a common characteristic of the costlier technologies of this type. Examples include the aseptic technique, vaccines, beta-blockers combined with aspirin, and antiretroviral treatment for HIV.

The second type includes technologies that, while effective in some indications, are prone to expanding their application across a population and to cases where their clinical utility is diminished. The decreasing marginal benefit dilutes the value derived from these technologies. Many diagnostic technologies (e.g. radiology and endoscopy) feature in this category. Cardiac catheterisation and angioplasty are other examples of a medical technology proven to benefit a certain category of patient, but whose application crept into patient types that could be better managed in other, often more conservative and less costly ways. Considerable geographic variation in the use of these technologies is often observed, partly driven by factors other than population health need. This is one of the reasons why even technologies that are cost-saving at individual level end up having an expansionary effect on aggregate expenditure: they are eventually applied to cases where they produce little benefit, thus undermining value.

The final type comprises technologies for which evidence of therapeutic benefit is weak or non-existent, and that are clinically equivalent to "watchful waiting" or less complex, conservative interventions. Many such interventions are costly in financial terms as well in the clinical risk posed by iatrogenic harm. They include some spinal surgery, a range of diagnostics such as liver function testing, and devices such as those that measure pulmonary artery pressure. Remarkably, provision (and reimbursement) of these interventions continues, despite decades of evidence for their lack of effectiveness in some cases.

The past indicates that the value of health care technology is undermined by its suboptimal and inappropriate application, diffusion and implementation. Similar benefit at lower cost could be generated from the therapeutic arsenal at society's disposal if more appropriate use was encouraged. Chapter 2 provides a number of examples. For example, wide variation in admissions to intensive care is observed, with little effect on clinical outcomes but a considerable inflation of costs. Aggressive medical interventions at the end of life can impose great financial costs with not only little benefit but – in many documented cases – disutility and suffering for patients and loved ones. Another example is antimicrobial resistance (AMR), to a large extent the result of unfettered application of the "miraculous" technology of antibiotics. Had more effort been made to ensure appropriate and prudent use of this technology – in both human and agricultural domains – the world would now perhaps not be facing the considerable cost of AMR.

The lesson for the future is that technology must be developed and applied intelligently, in a way that is based on evidence and with health benefits for individuals and populations the principal objective. The right policy settings can help maximise value derived from health technology. This will be critically important to ensure the financial and institutional sustainability of health care systems as more complex – and potentially costly – technology comes on stream in the next few years and decades. Enabling technology such as ICT (information and communications technology) is urgently needed to collect and provide better information for more rational deployment of treatment, interventions and health care system resources more generally.

2. Promises and challenges of new and emerging technologies

The flow of new technologies comes with many promises of future benefits for patients but also a number of challenges for policy makers. Some technologies blur the traditional frontier between medicines and medical devices or integrate digital technologies, requiring new regulatory pathways. Some are marketed at very high prices, impairing access to treatment and threatening the sustainability of current financing models.

2.1. New types of technologies challenge regulatory pathways

In the past, medical technologies were distinct from one another and used at discrete points of the care pathway. Today, technology categories increasingly converge in ways that profoundly alter the delivery of health care. Many of these technologies challenge regulatory systems, which traditionally address a single type of technology (medicines, medical devices).

Treatments are increasingly tailored to individual patients

Precision medicine (PM) holds the potential to radically transform medicine. Current research initiatives in this field are increasing the medical community's knowledge and capacity to predict, prevent and treat diseases (Box 1.2). So far, PM has mainly found concrete applications in the development of personalised or stratified medicines, which provide safer and more effective treatments to patients.

PM challenges regulatory pathways in many ways. First, new designs of clinical trials are tested out. In oncology for instance, trials where patients' treatment is selected according to the molecular characteristics of their tumour sometimes replace the traditional randomised controlled trial (RCT), which compare a treatment to a placebo. These trials have so far produced heterogeneous results, which suggests that prospective studies are still needed. In some cases, target populations are very small, trials cannot recruit hundreds of patients, and results must be inferred from very small samples. In addition, personalised medicines often target severely debilitating or life-threatening conditions for which no treatment is available. As a result, regulators are often under pressure to provide quick access to these medicines.

Box 1.2. **Precision medicine: some definitions**

Precision medicine (PM) is defined by the United Kingdom's Programme Coordination Group as "[refining] our understanding of disease prediction and risk, onset and progression in patients, informing better selection and development of evidence-based targeted therapies and associated diagnostics. Disease treatment and other interventions are better targeted to take into account the patient's genomic and other biological characteristics, as well as health status, medications patients are already prescribed and environmental and lifestyle factors" (Innovate UK, 2016). PM holds the potential to radically transform medicine, with a change of paradigm from "a medicine of organs (heart, liver)" to a medicine targeting cells, molecules, genes, etc. As an example, a few decades ago, blood cancers were grouped in five categories: chronic leukaemia, acute leukaemia, preleukaemia, indolent lymphoma and aggressive lymphoma. Today, medical science recognises 94 types of blood cancers (WHO, 2016), a refinement that contributed to the development of treatments that have improved five-year survival rates from virtually zero to as high as 82% for some subtypes (American Cancer Society, 2016).

Personalised or stratified medicines are pharmaceutical products whose approval is linked to the use of a biomarker[1] diagnostic test to determine the target population. Such a test is used to identify before or during treatment patients who are most likely to benefit from the corresponding medical product or patients likely to be at increased risk of serious adverse reactions. It is essential for the safe and effective use of the product. It is performed with an in vitro *companion diagnostic* device, whose use is stipulated in the instructions for use in the labelling of both the diagnostic device and the corresponding therapeutic product.

While biomarker diagnostics have been thought of so far in terms of "one test – one therapeutic strategy", the landscape is changing with the development of next-generation sequencing (NGS). NGS refers to a number of different modern sequencing technologies to sequence DNA and RNA much more quickly and cheaply than before. *Multiplex tests* – testing several biomarkers at the same time – are also being developed. For instance, three diagnostic tests in breast cancer now allow simultaneous testing for 12, 21 and 70 genes. NGS is expected to become more effective and potentially more cost-effective than current biomarker tests (Bücheler et al., 2014; Van den Bulcke et al., 2015) and may be preferred to individual biomarker tests associated with select treatments.

Whole genome sequencing (WGS – sequencing a person's entire genetic code) and *whole exome sequencing* (WES – limiting investigation to 1% of the genome) are also developing. In contrast with other types of tests, these tests are not designed to capture pre-defined data points (Evans et al., 2015). They can be used for several purposes and may also reveal incidental findings (information that was not sought), including "actionable" information (i.e. information that can be used to prevent or treat a disease). In France, the National Cancer Institute projects that by 2019, single gene tests will be totally replaced by multigene approaches for oncology patients (INCa, 2014).

1. A biomarker is a biological molecule found in blood, other body fluids, or tissues that is a sign of a normal or abnormal process, or of a condition or disease.

While controlled, comparative trials will likely remain the gold standard for pre-market evidence generation, these changes invite the development of new methods to assess the safety and efficacy of new medicines.

Second, as the safety and efficacy of personalised medicines depends on the performance and predictive value of the diagnostic test mentioned in their label, the approval of such medicines needs to take the latter into account. Today, regulatory requirements for the approval of biomarker diagnostic tests differ across countries but also depend on who develops and performs the test. In Europe and the United States, commercial in vitro diagnostics (IVD) need regulatory approval while laboratory-developed or in-house tests are not subject to the same level of requirements (Garrison and Towse, 2014). Without streamlined regulatory oversight of the quality and performance of all tests, health care systems may in turn struggle to effectively evaluate the costs and benefits of tests coming from varied sources and settings of care.

Finally, the development of multiplex tests and whole genome sequencing in clinical practice will require a number of adaptations to address technical and ethical challenges, such as: How will regulators and Health Technology Assessment (HTA) agencies determine the clinical utility of such diagnostic tools? What sort of patient consent should be sought and who is the owner of the information? Who will be responsible if "actionable" information provided by the test is not used to prevent or treat a disease in a given patient?

Mobile health applications are flooding the market

According to one estimate, more than 165 000 health apps were available in 2015, a figure that has doubled since 2013. These apps perform a constellation of functions: medication reminders, tracking movement and activity, monitoring fertility and progress of pregnancy, and analysing a person's speech to help in the management of mental health problems. Mobile health (mHealth) has the potential to improve health care by: continuous monitoring and timely response; interactions between patients and health professionals beyond traditional settings; and communication with systems that can provide real-time feedback along the care continuum, from prevention to diagnosis, treatment and monitoring. Such potential is welcome at a time of rising prevalence and incidence of chronic diseases and multimorbidity. As people's contact with the health care system shifts from short episodes of acute care to more sustained, long-term monitoring and management that requires a team-based approach, the utility of smartphones and portable devices will rise. In addition, mHealth favours patients' empowerment and engagement in the management of their own conditions. mHealth has the ability to put people at the centre of managing their health, to bring care closer to them, and to connect them with the right information, services and institutions at the right time.

But existing frameworks, processes and institutions are not adequately equipped to address these new technologies. Passive adoption of mHealth will not guarantee success in terms of either clinical outcomes or value for money. Successful integration of mHealth in health care systems requires a number of adaptations: the performance and clinical utility of mobile applications must be assessed for reliable and efficient use in health care, and financial incentives are needed to encourage take-up of mobile applications that are effective and cost-effective. In addition, exchanges of information must be protected by appropriate levels of security, and the expected individual and societal benefits balanced with privacy and security risks. Chapter 4 examines mHealth in more detail.

Combination products increasingly blur the line between drug and device technology

Many emerging medicines are "smart" combinations of drug and device technology. Examples include drugs containing nanotechnology to target tumours or clots, or "digital medicines" that deliver information on patient adherence. The common aim is to improve targeting of treatment with medicines, to enable them to reach the right area of the patient's body, for example, and to improve safety and effectiveness.

Combining the benefits of medicines and medical devices is not without risk. Evaluating such risks and benefits requires specialised expertise, which is why many countries have separate regulatory authorities for each technology type, or separate offices within the same agency. Evaluating evidence on a hybrid product therefore requires additional co-ordination and collaboration within and between health care systems.

Wearable devices and sensors employ digital communication tools

Traditional medical devices such as implantables (e.g. pacemakers) are employing digital communication tools to deliver and/or receive data, for example via a mobile application on patients' or providers' smartphone. Wearable devices and sensors can continuously transmit people's vital signs to their providers in real time, permitting more effective and tailored management of their health problems.

Such technologies combine the existing challenges in regulating medical devices with the emerging regulatory challenges surrounding mHealth, each discussed above. In particular, the performance of digital communication tools is paramount, as is adequate training and monitoring of users (providers and/or patients). This is true for any input to clinical decision making, but has become amplified as such treatment decisions become automated.

"3D printing" of devices is underway and bioprinting is emerging

3D printing is already commonly used in health care (for example, in dental care and joint replacement). 3D printing enables providers to create devices matched to a patient's anatomy, which in turn affects that device's safety and effectiveness. This causes disruption in the supply chain of such products, challenging not only the economic business model of the medical device industry, but also the regulation of these devices.

Issues around 3D bioprinting, currently in development, are even more challenging. 3D bioprinting applications engineer tissue from human cells. The ultimate goal of 3D bioprinting is seen as replacing damaged neurological tissue and entire organs to help meet the growing public health crisis of transplant organ shortages. However, this technology has other potential clinical applications – regenerative scaffolds and bones, bridge to transplant, in situ printing of cells directly onto a wound, or even potential cosmetic applications. While all bioprinted tissue is still currently experimental for human implantation, some tissues are beginning to enter clinical trials. A market is growing for bioprinted tissues to aid in research and development (R&D) – for example, studies of liver toxicity using 3D bioprinted liver tissue could be an eventual replacement for pre-clinical animal testing. This could potentially significantly reduce costs in the R&D process.

Regulatory considerations for 3D printing and bioprinting will largely hinge on the chosen model of dissemination. For example, in the case of 3D bioprinting, a key concern is defining the "product": is it the printer, the bioprinted tissue, or part of a surgical intervention? Most stakeholders expect that the existing regulatory pathway for cell/tissue products will apply, but the level of evidence required, and the detail to which the product is specified, need to be clarified as this technique moves towards human treatment.

2.2. The proliferation of high-cost medicines questions current pricing models

Payers are increasingly confronted with medicines with high price tags requested by manufacturers. Pharmaceutical spending is concentrating on specialty medicines.[3] While many specialty drugs offer considerable therapeutic value to patients and represent significant improvements over alternative treatment options, they usually have a much higher price than traditional drugs. A treatment for multiple sclerosis, for instance, now costs USD 60 000 per year, about ten times what it cost ten years ago (Hartung et al., 2015). A new gene therapy (Glybera®) entered the German market in 2014 at USD 1 million per cure. Notably, clinicians are refraining from using it because of its cost (Regalado, 2016).

Trends in oncology are particularly worrisome in this regard. The number of approvals for oncology indications is on the rise, with many more oncology drugs in the pipeline, while the prices of oncology treatments are soaring. In Australia for instance, the average reimbursement price per anticancer prescription drug increased by 133% in real terms between 1999 and 2012, while the price of all other prescription drugs increased by only 37%. As similar trends are observed in other OECD countries, the sustainability of current pricing models is questionable.

Trends in the orphan drug[4] market are also a subject of concern. The United States, the European Union, Australia and Japan have implemented policies to encourage development of medicines for rare diseases. These policies are a mix of incentives, such as tax credits on R&D expenditures, extended market exclusivity, regulatory assistance for clinical trials protocols, or reduced user fees for regulatory procedures. These incentives have undoubtedly fostered the development of orphan medicines, which now account for up to half of new molecular entities approved by the US Food and Drug Administration (FDA) every year. Orphan drugs, however, typically enter the market with very high prices, often exceeding USD 100 000. As a result, they are not available to all patients who need them. Among 60 orphan medicines with a marketing authorisation in Europe in 2010, almost all were available in France, the Netherlands and Denmark; two-thirds were available in Belgium, Hungary and Italy; but only one-third were available in Spain and Greece (Eurordis, 2010).

High-cost medicines do not always deliver commensurate health outcomes. The prices of medicines used for very severe conditions and/or diseases with no alternative treatment are too often disconnected from the health benefits they bring to patients. Many of these drugs are not cost-effective, according to standard thresholds.[5] A landmark study looking at 58 oncology medicines approved between 1995 and 2013 in the United States found that the average survival benefit was a little less than six months, while the treatment cost per life year gained – adjusted for inflation – increased by 10% per year (i.e. by USD 8 500 each year) to reach USD 207 000 in 2013. And these costs do not include the costs of other medicines or treatments used in combination nor the costs of dealing with adverse effects (Howard et al., 2015). For orphan medicines, incremental costs per quality-adjusted life year (QALY) gained often exceed USD 100 000 and even EUR 1 million in extreme cases (Schuller et al., 2015).

The approval of new treatments for hepatitis C in 2013 and 2014 raised a novel type of challenge in all OECD countries. These medicines represent a great medical advancement for patients, reaching cure rates of 95% or higher for specific population targets. Despite high prices, these medicines were assessed as cost-effective. However, the immediate budget impact of treating the entire population affected proved to be unaffordable for OECD countries and all payers decided to limit access to the most severely affected patients. For some countries, rationing access to highly effective treatments was a new practice and generated protests from both patients and clinicians. Beyond lack of access, the pricing strategy of the company marketing sofosbuvir (Gilead) raised a number of questions (see Box 1.3).

Box 1.3. **What is wrong with new treatments for hepatitis C?**

Gilead's pricing strategy raised legitimate questions and led to an investigation from the US Senate. Sofosbuvir (Sovaldi®) was initially priced at USD 84 000 for a standard 12-week course of therapy and sofosbuvir/ledipasvir (Harvoni®), launched a few months later by the same company, was priced at USD 94 500. In the United States, these two products contributed to a 12.2% increase in US prescription drug spending in 2014, in spite of access restrictions imposed by all payers. Yet only 2.4% of infected Medicaid beneficiaries got access to these treatments and the situation was even worse in prisons: while one-third of the 2.2 million prisoners are infected by hepatitis C, only 222 of them got access to these treatments in 2015 (Kapczynski and Kesselheim, 2016). In 2015, the list ex-factory price of a 12-week course of sofosbuvir across 26 OECD countries ranged from USD 48 999 in Japan to USD 84 000 in the United States. When adjusted for purchasing power parities, list prices appeared to be particularly high in Poland, Turkey, the United States and the Slovak Republic. By contrast, the lowest list prices were observed in Nordic European countries, Switzerland and the United Kingdom. Treating the entire population in these countries – assuming a 23% rebate in all of them – would cost from 10.6% of total pharmaceutical spending in the Netherlands to more than 150.0% of total pharmaceutical spending in New Zealand or Poland (Iyengar et al., 2016). While the price actually paid in each country is not transparent, treating the whole population would clearly be unaffordable in many countries, even with a 50% discount.

The US Senate report estimates the outlay for research and development for sofosbuvir at between USD 125.6 million and USD 942.4 million (estimates provided by Pharmasset – the initial developer of sofosbuvir – and Gilead, respectively). In return, Gilead earned USD 26.6 billion in the first 21 months of marketing for Sovaldi® (Kapczynski and Kesselheim, 2016), more than 25 times the initial R&D outlay.

Though Gilead made notable efforts to make these treatments available in low-income countries at highly discounted prices, affordability in high- and middle-income countries is a real issue. Even though countries may not want to treat all patients with a drug whose long-term effects are not yet known, current access sounds far too restrictive to doctors and patients. Many stakeholders condemn Gilead and believe that the company could reduce its price to widen access while still earning a sufficient return on investment. Though this reasoning seems at odds with the logic of value-based pricing (the medicine is cost-effective by the usual standard at the proposed price), it holds if one considers that the drug would be even more cost-effective at a lower price and that the total value created would be better shared between the company and society.

Debates on drug pricing mechanisms are flourishing on the international scene. Payers, doctors and patients increasingly question the rationale of companies' pricing strategies, which not only impair access but also do not seem sustainable. Whatever the perspective adopted, be it "fairness" or "value" (for patients and the general public), the outlook is discouraging. Well-meaning stakeholders acknowledge that trust between the pharmaceutical industry and other parts of society needs to be restored and pricing mechanisms revised.

2.3. Health care systems struggle to "pay for value"

As stated earlier, the ultimate objective of health care systems is to improve population health. Policy makers often act towards this objective under a budget constraint, which is more or less imposed on them. In addition, they are often expected to take into account the interest of the biomedical industry, whose knowledge-based activities are considered a strong economic asset in many OECD countries. This report primarily focuses on health policy. It considers that health policy should: 1) encourage the development and adoption of technologies (products and processes) that help improve population health; 2) ensure equitable access to these technologies; and 3) guarantee the sustainability of health care systems. This implies that technologies should be paid for at a price that offers value for money and is affordable.

Increasing pressure on public health spending, growing demand for health care, and the high pace of innovation require adaptations to the decision-making process to fund new technologies. Basically, societies cannot pay for everything and choices have to be made. If choices are not explicit, they might take the form of local rationing, the arbitrariness of which results in inefficiencies and inequalities. Therefore, policy makers need to ensure that they pay for new technologies that deliver value to patients, health care systems and societies.

Indeed, OECD countries increasingly refer to "value" to make decisions on coverage[6] and financing of health interventions. They increasingly use HTA to inform funding decisions and make public choices explicit. This is not, however, without ambiguity about the meaning of the term "value". In the extra-welfarist approach commonly used in health economics, value can be defined as the health outcomes achieved per dollar spent. In the pharmaceutical sector, for instance, value-based pricing[7] is envisaged as an interesting option to combine static efficiency (paying for good health outcomes today) and dynamic efficiency (providing the right incentives for future innovation). However, value-based pricing has proved difficult to implement in practice. In some market segments, such as oncology or rare diseases, prices are set at very high levels without commensurate benefits (Paris and Belloni, 2013). For medical services, providers' payments usually depend on the amount of resources engaged to produce them, without any reference to value. At best, "outcome-based payments" account for a small fraction of providers' payments (OECD, 2016).

The definition of value is a crucial issue. The underlying questions are: Do decision makers reflect "public preferences" when paying high prices for medicines that are not cost-effective? Is value limited to "health benefits related to incremental costs" or is it more than that? The response to these questions is ambiguous and depends on the perspective adopted (health care system or societal).[8] In the case of orphan medicines for instance, the extent to which the general public supports such decisions – reflecting a higher willingness to pay for patients with rare diseases – is not clear.

Researchers and stakeholders are exploring new methods to make more explicit the criteria and inputs used to determine value. In Europe, a range of stakeholders (payers, industry, experts, etc.) proposed a specific "value framework" to help assess the value of orphan medicines for reimbursement and pricing purposes (MoCA-OMP, 2014). This framework considers four criteria: the availability (or not) of therapeutic alternatives; the clinical effect of the medicine; the response rate; and the degree of uncertainty attached to evaluation. The framework suggests qualitative and quantitative benchmarks to assess the value of orphan medicines. More recent research, not specific to orphan medicines, also explores the possibility of using multicriteria decision analysis (MCDA) to make reimbursement and pricing decisions (Kanavos and Angelis, 2013). Such tools could potentially contribute to making coverage decisions, and the criteria on which they are based, more transparent and explicit. However, they do not have the ability to solve specific problems of unbalanced negotiation powers in certain therapeutic classes or affordability issues.

3. Appropriate diffusion and funding of value-adding technologies

To encourage appropriate diffusion of valuable technologies, OECD countries should: better prepare for new technologies; provide quick access to promising technologies for high unmet medical needs without compromising patient safety; strengthen the regulation of medical devices; adapt regulation to new health products; and use the potential of ICT to improve the safety and performance of new technologies and health care systems.

3.1. *Co-operative horizon scanning can be used to better prepare for new technologies*

As a first step towards priority setting and prudent allocation of scarce health resources, many countries are pro-actively thinking about medical technologies that are not yet on the market. Over half of OECD countries now deploy some degree of horizon scanning, most often to focus their immediate priorities for HTA. These early awareness and alert systems consider technologies in a two- to three-year horizon and some of them exhibit good practice by considering the broader governance impact of new technologies along the following dimensions: patient benefits, impact on process of care, regulatory considerations, purchasing and reimbursement considerations, utilisation/budget impact, legal and ethical considerations, and additional factors affecting appropriate dissemination of a new technology. International co-operation is common and developing in horizon scanning activities but opportunities exist to improve collaboration and shared work in this area to avoid duplication of effort.

Foreseeing technological changes in the medium to long term and assessing their potential impact on health care systems are more challenging tasks. The future of technologies considered at an early stage of their development is hard to predict and few countries actually conduct foresight studies in the health sector. Such studies, however, might be useful to envisage the impact of potentially disruptive technologies through scenarios, so as to envisage needed changes in regulatory frameworks and workforce planning and education.

Another area for improvement is the identification of unmet medical needs and priority for research. Such initiatives have recently taken place for Alzheimer's disease (OECD, 2015b) and AMR (Cecchini et al., 2015) – areas where a combination of scientific challenges and market failures led to failures in innovation (Box 1.4). It might be worth further identifying unmet medical needs to encourage research in neglected areas.

Box 1.4. Why are we not getting the technology we need? The case of AMR and dementia

Failure of the existing innovation model to produce health technology in areas of unmet need is illustrated by the emerging problems of antimicrobial resistance (AMR) and dementia.

AMR is now recognised as a top-order global health problem. Worldwide, AMR results in 700 000 deaths each year and if not addressed could escalate into a full-blown global health and economic crisis (Cecchini et al., 2015). While indiscriminate use of antibiotics is responsible for creating the problem, development of antibiotics to combat resistant

Box 1.4. Why are we not getting the technology we need? The case of AMR and dementia (cont.)

bacteria has slowed – the last major new class was discovered in 1987 (Butler et al., 2013). Given other policies to combat AMR (prevention; limiting antibiotic use), investment in this area has become unattractive. Incentives for private capital to develop new antibiotics are currently insufficient as the expected profitability is much lower than for other therapeutic categories, such as chronic diseases. In addition, cheap and effective diagnostic devices at the point of care are desperately needed, yet no such product has been developed. The same can be said for effective vaccines. The market is clearly not delivering in this important area.

Recent proposals suggest policy options to address this innovation failure (AMR Review UK, 2016; WHO, 2015; Cecchini et al., 2015). They aim to "delink" incentives from volume and comprise two categories:

- *Upstream interventions* target the early phases including basic research, which typically requires public funding due to the uncertainty of success, the time lags involved and the difficulties to appropriate returns. Examples include partnerships, grants and seed funding. While more financial risk is taken on by sponsors, enterprise participation is encouraged and it may be cheaper than downstream rewards (Spellberg et al., 2012).
- *Downstream mechanisms* – e.g. prizes or tax concessions – aim to boost the reward at the end of the development process. These reduce the risk to sponsors but they inflate the required amount because they essentially aim to replace returns through global product sales.

An ideal approach should combine up- and downstream mechanisms to encourage global innovation by lowering early development costs and boost the reward at the end of the development process. While countries have invested in the former, effective and large-scale action on the latter is still insufficient. Global research platforms may make research spending more cost-effective (Cecchini et al., 2015).

Dementia is emerging as another leading health priority across the world. Here the innovation problem is largely due to the complexity of the disease. This complexity results in high rates of research failure, necessitating alternative innovation models that reduce these risks. These include shared public-private funding, and a higher public investment in basic, upstream research (dementia makes up less than 0.5% of R&D budgets). Permitting early-phase clinical studies involving people with pre-symptomatic dementia must also be examined. As with AMR, global sharing of research data is crucial (OECD, 2015b).

Regulatory and reimbursement reform is another way to stimulate investment. Costs can be reduced by simplifying processes and harmonising them across countries. Clear reimbursement policies that ensure sufferers have access to effective interventions can reduce investor uncertainly. Industry, academia, regulators, payers and patient organisations each play important roles at various stages, and stronger collaboration between these groups is needed (OECD, 2015b).

AMR and dementia illustrate the problems with the current innovation system, which does not always deliver technology in the areas of greatest need. As global health burden patterns evolve and budgets tighten, governments and policy makers must become more pro-active and engage with industry throughout the development process to ensure that truly innovative products – in areas of health need – are developed to add value to patients, populations and the global community.

3.2. Quick access to promising technologies for unmet needs can be provided while still protecting patients

Market entry regulation needs to adapt to speed access to promising treatments for unmet medical needs, to improve safety and performances of medical devices and to address the specificities of new technologies.

Provide quicker access to promising medicines for unmet needs while mitigating patient risk

In the pharmaceutical sector, regulation of market entry is simultaneously perceived as costly and too stringent by pharmaceutical and biotech companies and some patients' associations, and as insufficient by public health experts. Both parties are right. On one hand, new drug approvals rely on demanding standards for producing evidence on safety and efficacy based on RCTs, which take several years to conduct and are costly. This sometimes delays access to promising medicines treating unmet medical needs, generating frustration for patients and clinicians.

On the other hand, current regulation is not entirely satisfactory. Several studies have shown that information communicated by companies responsible for conducting clinical trials is incomplete and biased towards good results. Too often, RCTs compare new products to placebos while in reality they will compete with existing treatments. In addition, patients recruited for RCTs are often not representative of the entire patient population, who, for example, may be affected by more than one disease, which in turn affects their response rate to the medicine.

Since the end of the 1980s and following pressure from the HIV patient community to expedite access to new treatments, regulatory agencies have implemented accelerated pathways to approve earlier and more quickly promising treatments for high unmet medical needs; i.e. severe diseases without any available treatments. Such treatments can be approved earlier in their development phase, with lower levels of evidence requirements, based on surrogate markers[9] instead of survival, for instance. In the United States and the European Union, conditional approval[10] can be granted on the condition that the company provides further evidence on the benefits of the medicine in real life.

Regulatory agencies are under pressure to do more. "Adaptive pathways" are under discussion in the United States and Canada and are being piloted in Europe. They consist of early approval based on incomplete clinical trial results, followed by post-marketing studies to be performed by companies. While it is reasonable to respond to patients with desperate needs for treatment, countries should consider several conditions to make the system work. First, patients must be adequately informed of the quasi-experimental status of products approved through such pathways. Second, regulatory agencies must be provided with the means to ensure that companies comply with their commitment to produce additional evidence within the agreed delay. The threat of withdrawal in case of non-compliance might be more effective than current systems of fines, which do not seem high enough to encourage compliance. Such an option would also clearly put the responsibility on firms in case of withdrawal. In addition, since adaptive pathways have the potential to significantly reduce the cost of producing evidence before market entry and provide companies with earlier returns on investments, payers and patients should benefit from these financial gains though lower prices and greater affordability. Finally, adaptive pathways should be reserved for exceptional circumstances and the generation of evidence before marketing authorisation should remain the standard rule.

Strengthen regulation of medical devices to improve safety and performance

The regulation of market entry for medical devices is often considered less stringent than that for pharmaceuticals. Evidence requirements for market entry vary across categories of devices according to potential risks for patients, but also across countries. Devices associated with higher risks for patients (such as those surgically implanted in a patient's body) are typically subject to higher scrutiny in all countries.

The regulation is nonetheless unsatisfactory in several respects. First, the high number of recalls after marketing authorisation suggests that evidence produced before market entry may not be sufficient. In Europe, where devices can be sold as soon as they get "CE marking"[11] from one of the dozens of notified bodies, safety problems are not uncommon. As notified bodies compete for user fees on the speed of their process and approval rates, they do not always apply the highest standards to grant approval. The fact that a vast majority of companies producing medical devices are small and medium enterprises is often invoked as a reason for not increasing approval standards, but this is not really acceptable from a risk management perspective.

Second, post-marketing surveillance systems,[12] which all primarily focus on safety issues, could do much more. The reporting of safety issues itself is incomplete, relying mainly on manufacturer reporting, with insufficient contributions from health care providers and patients. Post-marketing monitoring of performance is far from systematic. Yet national experiences of disease-specific registries have been very useful in identifying subperforming medical devices and influencing clinical practice and reimbursement policies. For instance, findings from Australia and the United Kingdom's orthopaedic registries showed that cemented hip prostheses were more performant than non-cemented ones. Similarly, a Swedish cardiac registry showed that drug-eluting stents – initially developed as a clinical improvement over bare-on-metal stents due to the slow release of a drug to prevent fibrosis – were actually less safe than bare-on-metal stents (Lagerqvist et al., 2007). Once the information becomes available, countries are more or less quick in making the best of it: while Sweden quickly adopted cemented prostheses in 98% of hip replacements, France only used them in 51% of cases in 2012. Such information is crucial to improve the quality of care and should diffuse more rapidly across borders.

Many countries have indeed acknowledged the need to more rigorously regulate medical devices. Revisions to the relevant EU legislation to strengthen the regulatory process were finally agreed upon and in the process of adoption at the time of writing (Council of the European Union, 2016). These revisions include: a more comprehensive description of risk classification and management; reinforcement of rules concerning clinical data; stricter pre-market control of high-risk devices; reinforced requirements for manufacturers to collect data on real-life performance of their device; and introduction of EU-wide standardised information for patients receiving implants (Hansson, 2016). These changes are expected to increase transparency and improve safety, notably through systematic reporting of clinical investigations, improved oversight of notified bodies by competent authorities, and how compliance of rules for clinical investigations comply with international standards to facilitate use of their results by other jurisdictions. Post-market vigilance will be improved through: an electronic system and a central database of incident reporting; requirements for manufacturers to establish a risk management system; introduction of a unique device identification (UDI) system; and better access to information for all stakeholders. The United States also introduced UDIs for devices to enhance traceability and monitoring. This information not only allows closer monitoring of devices but also offers great opportunities, when associated with electronic health records (EHRs), to produce real-world evidence (RWE) on the safety and comparative performance of competing medical devices. Countries should seize this opportunity and imagine ways to share evidence more effectively with their counterparts.

Adapt regulation to hybrid technologies and mobile applications

Countries need to respond to regulatory challenges posed by hybrid technologies, such as PM, wearable devices and 3D bioprinting. An example of regulatory response comes from the United States. In 2002, the US FDA created a special Office of Combination Products (OCP). The OCP's role is to ensure timely and effective pre- and post-market review of combination products by overseeing the timeliness of and co-ordinating reviews involving more than one agency centre. The OCP also streamlines submission of a single investigational application for a combination product, if appropriate, determining the need for separate marketing applications on a case-by-case basis. A sponsor may also choose to submit two marketing applications for a combination product to receive some benefit that accrues only from approval under a particular type of application (e.g. new drug product exclusivity, orphan drug status, or proprietary data protection when two firms are involved).

In Australia, the Therapeutic Goods Administration (TGA) recently recognised that some therapeutic products do not fit neatly within traditional categories. The TGA now provides a list of device/medicine boundary products that have been approved and identifies whether they have been classified as a medicine or a device. The TGA is also undergoing a broader review of its current regulatory pathways, which may help in providing assistance in determining the most appropriate regulatory pathway for these new therapeutic products. Challenges will remain in those countries where medicines and medical devices are regulated by different agencies. Progress in convergent medical technologies will require reshaping existing institutional structures to allow effective and timely regulatory reviews that cut across traditional disciplinary boundaries.

OECD countries also need to respond to specific challenges raised by developments in PMs and biomarker diagnostics. In the United States and Europe, reforms are under way or in discussion to harmonise regulatory requirements for IVD tests, be they developed by commercial sponsors or in laboratories.

In a similar vein, policy makers face distinct regulatory challenges regarding ICT, specifically mHealth applications. Some applications are embedded in medical devices and thus already subject to regulatory review. However, mobile applications available directly to consumers increasingly blur the line between wellness and medical advice.

To respond to the mHealth revolution in a manner that protects patients while not hindering appropriate innovation, health care systems should create a regulatory framework that ensures safety in terms of clinical risk and risks to privacy and security, encourages high-value innovation, and prevents ineffective, unsafe and low-value products from flooding the market and crowding out the more beneficial ones. Owing to the peculiarities of this domain – its rapid evolution, the entry of new actors and stakeholders, and the extension of the risk profile to data privacy – an innovative regulatory approach is required with appropriately nuanced processes, expertise and oversight. Some jurisdictions recognize this and are moving in the right direction.

3.3. A lifecycle approach for Health Technology Assessment can be adopted to inform coverage and funding decisions

HTA is increasingly used to inform coverage and funding decisions, but payers could do more to respond to challenges raised by earlier approval of promising technologies and to improve the performance and value of medical devices.

HTA methods, use, scope and role vary widely across countries and across technologies. While some countries systematically use HTA to inform coverage decisions (e.g. Australia, France), others only assess new technologies with uncertain effectiveness or high prices (e.g. England). HTA systematically includes an economic evaluation in some countries (e.g. Australia, Canada, England, Sweden) and only occasionally in others (e.g. France). In many but not all countries, medicines are more often subject to HTA than other technologies or procedures (Auraaen et al., 2016).

In most cases, HTA is performed once, at or just after market entry, relying on evidence existing at that time. It commonly informs one-off decisions to include new technologies in the range of benefits covered by health care payers. Only a few countries perform systematic or ad hoc re-assessment of technologies to adjust the range of benefits covered. Withdrawals from the "benefit basket" happen rarely and are most often due to obsolescence of clinical interventions or budgetary cuts, without much reference to HTA. Systematic re-assessment of all technologies after a given period of time would probably cost too much for the expected benefits, but ad hoc re-assessments, triggered by the production of new evidence or where initial assessment was inconclusive, are desirable.

Better articulate approval, Health Technology Assessment, coverage and funding decisions

For pharmaceuticals, the trend towards earlier approval based on lower levels of evidence complicates HTA expected to inform coverage or pricing decisions. For a number of recently approved medicines, HTA agencies struggled to assess clinical benefits, let alone cost-effectiveness, and were not able to provide conclusive assessments to decision makers. In such cases, payers face a dilemma: they can either delay decisions to reimburse a product or base their decisions on incomplete evidence.

Coverage with evidence development (CED), which conditions positive coverage decisions on further development of evidence, is used in several countries as an option for select medicines, devices and procedures. At the end of a specified period of evidence development, payers are expected to get more information from the company on effectiveness and sometimes cost-effectiveness of the technology, and to then decide whether to continue or stop coverage or to restrict coverage to subgroups of indications or populations. The Netherlands, Sweden, and the United States (Medicare), for instance, use such approaches. Results of these experiences are mixed but enough experience has been accumulated to draw some lessons. First, it is very difficult to stop coverage on economic grounds, whatever the results of the assessment, especially when the treatment concerns severe diseases with no alternative treatments. Second, in some cases, compliance with evidence development requirements is poor, suggesting that incentives are insufficient for companies to respect their commitments.

To deal with uncertainty and lack of evidence, payers increasingly use performance-based managed entry agreements (MEAs) for pharmaceuticals, linking the final price paid for a medicine to its performance in real life. In such arrangements, the effectiveness of the medicine observed in real life is compared with benefits claimed by the manufacturer. If observed outcomes are lower than expected, the company has to refund a share of the costs incurred. Most often, financial arrangements take the form of *ex post* rebates, but they can also consist of provision of free stocks, for instance. These agreements are widely used in Italy and England, mainly for oncology medicines. Here again, results are mixed. In Italy, the scheme was assessed as quite burdensome in terms of administration; the amount recouped by the National Health Service accounted for only 5% of total spending for the relevant indications, not reflecting high therapeutic success but rather difficulty in getting results from companies on post-marketing assessment. More generally, clinical results of performance-based MEAs – 40% of which concern oncology medicines in Europe – are usually not made available beyond involved parties. To date, the experience is that performance-based agreements do not increase knowledge on therapeutic benefits of new drugs. If decision makers and payers continue to rely on MEAs to manage uncertainty in spite of these contrasting results, their use should be limited until the associated challenges are overcome. In all cases, post-market evidence should be made available to the scientific community and international counterparts.

Finally, parallel or joint early dialogue (scientific advice) between regulatory agencies and HTA agencies could help pharmaceutical companies design and shape pivotal studies to answer (ideally) all questions; i.e. the demonstration of safety and efficacy for marketing authorisation and comparative effectiveness study by comparison to standard reference treatment for HTA. Such early dialogue is currently promoted at the European level, involving a network of HTA agencies and the European Medicines Agency. It could reduce development time and costs and accelerate access to treatment. A multistakeholder dialogue was engaged in Europe to move in this direction.

Use real-world evidence to adjust technology coverage

Collection of RWE could significantly improve the management of new technologies. Such evidence can be collected in two ways: through post-market studies designed to collect specific information on health outcomes, and potentially costs; or through routinely collected data. In both cases, assessment methods differ from that used in initial pre-market clinical trials and need to be refined. RWE cannot be expected to fill information gaps in situations where original pre-market evidence assessed a product's efficacy with a high-level of uncertainty. In addition, the effectiveness of a medicine in real life depends on a number of factors – including patient compliance – that usually do not affect clinical trials. However, RWE can be useful in helping to understand how a clinically effective product performs in different real-life circumstances. This information could, for example, be useful in revising posology, better targeting treatment (e.g. if it becomes clear that some patients with co-morbidities do not respond well), or revising cost-effectiveness estimates. These revisions could be reflected in coverage conditions.

New capacities in the generation and use of health care data offer great opportunities to fill information gaps – for both new and existing treatments. Information produced by clinicians, facilities, payers and patients themselves increasingly allows the generation of RWE; i.e. critical information on the safety and effectiveness of technologies in real life. An additional legal framework may be required to create incentives for doctors, patients and companies and to balance evidence generation with patient data protection. This will require adapting existing HTA agencies and methods. Instead of considering HTA as a one-off event, stakeholders should continuously draw upon RWE to monitor the use of medical interventions and their outcomes and to continually update coverage conditions and clinical guidelines (Figure 1.2).

Figure 1.2. **Lifecycle framework for successful integration of health technologies in health care systems**

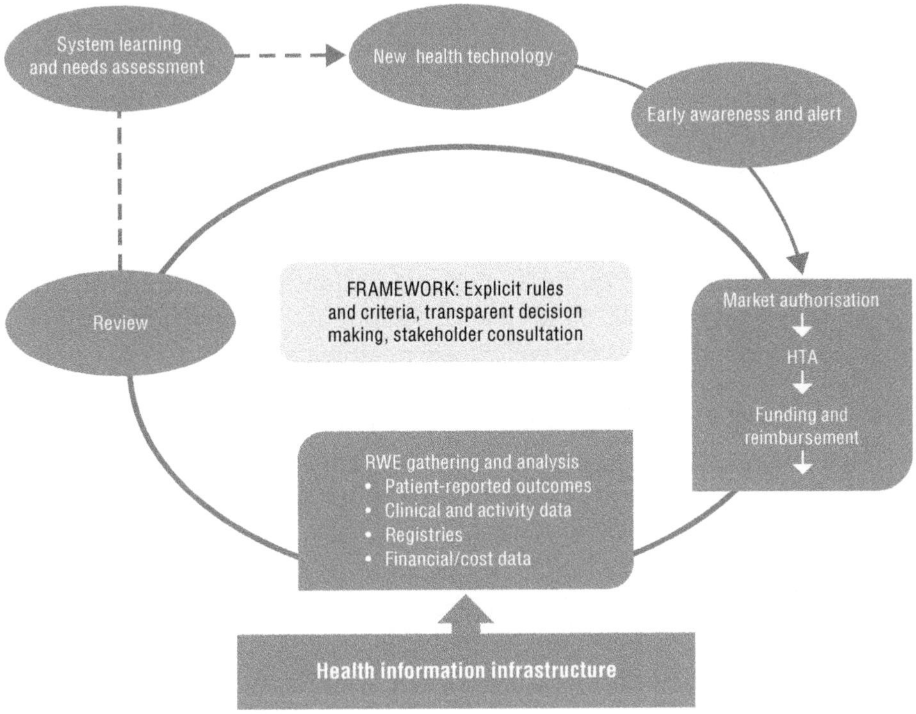

An open question is who will generate and fund the collection of such evidence. In some cases, the payer might be equipped and willing to bear the cost. In other cases, the promoter of the technology could be requested to do so. In any case, stakeholders should consider health data a public good and share both findings and data. International collaboration, including among experts, might be required to set high standards for the production of high-level evidence. At the EU level, several initiatives are targeted towards producing high standards for RWE generation (i.e. PARENT,[13] IMI GetReal[14]) and the European Network of HTA agencies (EUnetHTA) is working on methodologies to support post-marketing evidence generation.[15]

3.4. *Solutions are needed to manage access to and budget for high-cost medicines*

Countries need to find solutions to respond to the proliferation of high-cost medicines. They should first seek mechanisms to increase the negotiating powers of purchasers (payers and providers). Second, they should re-examine the incentives created by orphan drug legislation.

Seek mechanisms to increase purchasers' negotiating power

In pharmaceutical markets, the respective negotiation powers of purchasers and sellers need to be rebalanced. One option envisaged to increase purchasers' power in negotiations with global companies is joint procurement. Several countries in Europe and Latin America are working on such initiatives. This can only work if participating countries share a number of policy goals and characteristics, such as comparable income levels and/or willingness to pay. At a minimum, countries and payers should increase transparency and exchange of information to reduce the information asymmetry between them and global companies.

Payers are also seeking opportunities to foster competition in some therapeutic areas, such as oncology. Competition could occur at the level of providers or at the level of purchasers, through calls for tender for instance, provided that several medicines have the same indication and comparable effect on patients. This is not an easy task as providers and patients generally value choice and like having access to a wide range of therapeutic options. This is complicated by the fact that treatments are increasingly tailored to patient categories (i.e. PM), reducing opportunities for competition.

Finally, more radical options are proposed, such as compulsory licensing where affordability of essential treatments is impaired by pricing strategies. OECD countries, however, have been reluctant so far to use this option, even where it could be used (Kapczynski and Kesselheim, 2016), for fear of sending too negative a signal to investors and companies investing in R&D to develop new treatments.

Re-assess the relevance of incentives created by orphan drug legislation

OECD countries should assess whether incentives based on the extension of the market exclusivity period beyond original patent protection work as intended and are still relevant. Such incentives exist for all medicines and have been implemented to compensate developers for the length of the regulatory approval. Orphan medicines benefit from a further extension of market exclusivity and from a number of financial incentives, aimed to encourage their development and address market failures, such as tax credits, earlier and easier approval, waiver of regulatory user fees and extended market exclusivity.

The costs and benefits of incentives for orphan medicines, in particular, need to be examined. Incentives to invest in the development of treatments for rare diseases have been successful: the number of orphan medicines has continuously increased. The industry now envisages the development of orphan medicines as a good business opportunity, since all incentives are now combined with exceptionally high prices (EvaluatePharma, 2015). From payers' point of view, this is becoming a bitter pill to swallow. In spite of public support, including funding of basic research in addition to incentives mentioned above, orphan medicines are not available and affordable to all patients who need them. Moreover, companies are suspected of adopting "salami-slicing strategies" by marketing new medicines with narrow indications to claim an orphan drug status and a high price and then develop other indications (orphan or non-orphan). Finally, some orphan medicines perform very well – two of them are in the 50 top-selling medicines worldwide – which suggests that they may not need additional public subsidies to be commercially viable. Policy makers should launch a global assessment of the costs of public incentives for orphan medicines and of associated benefits, in terms of access to treatment and health benefits brought to patients.

3.5. Information infrastructure and governance can be constructed to realise health technology potential

Vast amounts of digital health data are generated by health care systems, and increasingly by individuals themselves, through the digital technologies mentioned above as well as by everyday activities such as social media and web browsing. An unprecedented amount of health-related data now flows across all areas of the economy, and advances in computer science enable them to be captured, stored and processed more effectively.

Health care systems are often thought of as data-rich and information-poor but emerging techniques and technologies – and more importantly, a new mindset of data as a valuable resource as opposed to a by-product – can enable the extraction of valuable information from these mountains of data.

Putting health data to work presents many opportunities to improve population health and individual outcomes. These opportunities can be grouped into four overlapping themes:

- *Improving patient care.* Information derived from health data can help providers in all settings manage uncertainty, and can enable more accurate, timely and co-ordinated decision making. It can also help evaluate and improve the effectiveness of therapies, care models and treatment protocols, and enable better personalisation and continuity. For example, data algorithms are improving the accuracy of personalised treatments for cancer, and accurately identifying people with chronic disease at risk of hospital admission.
- *Managing the health care system.* Analysis of health data can help monitor performance and drive greater transparency, accountability and continuous quality improvement. It can inform decisions regarding resource allocation and priority setting across health care systems. In the future, an integrated information system may enable funding and contract management based on health outcomes as opposed to volumes of services.
- *Enhancing surveillance and population health.* "Big Data" analysis especially can enable more accurate surveillance of population health care needs, help predict changing needs and help model new service configurations. For example, analysis of clinical, social care, environmental, socio-economic and commercial data combined with individuals' data on daily activities and/or sentiments can be deployed to predict acute exacerbations of chronic disease.
- *Enabling health research.* Better use of data enables research that is faster, deeper and of considerably larger scale than was previously possible. This should lead to richer evaluation of clinical and public health interventions, driving more productive investment in health. It can enhance prevention and treatment of complex diseases such as dementia.

Realising these opportunities can help establish the goal of a "learning health care system", leading to better health outcomes and more effective and efficient use of scarce resources. This includes providing the infrastructure and tools to evaluate the safety and utility of health technology in a consistent and cyclical fashion (Figure 1.2). However, to build such a 21st century information infrastructure, the right institutional and governance mechanisms need to be in place.

To generate useful information from health data, routine linkage of sources containing relevant data must be enabled, as no one dataset will contain all the necessary information. Health care systems still tend to capture data in silos and analyse them separately. Standards and interoperability are key policy issues that must be addressed – for example, in implementing an EHR (Box 1.5). In practice, interoperability means common protocols and ontologies that define the basic mechanisms by which users negotiate, establish, manage and exploit data. A 2013-14 OECD survey revealed that only a minority of countries regularly link all relevant health databases (OECD, 2015c).

A 2016 OECD survey of 30 countries revealed that most countries are investing in development of EHRs, but only some are actively progressing the possibility of putting the data to work to realise the opportunities listed above (more detailed results of the survey are

Box 1.5. **The electronic health record**

A key part of health information infrastructure is the electronic health record (EHR) – a comprehensive interconnected database that can capture and share a variety of information about people's health status, their history of encounters with the health care system, the results of all diagnostic and therapeutic interventions, and (ideally) their key social and demographic characteristics.

The critical functions of the EHR are that it puts information about people's health and their disease management within easy reach and provides them with the opportunity to contribute information to their record. The latter is important. For example, patient-reported measures on outcomes of care are valuable to providers, regulators, payers and researchers as well as other consumers.

Implementing an EHR is an industry-wide transformation, and mirrors the requirements of establishing a general health information infrastructure. It includes enactment of new legislation, for example to ensure the protection of information privacy; appropriate governance mechanisms; standards for both semantics and for the interoperability of EHRs across different settings; engagement of regional authorities, insurers and health care providers in the effort; collaboration with vendors and the private sector; and training and public education (OECD, 2013).

provided in Chapter 6). Nine countries exhibit both high governance readiness and high technical and operational readiness to harness EHR data. Others still have a way to go. These nine counties are overcoming challenges ranging from garnering adequate financial and human resources, to managing culture change, to effectively engaging the public, to ensuring data usability, quality, security and privacy protection. They are well-positioned to capitalise on the opportunity to develop world-class health information systems that not only support information needs regarding health care system quality, efficiency and performance reporting, but also create a firm foundation for scientific research and discovery.

Realising the potential of data requires not only investment in technical infrastructure but also human capital and expertise. Health care systems that are successfully modernising their information systems are recruiting and training data scientists, security experts and biostatisticians. It is also important to have health professionals and managers at ease with the fundamentals of data science and computing. Providers, policy makers and managers must have the requisite knowledge and skills to work with computer processing experts and ICT and legal professionals in developing and using the tools offered by digital technology (OECD, 2015a). This can go some way to overcome their reluctance and to help them embrace the opportunities of health data at all levels of the system.

Many OECD countries report legal barriers to the use of personal health data. As mentioned above, this includes enabling data linkages and developing databases (OECD, 2015c). A key problem is that the legislative instruments governing data, privacy and security pre-date the digital era; meanwhile, the lines between the various uses of health data are blurring, as is the case in the area of dementia (OECD, 2015b). Legal mechanisms enabling the use of health data need to be updated periodically.

Collection and use of personal health data present a number of important risks to the privacy of individuals. These can contribute to a loss of public confidence in government and its institutions. Yet equally significant risks to individuals and societies arise when health information assets are not developed, are unused, or are very difficult to use. The OECD developed a governance framework that contains technical, legal and political mechanisms to help realise the benefits and manage the risks of using health data in a transparent, explicit way (Figure 1.3) (OECD, 2015c). The OECD Council Recommendation on health data governance will assist countries with these challenges (OECD, 2017).

Figure 1.3. **OECD health data governance framework**

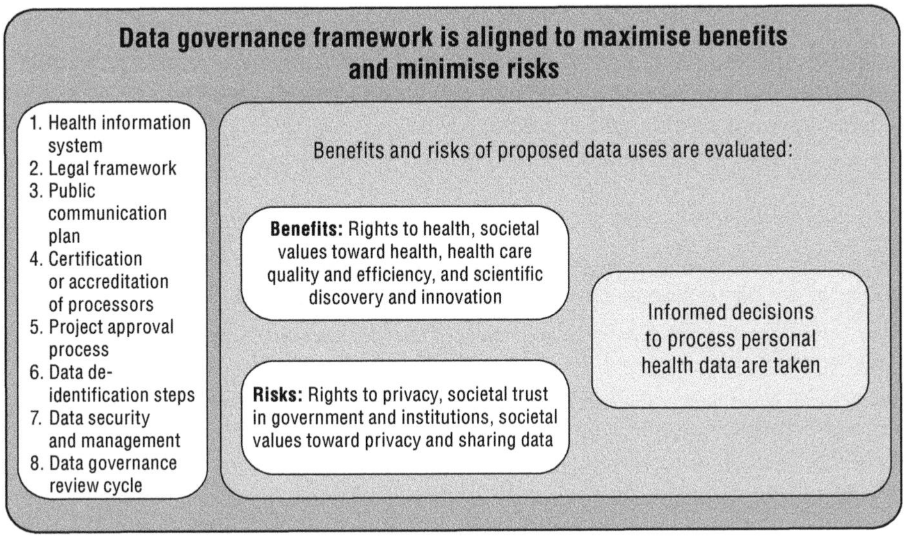

Source: OECD (2015), *Health Data Governance: Privacy, Monitoring and Research*, OECD Health Policy Studies, OECD Publishing, Paris, *www.oecd.org/publications/health-data-governance-9789264244566-en.htm*.

Conclusion

The sustainability of health care systems depends on intelligent adoption of technologies that enable gains in population-based outcomes. When technologies emerge that provide clear evidence of patient benefits in an affordable manner, they must be integrated into the health care system as soon as possible to improve its performance. Equally, policy makers must create the right institutions and mechanisms to ensure that technologies that do not deliver value to patients and societies are excluded from coverage and funding, and do not enter routine use across health care systems. This can be achieved by:

- Better preparing for new technologies through co-operative horizon scanning activities.
- Considering new incentives and mechanisms to address gaps in the pipeline of delivering innovations in areas with large unmet needs.
- Ensuring prompt access to treatments for severe diseases without alternative therapeutic options, without compromising safety, through conditional approval and/or coverage and assessment of products' performance in real life. This should be accompanied by clear messages to companies, patients and providers that new evidence may lead to coverage restrictions or price reductions – and by the necessary mechanism to do so.
- Adapting the regulatory framework to new types of products (hybrid technologies).
- Aligning economic incentives in health care systems to encourage take-up and diffusion of cost-effective technologies and appropriate use ("pay for value").
- Rebalancing negotiating powers of buyers and sellers in segments of the pharmaceutical market where prices are too high and re-examining the costs and benefits of incentives embedded in orphan drug legislation.

- Seeking opportunities for digital technologies and data analytics to improve care delivery, ensure secure and easy access to information by the appropriate parties, and improve population health outcomes via access to digital services.

In a context of unprecedented technological change, the overarching objective for policy makers should be, more than ever, to pay for value, thereby ensuring that new value-adding technologies are accessible to patients who need them, while discouraging or stopping to pay for innovations that do not provide value. Critically, this will require leveraging and mobilising new data and information systems at all points throughout the innovation and care process to increase ongoing generation and validation of knowledge about patient care, outcomes and efficiency.

Notes

1. This is the definition of value predominantly adopted in this report. For more detailed discussion on the use of the term value, see Box 2.1 in Chapter 2.
2. Chapter 2 provides a more detailed discussion of the past impact of health technology on health, expenditure and value.
3. These include most injectable and biologic agents used to treat complex conditions such as rheumatoid arthritis, multiple sclerosis and cancer and often require special handling or delivery mechanisms.
4. Orphan drugs refer to medicines developed for rare conditions. Countries use different thresholds to consider if a disease is rare: "rare conditions" are those that affect less than 1 in 1 500 people in the United States, less than 1 in 2 000 people in the European Union and less than 1 in 2 500 people in Japan.
5. In practice, economic evaluation most often consists of cost-utility analysis via estimation of an incremental cost-effectiveness ratio (ICER), i.e. the ratio of incremental costs to incremental benefits (measured in QALYs) of the new technology, by comparison with a reference treatment. In principle, this should go along with the definition of an ICER threshold, beyond which the assessed technology will not be funded through health coverage schemes (Culyer, 2016). Countries are often reluctant to set ICER thresholds. According to an OECD survey conducted in 2014-15, only five member countries (Hungary, Korea, Poland, the Slovak Republic and the United Kingdom) have published such a threshold.
6. Coverage in this report refers to funding by health coverage schemes, be they residence-based universal health coverage schemes or health insurance.
7. I.e. setting the price of medicine in relation to health gains.
8. Box 2.1 in Chapter 2 of this report reviews different conceptions of value in health care systems.
9. A "surrogate marker" is a laboratory measurement or physical sign that is used in therapeutic trials as a substitute for a clinically meaningful endpoint that is a direct measure of how a patient feels, functions or survives and is expected to predict the effect of the therapy.
10. Conditional approval consists of temporary approval of a medical product for a given period during which the company is required to provide further evidence of its safety and effectiveness.
11. CE stands for *Conformité Européenne*, and is a mandatory conformity marking for certain products sold in the European Economic Area. The CE marking represents the manufacturer's declaration that the product meets European standards, either via self-certification or working with an organisation called a "notified body", depending on the level of risk of the product. Medical devices are subject to such CE marking standards, as are products such as machinery, toys and radio equipment. National competent authorities in each country identify one or several "notified bodies" accredited to conduct "conformity [to EU Directive requirements] assessments". There were 59 notified bodies at the time of writing.
12. Post-marketing surveillance (PMS) is the practice of monitoring the safety of a pharmaceutical drug or medical device after it has been released on the market.
13. See *http://patientregistries.eu/*.

14. See *www.imi-getreal.eu/.*

15. See *www.eunethta.eu/activities/eunethta-joint-action-3-2016-20/work-package-5-life-cycle-approach-improve-evidence-gener.*

References

American Cancer Society (2016), *Cancer Facts & Figures 2016*, American Cancer Society, Atlanta.

AMR-Review, (2016), "Tackling Drug-resistant Infections Globally: Final Report and Recommendations", *Review on Antimicrobial Resistance*, chaired by Jim O'Neill, Wellcome Trust and HM Government, London.

Auraaen, A. et al. (2016), "How OECD Health Systems Define the Range of Good and Services to be Financed Collectively?", *OECD Health Working Paper*, No. 90, OECD Publishing, Paris, *http://dx.doi.org/10.1787/5jlnb59ll80x-en.*

Bücheler, M., B. Brüggenjürgen and S. Willich (2014), "Personalised Medicine in Europe – Enhancing Patient Access to Pharmaceutical Drug-diagnostic Companion Products", EPEMED, *White Paper*, Berlin.

Butler, M.S. et al. (2013), "Antibiotics in the Clinical Pipeline in 2013", *Journal of Antibiotics*, Vol. 66, pp. 571-591.

Cecchini, M., J. Langer and L. Slawomirski (2015), "Antimicrobial Resistance in G7 Countries and Beyond: Economic Issues, Policies and Options for Action", OECD Publishing, Paris, *www.oecd.org/els/health-systems/Antimicrobial-Resistance-in-G7-Countries-and-Beyond.pdf.*

Chandra, A. and J. Skinner (2012), "Technology Growth and Expenditure Growth in Health Care", *Journal of Economic Literature*, Vol. 50, No. 3, pp. 645-680.

Chandra, A. and J. Skinner (2008), "Technology and Expenditure Growth in Health Care", *NBER Working Paper Series*, Cambridge, United States.

Chernew, M. and J. Newhouse (2012), "Health Care Spending and Growth", *Handbook of Health Economics Vol. 2*, Elsevier.

Council of the European Union (2016), "Proposal for a Regulation of the European Parliament and of the Council on Medical Devices, and Amending Directive 2001/83/EC, Regulation (EC) No. 178/2002 and Regulation (EC) No. 1223/2009", *http://data.consilium.europa.eu/doc/document/ST-9364-2016-REV-3/en/pdf* (accessed 18 July 2016).

Culyer, A.J. (2016), "Cost-effectiveness Thresholds in Health Care: A Bookshelf Guide to their Meaning and Use", *Health Economics, Policy and Law*, Vol. 11, pp. 415-432.

Eurordis (2010), "Inventory of Access and Prices of Orphan Drugs across Europe", *www.eurordis.org/content/survey-patients%E2%80%99-access-orphan-drugs-europe* (accessed 15 November 2016).

EvaluatePharma (2015), *Orphan Drug Report 2015*, London.

Evans, B.J., W. Burke and G. Jarvik (2015), "The FDA and Genomic Tests – Getting the Regulation Right", *New England Journal of Medicine*, Vol. 372, No. 23, pp. 2258-2264.

Garrison, L.P. and A. Towse (2014), "Personalized Medicine: Pricing and Reimbursement Policies as a Potential Barrier to Development and Adoption", in Anthony J. Culyer (ed.), *Encyclopedia of Health Economics*, Vol. 2, Elsevier, pp. 484-490.

Hansson, E. (2016), "Update on EU Regulatory Developments", IMDRF 13-15 September, Florianoplos, Brazil.

Hartung, D. et al. (2015), "The Cost of Multiple Sclerosis Drugs in the US and the Pharmaceutical Industry – Too Big to Fail?", *Neurology*, Vol. 84, pp. 1-8.

Howard, D.H. et al. (2015), "Pricing in the Market for Anticancer Drugs", *Journal of Economic Perspectives*, Vol. 29, No. 1, pp. 139-62.

INCa – French National Cancer Institute (2014), *Scientific Report 2013-2014*, Paris.

Innovate UK (2016), "Mapping the Precision Medicine Landscape", *www.gov.uk/government/uploads/system/uploads/attachment_data/file/483560/Precision_Medicines_Booklet_Final_Web__002_.pdf* (accessed 19 October 2016).

Iyengar, S. et al. (2016), "Prices, Costs, and Affordability of New Medicines for Hepatitis C in 30 Countries: An Economic Analysis", *PLoS Medicine*, Vol. 13, No. 5.

Kanavos, P. and A. Angelis (2013), "Multiple Criteria Decision Analysis for Value-Based Assessment of New Medical Technologies: A Conceptual Framework", *Working Paper* No. 33/2013, LSE Health, London.

Kapczynski, A. and A.S. Kesselheim (2016), "Government Patent Use': A Legal Approach To Reducing Drug Spending", *Health Affairs*, Vol. 35, No. 5, pp. 791-797.

Lagerqvist, B. et al. (2007), "Long-Term Outcomes with Drug-Eluting Stents versus Bare-Metal Stents in Sweden", *New England Journal of Medicine*, Vol. 356, pp. 1009-1019.

MoCA-OMP – Working Group on Mechanism of Coordinated Access to Orphan Medicinal Products (2014), "Transparent Value Framework, Process on Corporate Social Responsibility in the Field of Pharmaceuticals Platform on Access to Medicines in Europe", Brussels.

OECD (2017), "Recommendation of the Council on Health Data Governance", OECD Publishing, Paris.

OECD (2016), "Better Ways to Pay for Health Care", *OECD Health Policy Studies*, OECD Publishing, Paris, *http://dx.doi.org/10.1787/9789264258211-en.*

OECD (2015a), *Data-driven Innovation: Big Data for Growth and Well-being*, OECD Publishing, Paris, *http://dx.doi.org/10.1787/9789264229358-en.*

OECD (2015b), *Dementia Research and Care. Can Big Data Help?*, OECD Publishing, Paris, *http://dx.doi.org/10.1787/9789264228429-en.*

OECD (2015c), *Health Data Governance: Privacy, Monitoring and Research*, OECD Publishing, Paris, *http://dx.doi.org/10.1787/9789264244566-en.*

OECD (2013), *Strengthening Health Information Infrastructure for Health Care Quality Governance*, OECD Publishing, Paris, *http://dx.doi.org/10.1787/9789264193505-en.*

Paris, V. and A. Belloni (2013), "Value in Pharmaceutical Pricing", *OECD Health Working Paper*, No. 63, OECD Publishing, Paris, *http://dx.doi.org/10.1787/5k43jc9v6knx-en.*

Regalado, A. (2016), "The World's Most Expensive Medicine is a Bust", *MIT Technology Review*, 4 May, *www.technologyreview.com/s/601165/the-worlds-most-expensive-medicine-is-a-bust/.*

Schuller, Y., C.E.M. Hollak and M. Biegstraaten (2015), "The Quality of Economic Evaluation of Ultra-orphan Drugs in Europe – A Systematic Review", *Orphanet Journal of Rare Diseases*, Vol. 10, p. 92.

Spellberg, B. et al. (2012), "The Critical Impact of Time Discounting on Economic Incentives to Overcome the Antibiotic Market Failure", *Nature Reviews Drug Discovery*, Vol. 11, No. 2, p. 168.

Van den Bulcke, M. et al. (2015), "Next Generation Sequencing Gene Panels for Targeted Therapy in Oncology and Haemato-oncology – Synthesis", *KCE Reports* No. 240Cs, Health Technology Assessment (HTA), Belgian Health Care Knowledge Centre (KCE), Brussels.

WHO – World Health Organization (2016), *International Classification of Diseases, 10th Edition* (ICD-10), Version 2016. Geneva, *http://apps.who.int/classifications/icd10/browse/2016/en* (accessed 6 June 2016).

WHO (2015), *Antimicrobial Resistance: Global Report on Surveillance*, World Health Organization, Geneva.

New Health Technologies: Managing Access, Value
and Sustainability

Chapter 2

The past and potential future impact of new health technology

by
Luke Slawomirski, Allison Colbert *and* Valérie Paris

The proliferation of health technology over the past century has profoundly influenced service delivery and health outcomes. It has also been a dominant factor in the growth of health care expenditure observed in the majority of OECD countries over this time. Has the expenditure growth been "worth it" in terms of health benefits? Could more value have been generated by allocating resources in alternative ways? These questions are ever more important given the modern context of fiscal limitations, demographic changes and rising community expectations. This chapter examines the historical impact of health technology and applies these learnings to the future management and integration of emerging technologies such as precision medicine, combination products, mobile health and 3D bioprinting. It discusses the need for and utility of efforts such as horizon scanning and foresight studies to help health care systems prepare for the types of health technology that are still some way off but have the potential to both disrupt and revolutionise health care delivery.

We thank Léa Maitre for her contribution to initial research on horizon scanning and foresight studies. We thank country delegates and experts, as well as BIAC members, for their comments on earlier versions of this chapter and during the expert meeting of 22 March 2016. Among them, we acknowledge in particular suggestions and material provided by Andrew Stevens (Birmingham University) and Iñaki Gutiérrez Ibarluzea (Osteba).

Introduction

Technology has had a profound impact on medicine and health care. In the past, clinical activities were "limited to identification of illness, the prediction of the likely outcome, and then the guidance of the patient and [their] family while the illness ran its full, natural course" (US Department of Health, Education, and Welfare, 1976, p. 3). Today's health care landscape is vastly different. A bewildering array of technologies is at the disposal of providers and health care systems. Technology has become deeply ingrained in, and almost synonymous with, humans' conception of disease and wellness, and in modern medical culture. Now, emerging and future health technologies are growing in complexity and sophistication. Not only are the formerly discrete technological categories converging in a range of ways, the adoption of digital innovation into health care provision and health care systems is also generating a range of opportunities as well as challenges for policy makers, regulators, payers, providers and patients.

This chapter looks first at the past and then at the future. Section 1 explores the impact that adoption and diffusion of health technology has had on health, welfare and health care expenditure. It seeks to examine whether the numerous technologies and innovations that entered routine use over the past century have been "worth it" – have their benefits outweighed the costs? Section 2 describes the challenges brought by the direction health technology is taking, focusing on converging, hybrid and digital innovations that are fundamentally changing, and in some cases disrupting, the health care landscape.

Section 3 discusses the challenge of promoting development and diffusion of high-value technologies in a sustainable manner. The section explores existing national and international initiatives around horizon scanning and technology foresight. It discusses potential ways to improve the capacity, efficiency and impact of these systems to better prepare for the broader impact of new technology on care delivery and to promote high-value technology that citizens need. This sets the scene for a more detailed examination of specific technologies – pharmaceuticals, precision medicine, medical devices and digital technology – in subsequent chapters of the report.

Box 2.1. **Value in health care**

"Paying for value" is one of the most overused tropes in health care today. It is also the least well understood, because its meaning is manipulated by each stakeholder (Chandra and Goldman, 2015).

The terms "value" and "value-based" (payment, pricing, reimbursement) blossomed in health care analyses and policy in the 2000s. In a broad sense, a "value-based" health care system is a system whose activities are oriented, organised or funded so as to maximise benefits for patients and/or the society for a given amount of resources invested (or to minimise costs for a given amount of benefits). It is difficult to disagree with this general proposition as an overarching goal for policy makers. However, patients, health care providers,

Box 2.1. **Value in health care** *(cont.)*

payers, the biomedical industry, policy makers, and the public, pursue a range of objectives that tease out the inherent tensions in this broad definition. The definition of value therefore depends very much on 1) how "benefits" are defined and measured and 2) the perspective adopted: the patient, the health care system, or society.

In ***economic evaluation,*** which is often part of health technology assessment that informs coverage decisions, three approaches are used to examine the value of new technologies (Hurley, 2000, Drummond et al., 2005):

- In the extra-welfarist approach, the objective of the health system is to maximize health outcomes from a constrained health care budget. Health improvements (e.g. life year gained) are the only outcome taken into account. Health improvements may be weighted by "health states preference scores" (or utility derived from different states of health) in aggregate measures such as "quality-adjusted life years" The most common economic evaluation methods (cost-effectiveness and cost-utility analysis) are based on this approach, and are mainly used to make decisions (funding, reimbursement and pricing) on new technologies. They compute a ratio of incremental costs to incremental benefits of using the new technologies, compared to existing alternatives. A new technology is considered to generate value when a) it is cost-saving or when b) its cost per QALY is below a pre-defined threshold (Culyer, 2016). How this threshold should be defined is the subject of ongoing debate.
- In the welfarist approach, the best way to measure the outcome of a "programme" (technology) is the amount individuals are willing to pay for it. If willingness to pay (WTP) is higher than costs, the programme (technology) should be implemented or the service supplied. This approach is often used for the evaluation of public investment projects (in cost-benefit analysis) or to measure the impact of environmental nuisances (e.g. pollution). Different methods can be used to assess consumers' WTP and derive a figure, such as the Value of the Statistical Life, which is then used to monetize the societal impact of the object of enquiry (OECD, 2012). This approach is not commonly used in economic evaluation of health care interventions. Yet, it has often been deployed in economic studies evaluating the societal value of technological progress retrospectively (e.g. Murphy and Topel, 2006), and more recently to estimate the societal value of using new hepatitis C medicines (Van Nuys et al., 2015). In the latter case, the model used allows going beyond the incremental costs (and savings) and health gains for an individual patient and measuring the impact of reduced transmission of the virus.
- An intermediary position rejects the WTP as a relevant measure of outcomes but suggests adopting a broader social perspective – not limited to health system and budget – and considering a wider range of costs and consequences. This is referred to as the "decision-maker" approach (Drummond et al., 2005).

The extra-welfarist approach, although commonly used, is often criticised for its theoretical, methodological and ethical shortcomings. One of the main arguments concerns the fact that it may not adequately reflect public preferences. By design, QALYs are of equal value regardless of the recipient ("a QALY is a QALY is a QALY"). In practice, this means that a QALY gained has the same value, whatever the condition or the personal characteristics of the population treated: age, sex, severity of disease, level of deprivation, or other characteristics. For instance, a QALY gained at 8 years is given the same weight than a QALY gained at 88 years. Decision makers, who are unlikely to be indifferent to these criteria, account for them – most often implicitly. For instance, accepting to pay for orphan or oncology medicines or implement programmes which do not meet cost-utility thresholds

Box 2.1. **Value in health care** *(cont.)*

(see Chapter 3 of this publication). New approaches to assessing the value of health care interventions are being proposed and trialled, including multi-criteria analysis (Angelis and Kanavos, 2014). Such methods allow an explicit consideration of stakeholder and public preferences in trade-offs.

Another approach, popularised by Porter (2010) aims ***to promote value in the provision of health care services***, through competition between providers. "Achieving high value for patients must become the overarching goal of health care delivery, with value defined as the health outcomes achieved per dollar spent" (Porter, 2010). The key difference with the extra-welfarist approach resides in the outcomes measurement method. Extra-welfarism applies a unifying measure (e.g. QALY), while the managerial approach assess outcomes using a combination of traditional metrics (e.g. survival), as well as condition-specific patient-reported measures (e.g. incontinence), the (dis)utility of the care process or treatment (e.g. e diagnostic errors, ineffective care, treatment-related discomfort, complications, adverse effects); the sustainability of health or recovery and the nature of recurrences; as well as long-term consequences of therapy (e.g. care-induced illnesses), without trying to aggregate them in a single metric. Monitoring these outcome sets against the costs of care is thought to enable payers and providers to assess and improve value and performance of providers. Proponents of this approach recommend adjusting payments based on observed outcomes, and to supplant fragmented payment models (e.g. fee for service) with "bundled" payments for entire cycles of care. It is therefore more suited to compare processes for a specific disease as opposed to comparison of the "value of health care" across diseases.

This chapter and this report may adopt different conceptions of value, depending on the context and the available literature, to reflect current analyses and debates. In most cases it refers to the quantity of health outcomes obtained for the resources invested ("per dollar spent") within the perspective of the health care system.

1. The past impact of technology on health, expenditure and value

This section explores the past impact of technology on health, welfare and expenditure. The aim is to answer the question of whether development and dissemination of health technology – particularly over the past century – resulted in added value, or if the resources devoted to developing and using increasingly expensive diagnostic and therapeutic interventions could have been better invested elsewhere in the health care system, or in other sectors of the economy. The focus is predominantly on biomedical technology – the subset of health technology that involves products such as drugs or devices used to treat disease. It does, however, include several examples of enabling technologies that address the way health care is deployed. The aseptic technique, discussed below, is one such example.

This question is difficult to tackle empirically. Technology varies greatly in terms of its complexity and cost, as well its impact on health. A diverse stream of technologies and innovations – from targeted medical products to diffuse, enabling innovations – has inundated the health care landscape for close to a century, making it difficult to measure change at aggregate level, and to determine an aggregate measure of technological progress. The situation is further complicated when new uses are found for existing technologies – a common occurrence (Gelijins and Rosenberg, 1994; Chernew and Newhouse, 2012).

Even if it were possible to accurately measure technological progress over time, the question remains, to what extent this contributes to health outcomes for individuals and for populations? Many factors determine health and illness; only some of these reside in the biomedical domain, and assessing the true impact of medical technology on health outcomes such as mortality and quality of life needs to account for 1) their amenability to medical care, and 2) non-medical determinants (Nolte and McKee, 2004), something that some studies fail to do (Lichtenberg, 2013). Another difficulty concerns generalisability. The impact of health technology depends on historical and contextual factors that differ between countries and health care systems.

The technologies examined in this section are mostly biomedical – drugs, devices, procedures and diagnostics. Impact is studied in aggregate as well as at a disease-specific level. Process innovation features to a lesser degree. Analysis of diffuse, enabling technologies, in particular eHealth, is lacking due to the paucity of available literature. First, the impact of a variety of health technologies on health outcomes is examined, then the effect on health expenditure, followed by a discussion on whether investment in technology has been "worth it", both in broad terms and within specific disease categories.

The overall finding is that technology has contributed significantly to human health and welfare, but its diffusion has been a significant driver of expenditure growth. This is due to the rising (real) cost of technology but also because new technology has expanded the volume of services provided, instead of substituting for existing processes and procedures. In many cases, the benefits have outweighed the costs. However, a considerable number of effective technologies are deployed unnecessarily and inappropriately. Many ineffective products and procedures continue to be used. This varies widely between technologies and disease categories, and over time. Based on the available peer-reviewed literature, the cost-effectiveness and value of new medical technology has progressively diminished over the past century (a fact acknowledged even by researchers finding good aggregate value from this expenditure), through a combination of rising prices and lower incremental benefits – that is, systems are paying progressively more for new technology and getting less health in return at the margin.

Three key lessons can be drawn for policy makers wanting to maximise the value derived from health technology:

1. Regulators and payers need to be more prudent and discerning. To ensure intelligent adoption of health technology, benefits need to be consistently judged against costs and compared to the available alternatives.
2. Mechanisms should be instituted to decommission existing technologies that have been superseded or whose comparative effectiveness is not supported by evidence.
3. System incentives must be aligned to ensure technology is deployed appropriately. Unnecessary, non-beneficial use must be discouraged.

1.1. *Medical technology has had a profound impact on human health and welfare*

Some of the greatest, paradigm-shifting technological innovations in health concern infectious diseases. In the mid-1800s, Hungarian physician Ignaz Semmelweis demonstrated that disinfecting the hands before undertaking obstetric procedures could reduce maternal mortality from puerperal fever by a factor of six (Lane et al., 2010). This led to Joseph Lister's recommendation for physicians (particularly surgeons) to practice aseptic technique and to swab wounds with carbonic acid, resulting in vastly reduced surgical mortality (Chandra and Skinner, 2012). Subsequent research in microbiology and development of germ theory led to the development of penicillin, and finally to the mass production of antimicrobial agents that have saved hundreds of millions of lives. For example, mortality from certain types of bacterial meningitis reduced from close to 100% at the beginning of the 20th century to below 20% at the end (Swartz, 2004). Another example are vaccines, which have greatly reduced the incidence of communicable diseases in many parts of the world. Vaccines must be cited as a major technological advance in medicine and public health.

The emergence of antimicrobial resistance (AMR), brought about by indiscriminate and inappropriate use of antibiotic technology over the past decades, however, has distorted the benefits and the costs of this near-miraculous technology, however. While antibiotics were historically inexpensive, their true cost – brought to bear through AMR – is the result of indiscriminate and inappropriate use.[1]

In response to the rising morbidity and mortality burden of ischaemic heart disease (IHD) in developed countries, considerable effort has been devoted to addressing this public health problem. Interventions developed to combat IHD fall into three categories: 1) preventive population-level interventions aimed at reducing risk factors;[2] 2) medicines aimed at prevention as well as management of IHD (e.g. aspirin, beta blockers and statins); and 3) invasive interventions (angiography, angioplasty and coronary bypass).

IHD mortality has reduced considerably since the 1970s with a concomitant increase in survival and added life years. Decades of research provide insights into the relative influence of the three technologies. A longitudinal study by Ford and colleagues suggests that the first group – public health – accounted for 61% of the mortality reduction in the United States. Twenty per cent was attributed to conservative management with medication and other non-invasive modalities, while the "high-tech" invasive (and expensive) interventions accounted for only 7% of the gains (Ford et al., 2007). In short, it appears US citizens may have benefitted more from behavioural interventions than from complex medical technology (Garber and Skinner, 2008). This is not to negate the contribution of invasive coronary interventions, whose effectiveness in acute and severe IHD patients has been established (Hartwell et al., 2005). The issue concerns appropriate and evidence-based deployment of the technology. For *stable* IHD (the most common presentation), conservative management results in survival rates identical to those of invasive treatment (Sedlis et al., 2015). In many cases, patients undergoing procedures have worse outcomes than those managed with medication (Jena et al., 2015). On the other hand, unmet clinical need for invasive coronary intervention has also been observed (Chew et al., 2016).

Medical technology has played a considerable part in reducing infant and maternal mortality. Lister's aseptic technique is an early example of a simple but highly effective intervention. More recently, targeted prenatal care and maternal influenza shots have been very effective at reducing neonatal mortality. More sophisticated technology such as ventilators and artificial surfactants to assist development of the lungs, developed in the 1950s, have improved the survival and life expectancy of low-birth-weight infants (Cutler and Meara, 2000). Here, the majority of these gains can be attributed to technological improvements as opposed to changes in maternal behaviour.

Another example of effective biomedical technology includes antiretroviral therapy for HIV. An important factor in the aggregate effectiveness of these drugs is the low risk of inappropriate use. HIV diagnosis is binary and the drugs have serious side effects. No physician would prescribe them without a diagnosis. The population in need is clearly defined and the use of the drug is unlikely to expand to recipients who will not benefit and who may be harmed by the treatment (Chandra and Skinner, 2012). A similar example is cataract removal, which has benefited from many technological advances since it was first performed surgically in 1748. It can now be performed highly effectively in several minutes with minimum invasiveness and side effects (Bellan, 2008; Asacaso and Huerva, 2013). The target population is well-defined, preventing inappropriate deployment of the technology.

Defining the patient population is more challenging with other technologies. Intensive care is an example. Intensive care units (ICUs) are perhaps the modern embodiment of high-tech health care. They enable successful treatment of the gravely ill, those suffering multiple trauma, and patients who suffer serious complications of care. However, defining what patients should receive this type of care has proven difficult. Chang and Shapiro (2016) found wide variation in ICU utilisation in patients admitted to 94 US hospitals between 2010 and 2012 for four conditions that require clinical judgement regarding whether ICU admission is necessary: diabetic ketoacidosis, pulmonary embolism, upper gastrointestinal bleeding and congestive heart failure. ICU utilisation was not associated with risk-adjusted patient mortality across all four conditions, but resulted in higher costs and likelihood to use invasive interventions.

Intensive, technology-laden care is often used to prolong the lives of the terminally ill, despite the patient's preferences (Somogyi-Zalud et al., 2002). Inappropriate use of medical technology has been shown to have deleterious consequences on the quality of life of these patients and their families (Temel et al., 2010). A systematic review found that non-beneficial ICU admission near the end of life can be as high as 10%. The review also found that 33% of cancer patients in the last six weeks of life receive chemotherapy – another prominent medical technology with deleterious side effects that can impede a dignified and peaceful death (Cardona-Morrell et al., 2016). In the United States, a two-fold regional variation in intensity of care in the last months of life in cancer patients was observed, with the difference unlikely to be explained by patient preference (Morden et al., 2012; Barnato et al., 2007). Internationally, the variation is more striking. Eleven per cent of Americans over 85 die in ICUs compared to 1.3% in the United Kingdom (Wunsch et al., 2009). Such variation raises questions about how appropriately such medical technology is deployed in these situations.

Diagnostic imaging is another medical technology that has undergone great advances since Wilhelm Roentgen developed the medical X-ray. More recent developments include magnetic resonance imaging (MRI) and computed tomography (CT) scanning. These provide major advances in the timely and accurate detection of pathology such as cancer. The benefits of targeted radiologic screening have been established. However, use of several imaging technologies involves radiation exposure (a CT scan delivers 1 000 times the nuclear radiation of a plain X-ray). There is also a tendency to scan an expanding cohort of patients, resulting in direct expenditure and other costs (e.g. patient anxiety), as well as triggering additional, unnecessary treatment. A recent study suggests that commonly used statistical packages to analyse functional MRI (fMRI) to measure brain activity can produce false results in up to 70% of investigations (Eklund et al., 2016).

Technological advances have resulted in a rapid expansion in the number of diagnostic tests available. These tests vary greatly in terms of their clinical risks, costs and benefits. Many are useful in detecting pathology for which effective treatment exists, others are not. For example, testing for c-reactive protein, vitamin B12, vitamin D, folate, liver function and electrocardiogram for angina contribute little towards better care and outcomes (Elshaug et al., 2012). Similar to imaging, many tests are prone to overuse. A 30-fold geographic variation in colonoscopy rates was observed in Australia (ACSQHC, 2015) and is unlikely to be explained by varying clinical need.[3] Vaccarella et al. (2016) observed striking increases in the rate of thyroid cancer in eight countries since the 1980s without concomitant increases in associated mortality (most pronounced in South Korea, where incidence in adults has increased five-fold since 1993). This suggests overdiagnosis of this condition. They attribute this trend to new diagnostic techniques enabling the detection of small papillary lesions that tend to remain asymptomatic but can lead to aggressive and harmful treatment.

Then there are technologies that are shown to be ineffective and for which risks outweigh benefits in the overwhelming majority of cases. An example is the pulmonary artery catheter (PAC), developed in 1970 to assist in haemodynamic management. Not long after it entered routine use, studies began to show that the PAC did not improve patient outcomes and, in fact, some patients fared worse as a result. Yet the PAC is still used in some hospitals today (Dalen, 2001; Binanay et al., 2005; Harvey et al., 2006; Rajaram et al., 2013). Other technologies that continue to be applied despite no evidence of their effectiveness include: spinal fusion for non-specific low back pain (Atkinson and Zacest, 2016); vertebroplasty following osteoporotic vertebral fractures (Buchbinder et al., 2009); and arthroscopic debridement for degenerative knee pain (Shivonen et al., 2013). These risky, expensive interventions are still performed in many health care systems (OECD, 2014; ACSQHC, 2015).

1.2. Health technology contributed to health care expenditure growth

Health spending has outpaced economic growth across the OECD for several decades (Figure 2.1). Adoption and diffusion of health technology is often cited as the dominant factor. A considerable amount of empirical and theoretical research is devoted to this subject (Chernew and Newhouse, 2012; Weisbrod, 1991; Sorenson et al., 2013). The US health care system is the focus of most of this research, perhaps appropriate given both the remarkable expenditure growth and the increased adoption and diffusion of medical technology in that country since 1970 (Chandra and Skinner, 2012). However, similar conclusions have been reached from analyses of other national health care systems (Productivity Commission, 2005).

Figure 2.1. **Per cent of GDP spent on health care in selected countries, 1970-2015**

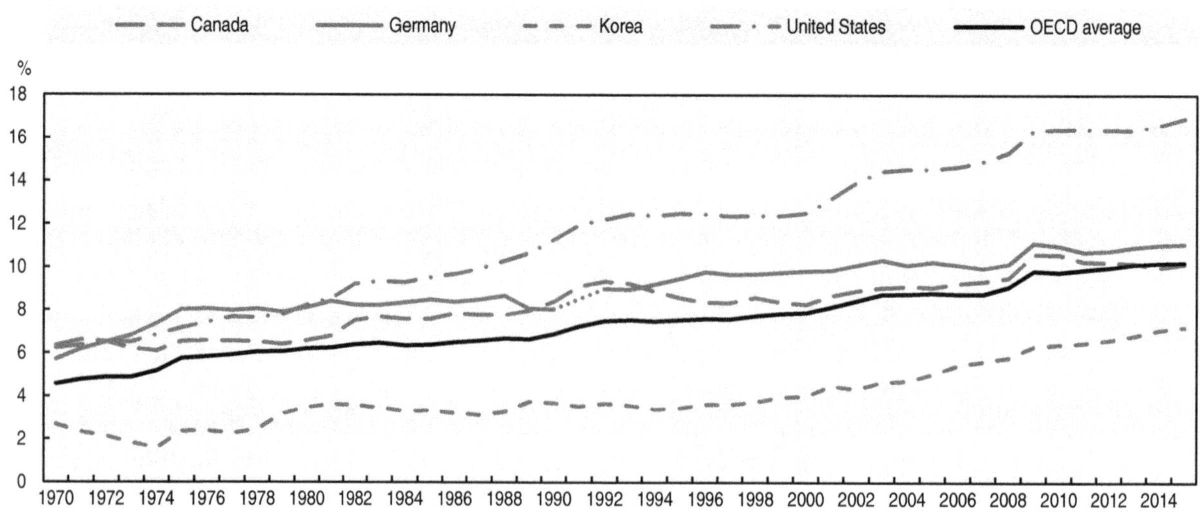

Note: The OECD average includes 18 countries.
Source: *OECD Health Statistics 2016.*

StatLink http://dx.doi.org/10.1787/888933442854

Technology can potentially influence the use of resources in six ways, by: 1) substituting for an existing intervention; 2) targeting an existing intervention more accurately; 3) intensifying the level of treatment for a given condition; 4) expanding the number of treatable conditions and patient types; 5) broadening the definition of disease; and 6) changing processes and the delivery of care (Sorenson et al., 2013). The interest of enquiry here is *growth*, as opposed to the expenditure level at a given time. The fact that in 2015 US expenditure on health care was double that of the OECD average is of lesser import in this discussion than the observation that four decades ago it was not dissimilar to that of other developed economies.

Studies of technology as a driver of expenditure growth typically take one of two broad approaches: aggregation or bottom-up (Chernew and Newhouse, 2012). Aggregation methods attempt to capture the overall effect of all "health care technology" on expenditure growth. The most common *residual* approach estimates the impact on spending growth of variables that are more easily measured: population ageing, morbidity, insurance coverage, physician density and per capita income. The remainder is attributed to technology. A variant is the *proxy* approach, which attempts to measure the contribution of technology using proxies, for example the concentration of high-tech medical equipment (Chernew and Newhouse, 2012; Lamiraud and Lhuillery, 2015). A key drawback of these methods is the potential to wrongly estimate the impact of technology if other factors are incorrectly specified or inaccurately modelled. An advantage of aggregation methods is that they potentially capture the impact of diffuse technology that is not easily attributed to any one disease type or clinical specialty, such as eHealth.[4]

The bottom-up approach attempts to directly assess how specific technologies contribute to expenditure growth. These studies tend to focus on particular diseases. While this captures more accurately the effects of a specific technology, as the technology expands to other clinical purposes its effects are not captured. Nevertheless, these studies tend to focus on high-impact illnesses and yield some valuable insights. Great variability exists in how technology and innovation have affected expenditure growth across various diseases. For example, introduction of coronary care units and bypass surgery – both landmark medical innovations – added 33% to the treatment cost of acute myocardial infarction (AMI). Similar increases were also observed with the introduction of caesarean sections for childbirth. However, the impact of "little ticket" technologies – those with low unit prices but broad application (e.g. lab tests; X-rays) – has also been considerable (Scitovski, 1985; Scitovski and McCall, 1976).

Importantly, the introduction of many technologies that enabled treating a specific pathology more efficiently (with fewer inputs) increased expenditure in aggregate, as providers responded to the surplus capacity by treating more cases. Laparoscopic cholecystectomy, which enabled the procedure to be conducted as a day-case not necessitating an overnight hospital admission, is a good example (Legorreta et al., 1993; Steiner et al., 1994). On the other hand, preventive technologies such as vaccines have resulted in dramatic reduction in costs through a reduction in illness and care avoided. In most cases, however, technologies have been *additive* rather than substitutive in existing clinical practice (Showstack et al., 1982), thus placing upward pressure on expenditure growth. Studies examining a range of clinical specialty areas found that those with greater adoption and use of new technologies, such as cardiology and orthopaedic surgery, exhibited greater spending growth (Holahan et al., 1990).

Despite the limitations, these studies of health expenditure growth have advanced discussion on the impact of technology. Overall, adoption and diffusion of health technology across a health care system exerted an expansionary effect on the provision of health care, and was therefore an important driver of expenditure growth. Estimates vary, but depending on the data, modelling techniques and assumptions, the estimated contribution of technological progress to spending growth ranges from 20% to 70% (Chernew and Newhouse, 2012).

The economics of health care systems go some way to explaining this. In the medium run, the supply of human capital and infrastructure in a health care system is fixed due, among other things, to its inherent complexity, barriers to entry, and the investment – including time – required to train providers. Fixed capacity is rapidly filled and new technologies, as well as new applications of existing ones, serve as a way to fill it: cardiac catheter labs will be used, ICU beds filled. This may explain why even cost-reducing technologies, in practice – by freeing up capacity – often increase aggregate expenditure as more patients are treated. For example, evidence suggests that the availability of more sophisticated technology (e.g. MRI scanners, cardiac catheter labs for angioplasty) does not substitute for or offset the use of other technology (CT scanners, bypass grafting), supporting the observation that new medical technology has, in general, an expansionary effect on resource use and expenditure (Baker et al., 2003).

Studies of the influence of technology shed light on the influence of other factors on expenditure growth. Population ageing exerts a smaller than expected effect, whereas changes in clinical practice exert a strong influence on expenditure growth (de Meijer et al., 2013; Dormont et al., 2006). Rising individual and national income have been shown to be strong contributors to expenditure growth through demand for, and supply of, greater insurance coverage (Smith et al., 2009). The interplay is dynamic and complex. New technologies generate consumer demand for care – and demand for insurance to cover it. This care may be more intensive and more costly, with little incremental benefit – particularly if promoted aggressively by developers and providers. Payers, both public and private, often acquiesce to the demand through political or market mechanisms.[5] In turn, expanding insurance provides more incentive to develop new, expensive technologies (Sorenson et al., 2013).

The effect of health technology can therefore not be seen as purely exogenous. A complex, dynamic interplay arises between several drivers: rising income, insurance, funding, disease patterns, regulation, and clinical practice style and medical culture (Figure 2.2). The conclusion – as foreshadowed above – is that it is not technology per se that drives expenditure growth, but its *deployment and use* by health care providers and patients. This, of course, is not independent of context, which may include drivers such as income levels and consumer demand for more "health" derived through medical interventions. Health care system characteristics such as resource scarcity, budgeting, and funding and remuneration models will also influence policy and practice (Lambooij et al., 2010), and thus diffusion of certain types of technology and innovation over others.

Remuneration and pricing for the use or application of technologies is an important factor of aggregate and expanding expenditure. Remuneration drives diffusion and uptake of technology in combination with funding models, insurance, regulation and demand, and thus contributes to the impact of technology on expenditure level and growth. Among a sample of OECD countries,[6] remuneration for a CT scan, hip replacement and the drug Plavix varies seven-fold, five-fold and ten-fold, respectively. Within the United States,

Figure 2.2. **Technology and the drivers of health care expenditure growth**

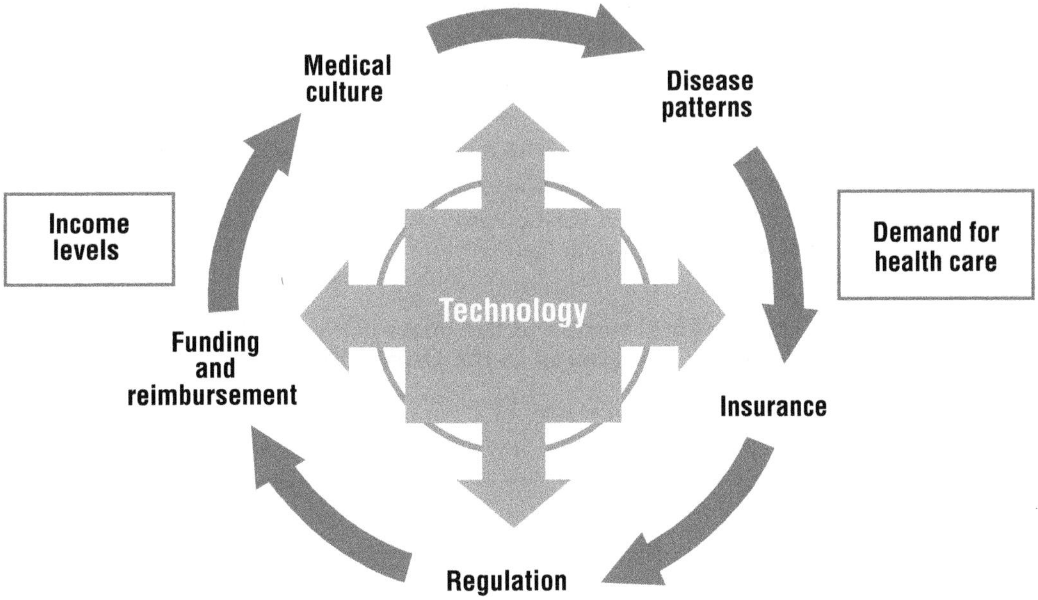

reimbursement for CT scans varies 17-fold (Reinhardt, 2012). The same on-patent oncology drugs, for example, are priced at considerably higher levels in the United States than in other countries (Goldstein et al., 2016). Policy makers exert influence over remuneration for technology and therefore over its use and impact on expenditure growth.

1.3. *The value of medical technology has declined over time*

So far it has been established that health technology: 1) has a variable impact on health outcomes depending on the specific innovation, disease or illness, and how the technology is deployed; and 2) is a significant driver of the growth in expenditure on health care. The next question concerns value and the achievement of health care system objectives. In other words, have the resources invested in development,[7] diffusion and use of medical technology been "worth it" in terms of outcomes for population health and welfare?

Considerable empirical work has examined the value of biomedical technology, adopting a range of approaches to define and estimate the outcomes and costs. This section considers the evidence of value, based on aggregate studies of medical technology, disease-specific analyses and pharmaceuticals.

Aggregate studies of value suggest a declining trend

Murphy and Topel (2006) estimated the social value (based on willingness to pay) of increased life expectancy in the United States between 1970 and 2000 to be USD 95 trillion – approximately three times the health care expenditure over that period. Notably, two-thirds of this value was generated in the 1970s, a decade during which the longevity gains were higher, and expenditure lower, compared to subsequent decades.

Cutler et al. (2006) estimated the cost per life year gained in the United States from 1960 to 2000, assuming that 50% of longevity gains were attributable to health care. During the whole period, life expectancy (at birth) rose by almost seven years and (real) lifetime per-capita health care expenditure increased six-fold. Expenditure in four age groups was calculated for each of the four decades (the 1960s, 1970s, 1980s and 1990s). The *average* cost per year of life gained over the entire period (in 2002 USD) increased with age: USD 19 900 at birth, USD 31 600 at 15, USD 53 700 at 45 and USD 84 700 at 65 years. Similar to Murphy and Topel's findings, the 1970s was the most "productive" decade in terms of value (expenditure per life year gained). The cost had risen five-fold by the 1990s. The same temporal pattern was observed for the other age groups, but was more pronounced in those aged 65 and over (Figure 2.3). The authors concluded that, on average, the cost per life year over the period offered reasonable value but warned of the upward trend in more recent decades, and high relative costs in older patients (Cutler et al., 2006).

Figure 2.3. **Longitudinal trends in the costs per year of life gained in four age groups in the United States**

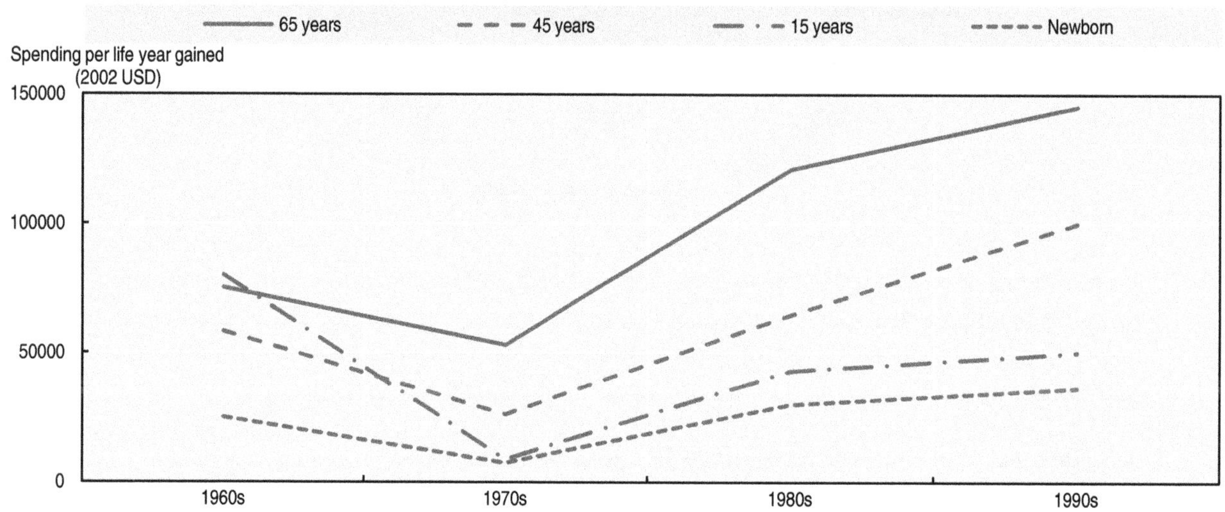

Source: Adapted from Cutler, D., A. Rosen and S. Vijan (2006), "The Value of Medical Spending in the United States, 1960-2000", *New England Journal of Medicine*, Vol. 355, No. 9, pp. 920-927.

StatLink http://dx.doi.org/10.1787/888933442865

The authors assumed that 50% of the life expectancy gains were attributable to medical interventions.[8] Notably, while future expenditure was discounted, this was not done for life years gained. This is problematic – treating benefits equally regardless of how far into the future they are realised creates the mathematical implication that all health expenditure should be delayed indefinitely (Keeler and Cretin, 1983). Discounting future longevity gains in this study would inflate the cost per life year gained. Results for the 45-year-old cohort are provided as an example in Figure 2.4 (Garber and Skinner, 2008). This supports the observation that the costs of longevity gains may be trending towards the unfavourable.

Aggregation studies make a significant assumption in attributing a "flat" contribution rate across all technology types and diseases. This may be overly simplistic. As noted throughout this section, the relative contribution of technology to longevity compared to other determinants of health and disease differs considerably between technologies and clinical areas. Diffuse technology that improves processes and delivery of care (e.g. digital technology) will have a very different cost/benefit signature from a clinical intervention to treat diabetes or from an organ transplant. For example, using an Italian primary care dataset, Atella and D'Amico (2015) disentangle the effect of patient-related risk factors,

Figure 2.4. **Cost per life year gained for the 45-year-old cohort in Cutler et al. (2006) using undiscounted and discounted future life years**

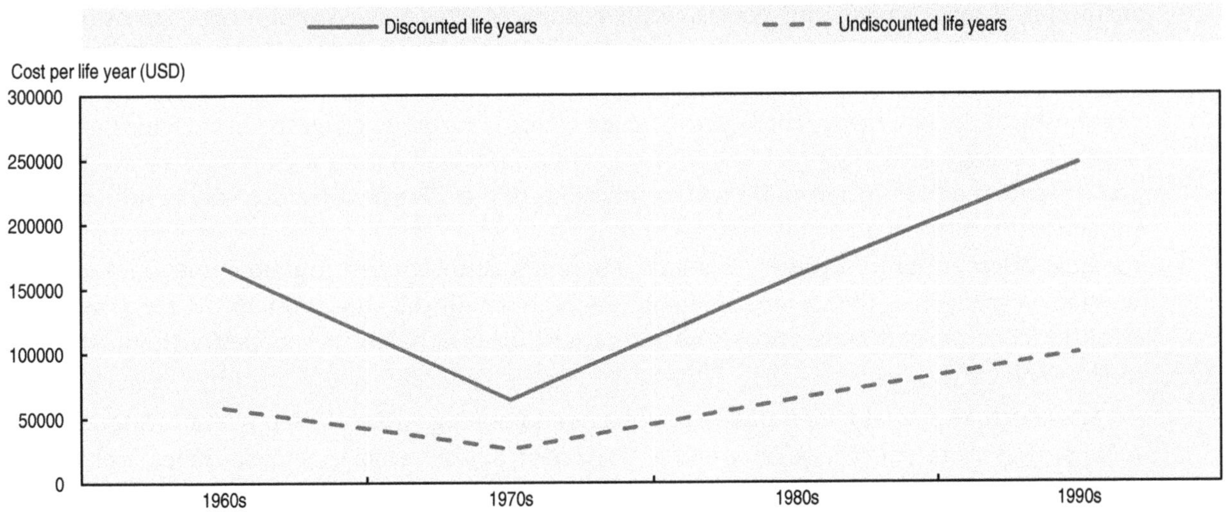

Source: Based on Garber, A. and J. Skinner (2008), "Is American Health Care Uniquely Inefficient?", *Journal of Economic Perspectives*, Vol. 22, No. 4, pp. 27-50.

StatLink http://dx.doi.org/10.1787/888933442873

physician input and technology (cholesterol-lowering drugs) in the treatment of hypercholesterolemia. In this patient group, medication has by far the greater effect on patients' speed in recovering optimal cholesterol levels.

On the other hand, these studies use life expectancy as their outcome measure and do not consider quality of life. Because much of modern health care aims to improve function, well-being and comfort as well as longevity, these studies may underestimate the value of technology.

Disease-specific analyses support this finding

Turning to specific clinical areas, the control of infectious diseases has delivered exceptional value – a dramatic reduction in mortality at a low cost. Yet some technologies have been more successful than others. Sanitation and hygiene initiatives such as waste management and ensuring a clean water supply have been incredibly cost-effective (Hutton and Haller, 2004; Varley et al., 1998).[9]

Cutler and Meara (2000) evaluated the benefits from the care of low-birth-weight infants in the United States from 1950 to 1990. During this period, inflation-adjusted spending on low-birth-weight infants rose by USD 40 000 per birth. Applying a value per life year gained of USD 100 000, and factoring in the costs of care for surviving infants in later life, the authors estimated a five-fold return on this expenditure – impressive although, as acknowledged by the authors, still not as cost-effective as neonatal care and influenza shots (Cutler and Meara, 2000).

Cutler and McClellan (2001) examined the costs and benefits of technologies used in the United States for the period 1950 to 1990 to treat five conditions: heart attack, depression, low-birth-weight, cataracts and breast cancer. Valuing a life year at USD 100 000, they concluded that with the exception of breast cancer, the cost of longevity gains in all clinical areas was below this threshold. Breast cancer failed to meet the cut-off due to the comparatively low cost-effectiveness of screening younger women. Screening of women over 65, however, was demonstrated to be highly cost-effective (Cutler and McClellan, 2001). In these analyses at the disease level, authors attribute the majority of longevity gains to the medical interventions targeting these specific conditions. This may be appropriate. Survival of low-birth-weight infants, for example, is predominantly a result of medical care and not maternal behaviour. On the other hand, AMI (as opposed to IHD) is more complex. A person presenting to the emergency room with a heart attack is certainly given the best chance of survival by aggressive, high-tech medical intervention. Behavioural interventions or even conservative medical management will, at this stage of the disease trajectory, exert a minor influence (the authors do report that the findings hold when 70% of survival is attributed to medical intervention). However, this analysis raises some interesting questions. Is the disease progression a *fait accompli*, or should the cost-benefit calculus consider the range of health technologies that can prevent and manage disease before it becomes a medical emergency?

Research and development (R&D) to prevent and manage IHD resulted in a number of technologies of varying complexity and invasiveness. These range in clinical indications, level of risk and financial cost. Analysing US data from the early 1980s to the late 1990s, Cutler and McClellan (2001) and Cutler (2007) examined the high-cost interventions to treat AMI. These include cardiac catheterisation (an invasive diagnostic procedure), angioplasty, stenting and bypass surgery. All gains in longevity are attributed to these interventions. The authors concluded that aggregate expenditure on these interventions was "worth it". This conclusion can be contested when data are examined for temporal trends and regional variation. Skinner et al. (2006) compared Medicare billing data with survival gains in AMI patients between 1986 and 2002, at the regional level. They found that medical expenditure growth was not correlated with increases in risk-adjusted survival (Figure 2.5). This prompts further reflection on the use of low-cost, highly effective technologies instead of their high-cost counterparts.[10] They also observed a plateauing of survival gains beginning in 1996 (Skinner et al., 2006).

Figure 2.5. **Changes in survival of AMI patients and in Medicare expenditure by US hospital referral region, 1986-2002**

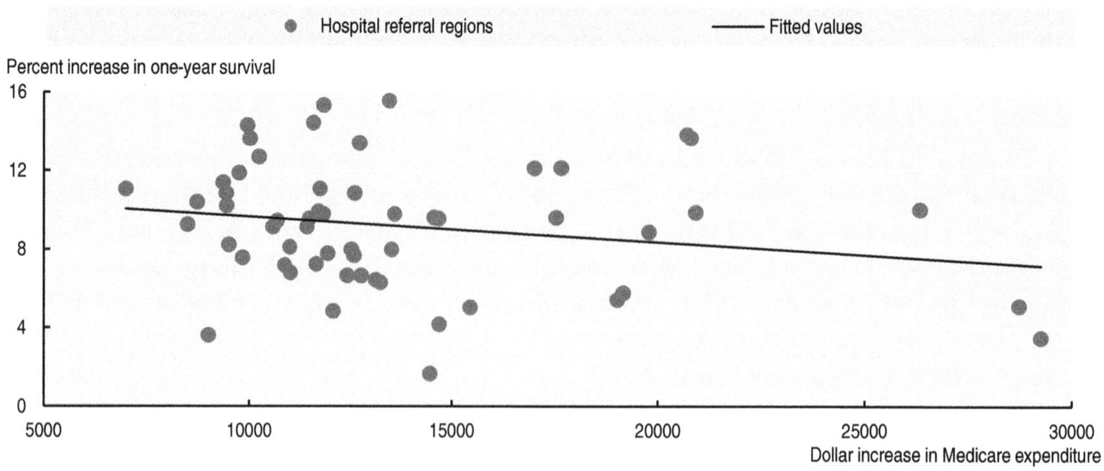

Source: Adapted from Skinner, J., D. Staiger and E. Fisher (2006), "Is Technological Change in Medicine Always Worth It? The Case of Acute Myocardial Infarction", *Health Affairs*, Vol. 25, pp. w35-w47.

StatLink http://dx.doi.org/10.1787/888933442888

Other studies show that prevention and conservative medical management have had a more significant impact on IHD mortality than invasive interventions (Ford et al., 2007; Sedlis et al., 2015; Jena et al., 2015). These are also considerably cheaper than their invasive, high-tech counterparts. The evidence suggests that costly coronary interventions are often needlessly used with no impact on longevity compared to more conservative management. Better value can thus be derived through broader application of "low-tech" care, as well as more appropriate, evidence-based use of more expensive, invasive interventions.

The value of pharmaceutical care varies

As discussed further in Chapter 3, pharmaceuticals account for one-fifth of health care expenditure (OECD, 2015a). The value of using pharmaceuticals varies immensely. This is due to the inherent effectiveness of drugs, their price and how they are used. Antiretroviral treatments for HIV bring high value in spite of relatively high prices, because they bring high benefits to patients and are not used in the non-infected population (Chandra and Skinner 2012). Sofosbuvir, which cures hepatitis C in 95% of recipients, is another example. It was assessed to be cost-effective, even at a price of USD 84 000 per treatment (Chhatwal et al., 2015). Some cheap drugs such as aspirin and beta blockers – highly effective in managing IHD – are also of high value when used appropriately.

In some pharmaceutical classes, cost-effectiveness gradually declined over time. Cancer drugs are an example. New-generation cancer drugs extend life by a matter of months, but prices are rising. In the United States, entry prices of oncology medicines per life year gained multiplied four-fold between 1995 and 2013 in real terms, with no significant improvement in benefits or side effects (Howard et al., 2015).

Pricing and reimbursement exert a strong effect on the diffusion and adoption of medical technology – both in terms of the amount (price) as well as payment model (prospective payment; fee-for-service) (Gelijins and Rosenberg, 1994; Chandra and Skinner, 2012). For instance, US physicians have incentives to favour prescribing oncology medications that require clinical administration over equally effective drugs that patients can self-administer because they have the potential to earn profit (Newcomer, 2012). The challenge for policy makers is to create the right incentives for appropriate use while discouraging inappropriate or blanket application.

The value function of health technology seems to be flattening

Ongoing debate exists about the overall value added by health technology over the past 50 years. Temporal trends suggest that the days of conventional, biomedical technology delivering high levels of value may be in the past. Even investigators concluding in favour of the return on investment of health care expenditure (e.g. Cutler) concede that the trajectory of the cost-benefit function is not favourable and may lead to sustainability problems. Chandra and Skinner (2008) note that *"[o]n average, we may have gotten good value from health care in the past, but the trend for average value in the future is perhaps more tenuous"* (p. 29). The analyses presented above suggest diminishing marginal returns of technology across a range of common conditions. The impacts on social welfare of continuing to introduce new technology, and expanding the use of existing technology without regard for real-world utility, may need to be questioned.

This is especially the case when the scope of analysis is expanded beyond health care systems. Welfare can be generated in other sectors of the economy. The growing share of countries' gross domestic product (GDP) spent on health care – much of which is driven by development and diffusion of medical technology – may crowd out other areas of public or private spending generating welfare, such as education, welfare support and social care.

This is more than simply theoretical, Paretian conjecture and questions about macro-level allocative efficiency are frequently voiced (Garber and Skinner, 2008).[11] Sorenson et al. (2013) make this point succinctly: "*It would be prudent to debate the opportunity costs of funding new (and increasingly expensive) technologies. Even in cases where medical technologies are cost-effective, available resources may be better allocated to other equally or more cost-effective investments outside of the health care sector, such as the environment or education*" (p. 230). To ensure a better welfare return across entire economies, policy makers need to look beyond health care when assessing the value of health technology and when setting cost-effectiveness thresholds.

1.4. Health technology's value can be enhanced with better policy and practice

Using the lens of value, three broad types of medical technology emerge, based on their effectiveness as well as their application (Chandra and Skinner, 2008, 2012). These are summarised in Table 2.1. The first type comprises "high-value" technologies. Many of these are relatively inexpensive and include the public health interventions described above.[12] Effective, relatively cheap products such as vaccines, aspirin and beta blockers feature here. They also include process innovations that reduce clinical risk and enhance efficiency – sterilisation of surgical equipment, for example. Some digital technologies such as mobile health (mHealth) and modern ICT-enabled Telehealth[13] designed to offer more efficient care and/or management of disease *may* also be in this category. However, as discussed in Chapter 6, a vast array of innovations are in this class, and concrete evidence for their utility is still lacking.

Table 2.1. **The value framework for health technology**

High-value technology (type A)	Process innovation • Aseptic technique; Wound sterilisation Low-cost, highly effective • Aspirin and beta blockers • Vaccines • Public health and preventive interventions High-cost, highly effective, clearly defined target population • Antiretroviral treatment • Cataract removal • New-generation hepatitis C medication
Effective technology with a risk of expanding use (type B)	Effective for some patients, but broad application diminishes marginal and overall benefit • Diagnostic imaging • Cardiac catheterisation and angioplasty • Laparoscopic surgery • Intensive care (end of life)
Low-value technology (type C)	Little evidence of effectiveness or low effectiveness • Expensive substitutes (e.g. robot-assisted surgery for some indications) • Spinal surgery in low back pain • Many diagnostic tests • Many high-cost cancer drugs • Pulmonary Artery Catheterisation (PAC)

Source: Based on Chandra, A. and J. Skinner (2012), "Technology Growth and Expenditure Growth in Health Care", *Journal of Economic Literature*, Vol. 50, No. 3, pp. 645-680; and Chandra, A. and J. Skinner (2008), "Technology and Expenditure Growth in Health Care", *NBER Working Paper*, Cambridge, United States.

High-value technology does not necessarily need to be low-cost. Surfactants and ventilators to improve survival of low-birth-weight infants, cataract surgery, new-generation hepatitis C medications, and antiretroviral treatments for HIV (all interventions that cannot be classified as low-cost) can be in this category (type A) because they bring high health benefits to well-targeted populations.

Type B covers interventions that are effective for some indications but whose use expands to a growing number of patients and indications where they produce less certain benefit. This results in diminishing incremental value. Diagnostic imaging is a good example. Used prudently and appropriately, these technologies are highly cost-effective, but a broadening of the patient population sees a sharp decline in marginal benefit and therefore value. Intensive care is highly effective in many cases but detrimental to patient welfare if misused, for example at the end of life. The suite of invasive methods for treating IHD, particularly angiography and angioplasty, features in this second group.

The third type of technology in this value framework includes interventions for which little evidence of effectiveness has been produced despite repeated investigation and clinical use (as opposed to new, innovative products that take time to evaluate properly). These do not generate any benefit or value. The PAC was used for three decades beginning in 1970. In the United States, an estimated USD 20 billion was spent on its use throughout the 1990s, for very little clinical utility (Dalen, 2001). Equally, little value is derived from substituting expensive technologies for effective, existing interventions. Robot-assisted surgery is a good example, where in many cases little or no additional benefit is gained for a higher cost (Breeden, 2013; Bochner et al., 2014). Type C also includes a variety of diagnostic tests that individually may be cheap but in aggregate present a considerable cost burden to the health care system. If calculating value based solely on the cost per life year or per quality-adjusted life year, many new and expensive cancer drugs – which extend life by weeks and months – would fall into this category.

The hypothetical value functions of the three technology types are illustrated in Figure 2.6. The x-axis indicates the number of patients subjected to the intervention and therefore the aggregate cost of the technology or intervention. The cumulative benefit is plotted on the y-axis. The blue curve represents type A technologies, whose benefit grows in a linear fashion (each additional use produces the same benefit as the previous one). The black curve represents type B technologies – the value diminishes with each additional use as the intervention is applied to recipients who do not benefit from it. Type C technologies are represented by the dotted curve. Here the benefit strays into negative territory given the inherent clinical risk of these interventions, which are often invasive or have deleterious side effects.

Historically, type A and appropriate use of type B technologies and innovations delivered the most value in aggregate. This is undermined by inappropriate use of type B and continued deployment of type C technologies. Again, the conclusion is that how technology is deployed is crucial in determining value.

This is an encouraging conclusion. It means that the value to be derived from health technology can be captured with the right policy settings. The challenge for policy makers, regulators and payers is to structure incentives across the system to promote appropriate use and discourage inappropriate application of technology. This challenge extends to providers, who must partner with their patients in providing safe interventions appropriately and based on the available evidence. Broadly speaking, technologies in the type A category should be promoted, policy levers implemented to ensure only appropriate use of type B technologies, and funding and use of type C technologies systematically

Figure 2.6. **Theoretical value functions of technology types A, B and C**

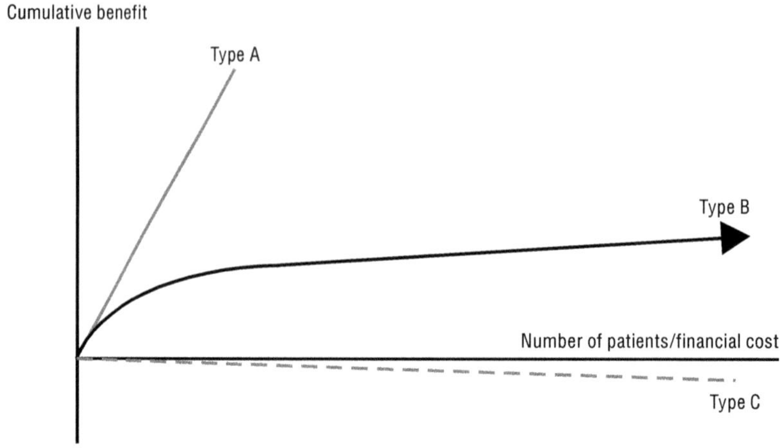

Source: Based on Chandra, A. and J. Skinner (2008), "Technology and Expenditure Growth in Health Care", *NBER Working Paper*, Cambridge, United States.

re-evaluated. All of this must be underpinned by robust, transparent and ongoing empirical evaluation of the effectiveness, benefits and costs of existing and new technologies.[14] A range of financial, regulatory and behavioural levers can be deployed to achieve this – and evidence is emerging that policy can affect utilisation of health technology (Lee and Levy, 2012). These issues are discussed in more detail below and in subsequent chapters.

2. Challenges and opportunities of accelerating technology development

An important question is whether these lessons from the past will hold true for emerging technologies in health care. Indeed, headlines regarding exponential advances in technology could lead one to believe that health care systems are in the midst of a revolution into the realm of science fiction: artificial intelligence, sensors, robotics, 3D printing, "Big Data", genomics, stem cells and more. However, such potentially miraculous patient benefits generated by these innovations are feared to come with correspondingly astronomical costs.

The nature of innovation in health care systems is becoming more complex. In the past, medical technologies were distinct from one another and used at discrete points of care pathways. Today, technology categories increasingly converge in ways that alter the delivery of health care. For example, treatment pathways are becoming tailored to individual patients via combinations of drugs and diagnostics known as precision medicine – discussed elsewhere in this report. Medical devices (also treated elsewhere in this report) increasingly employ digital communication tools to deliver and/or receive data, for example via a mobile application on a patient or provider's smartphone. Biopharmaceuticals are becoming "smart" combinations of drug and device technology, such as drugs containing nanotechnology to target tumours or clots, or digital medicine to deliver information on patient adherence.

Emerging and converging technologies raise profound ethical, legal, social and cultural questions. Existing processes and settings of care, regulatory pathways and reimbursement systems risk becoming obsolete. To adapt to the challenges of new innovations, and to make adoption of technology sustainable into the future, payers are increasingly seeking to pay for value demonstrated in real-world settings. At the moment, health care system discussions of value come later in the technology lifecycle, usually after regulatory approval/licensing. As discussed in Chapters 3 and 4, these mechanisms should potentially be restructured to develop and use real-world evidence (RWE) to facilitate paying for value.

In this context, policy makers, regulators and the public need to better understand the opportunities and challenges of emerging and converging technologies to facilitate responsible decision making in, for example, regulatory policy development, public and private funding, and product adoption. Such early dialogue can help truly innovative and valuable converging technologies from being bound with long development processes and regulatory complexity, to best balance the risk and ethical responsibilities with therapeutic opportunities. This could help ensure targeting to patients who receive the greatest benefits from resource-intensive and often high-cost interventions, and potentially entice investors in the development of low-cost, high-value products.

This section provides an overview of key technology trends likely to transform health care in the next five to ten years, highlighting their potential benefits as well as challenges they raise to regulators and payers. Many of these technology trends are discussed in additional detail in other chapters of this report, so a synopsis of key issues is presented here. These technology trends were identified in a review of foresight or horizon-scanning studies that aimed to elucidate the use of both horizon-scanning and technology foresight mechanisms by various stakeholders within OECD member countries (see Box 2.2). Further discussion of these early awareness and alert systems and their methods, use and impact is in the following section.

Box 2.2. **Identifying future technologies with potentially high impact on health care systems**

To identify emerging and future technologies likely to impact health care systems, the OECD reviewed technology foresight and horizon-scanning studies and other literature focused on technologies with a high potential to transform health care in the next five to ten years (2020–25). These studies typically use a set of criteria to prioritise technologies for further scrutiny, including:

- potential health benefit: population level (size of population affected) and/or patient level (e.g. high mortality rate)
- potential for technical realisation
- potential acceptance by health care systems and society
- incremental benefit in comparison to current alternatives
- potential to trigger system changes (service reorganisation, structural changes, new educational needs, regulatory issues)
- unit cost or budget impact (in some cases)

These methods are examined in more detail in the following section.

2.1. *Precision medicine enables treatments tailored to individual patients*

Precision medicine holds the potential to radically transform medicine. Current research initiatives in this field are increasing the medical community's knowledge and capacity to predict, prevent and treat diseases. So far, precision medicine has mainly found concrete applications in the development of personalised or stratified medicines, which provide safer and more effective treatments to patients. The use of genomic, epi-genomic, microbiome, exposure and other data will increasingly define patterns of disease and treatment, including drug/diagnostic combinations that target specific treatments to individuals who can benefit from them.

Precision medicine challenges regulatory pathways in many ways. First, it changes the design of clinical trials. In oncology for instance, the traditional randomised controlled trial comparing a treatment to placebo is increasingly being replaced by trials where patients' treatment is selected according to the molecular characteristics of their tumour. In some cases, target populations are very small and trials cannot recruit hundreds of patients. Results have to be inferred from very small samples. These changes require development of new methods to assess safety and efficacy. In addition, emerging personalised medicines often target severely debilitating or life-threatening conditions for which no treatment is currently available. As a result, regulators are often under pressure to provide quick access to these treatments.

Second, as the safety and efficacy of a personalised medicine depends on the performance of the diagnostic test mentioned on its label, approval of the medicine needs to take the latter into account. Today, regulatory requirements for the approval of biomarker diagnostic tests differ across countries but also depend on who develops and performs the test. In Europe and the United States, commercial in vitro diagnostics need regulatory approval while laboratory-developed or in-house tests are not subject to the same level of requirements (Garrison and Towse, 2014). Without streamlined regulatory oversight of the quality and performance of all tests, health care systems may struggle to effectively evaluate the costs and benefits of tests coming from varied sources and settings of care.

Finally, development of multiplex tests and whole-genome sequencing in clinical practice will require a number of adaptations to address the following challenges: How will regulators and Health Technology Assessment (HTA) agencies determine the clinical utility of such diagnostic tools? What sort of patient consent should be sought to know what to do with incidental findings? Who will be responsible if "actionable" information provided by the test has not been used to prevent or treat a disease in a given patient?

As discussed in Chapter 5, one of the big challenges for this discipline is how to best transfer R&D results to routine care ("bench to bedside"), and conversely, how to ensure that information collected on routine care processes and outcomes can effectively feed further research.

2.2. *Combination products increasingly blur the line between drug and device technology*

Many emerging medicines are "smart" combinations of drug and device technology. Examples include drugs containing nanotechnology to target tumours or clots, or "digital medicines" that deliver information on patient adherence. The common aim is to improve targeting of treatment with medicines, to enable medicines to reach the right area of the patient's body, for example, and to improve safety and effectiveness.

A key forecasted application of the technology trend of combination device/drug products is smart drug delivery systems, which are drug eluting systems enabled with some degree of diagnostic/computing capability to target the release of therapy at a certain location or when a certain set of diagnostic criteria are met. They are seen as holding particular promise for patient-centred treatment, such as improved care for tumours.

The *WHO Health 2020 Report* cites nanotechnology as one of three key technology trends likely to affect the WHO European region (the others being genomics and self-management), particularly when used for more targeted drug therapies or smart drugs, noting that they have "already been shown to cause fewer side effects and be more effective than traditional therapies" (WHO, 2013). That said, rapid developments in these fields in academia have yet to see matching industry investigation needed for widespread adoption.

In addition, combining the benefits of medicines and medical devices is not without risk. Evaluating such risks and benefits requires specialised expertise, which is why many countries have separate regulatory authorities for each technology type, or separate offices within the same agency. Evaluating evidence on a hybrid product will therefore require additional co-ordination and collaboration within and between health care systems. Potential regulatory issues include questions about the impact of new delivery systems on pharmaceutical safety and efficacy.

Combining key concepts from computer science with chemistry and biology into a new form of therapy will necessitate closer interaction between the pharmaceutical and medical device industries, while the growing prominence of eHealth will require greater collaboration with the digital industry and associated expertise.

2.3. Mobile health is developing rapidly but has yet to attain mainstream adoption

Mobile health (mHealth) describes the practice of medicine and public health supported by mobile devices. mHealth innovation includes software applications (apps) and portable devices, as well as any technology that enables telehealth.[15] It can also encompass a combination of these modalities. mHealth was enabled by the invention of the Internet and related technology (broadband and Wi-Fi), as well as more recent innovations such as the smartphone, and has opened a new frontier in promotion of health and management of disease. A smartphone can be connected to the Internet as well as a telecommunications network, and combines the features of a cell phone with that of a range of other portable devices: camera, voice recorder, email and calendar platform, web browser, media player and a GPS navigation unit. Modern smartphones even have motion detectors useful to, for instance, enable detection of falls in the elderly. Its utility-bearing features have been harnessed by many industries.

The mHealth market is growing fast. According to one estimate, more than 165 000 health apps were available in 2015, a figure that has doubled since 2013 (IMS Institute for Healthcare Informatics, 2015). These apps perform a constellation of functions: medication reminders, tracking movement and activity, monitoring fertility and progress of pregnancy, and analysing a person's speech to help in the management of mental health problems.

mHealth's potential can be realised in three ways. First, enhanced monitoring improves information and timeliness of response, raising the quality and co-ordination of care. Second, unnecessary use of health care resources may be avoided by preventing hospital and physician visits – as is already being demonstrated in diabetes management (Nundy et al., 2014). Third, through its scalability and connectivity, mHealth can broaden access to care, taking it beyond traditional settings. It offers a wide range of smart modalities by which patients can interact with health professionals, or with systems that can provide helpful, real-time feedback along the care continuum, from prevention to diagnosis, treatment and monitoring (Figure 2.7).

Figure 2.7. **mHealth's potential uses**

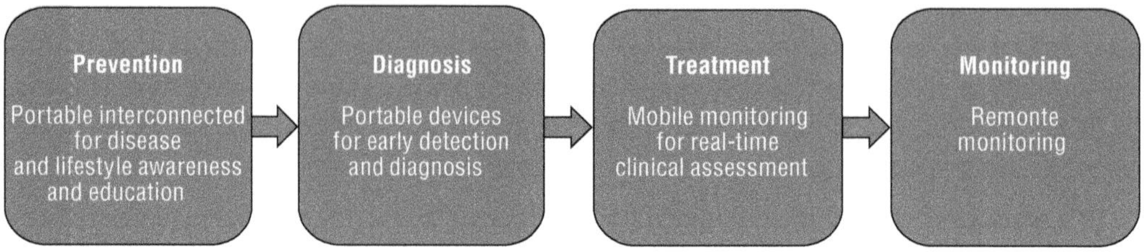

Source: OECD (2015), *Data-driven Innovation: Big Data for Growth and Well-being*, OECD Publishing, Paris, *http://dx.doi.org/10.1787/9789264229358-en.7.*

Smartphone apps can assist providers and practitioners with a range of administrative and clinical activities as well as collaboration with patients and colleagues. These are particularly useful to clinicians working on busy hospital wards where computer terminals are scarce, or to practitioners working in mobile or home-based care (Kuo et al., 2016). Apps can range from simple communication enablers (reminders, alerts, instant messaging) to information and processing software, enhanced by Internet connectivity. These include clinical guidelines, protocols, dosing and treatment algorithms, as well as instant access to patient records and diagnostic results. If well-designed with the user in mind and integrated into a functioning and reliable information infrastructure, such innovations can enhance quality of health care, and the smartphone or tablet may become the "workstation-of-choice" for providers (Weinstein et al., 2014).

Such potential is welcome at a time of rising prevalence and incidence of chronic diseases and multimorbidity. As people's contact with the health care system shifts from short episodes of acute care to more sustained, long-term monitoring and management that requires a team-based approach, the value of the smartphone and portable devices will rise. In addition, mHealth can potentially favour patients' empowerment and engagement in the management of their conditions. mHealth has the ability to put people at the centre of managing their own health, to bring care closer to them, and to enable access to the right information, providers and services.

For example, smartphone apps enable a diagnosis from a dermatologist using a photograph of a skin condition and, if necessary, a prescription to be sent to a local pharmacy. The service is said to be cheaper and timelier than a traditional, face-to-face, consultation (Dermio, 2016). A recent study using a cohort of Kenyan diabetic patients concluded that a visual acuity test conducted using a smartphone is accurate and repeatable, and that its results are consistent with those of conventional clinical testing (Batsawrous et al., 2015).

An important distinction between mHealth and conventional medical technology (drugs and devices) is that it does not involve introduction of new biomedical interventions or procedures. Rather, it improves communication (a reliably consistent factor in high-quality care), and may enable existing clinical activity to be performed more effectively and efficiently. Health care is an inexact science, and this technology simplifies the processes of managing the complexity that underlies human disease, especially in managing chronic illness.

Parallels can be found in other industries. Digital technology did not create cars, music or commercial aviation. However, digital innovations such as car-sharing platforms, music-streaming apps, and flight-booking websites make utilisation of these pre-existing services more efficient, effective and convenient for consumers. In this sense, mHealth (and other applications of digital technology discussed in Chapters 4 and 6) has the potential to add value (manage costs as well as improve outcomes) – if implemented well in terms of regulation, coverage and funding.

A related advantage of smartphone apps is their negligible marginal cost and their scalability. Once programming is completed and the app tested and verified, the number of times it can be downloaded and used is virtually unlimited. There is no need for hardware as users will generally not purchase a smartphone only to use health and wellness apps. Any improvements or corrections to the software are automatically updated on the user's smartphone via the Internet. More importantly, an app can be used over and over, incurring only a one-off expense to the consumer. Some health apps, however, charge a monthly user fee and those enabling telehealth deploy a FFS model (Duffy, 2015). In 2016 a Massachusetts company offered to test and place individuals' entire genome on their smartphone for USD 999 (Regelado, 2016).

The regulatory and funding implications of mHealth are discussed in Chapter 4. Existing frameworks, processes and institutions are not adequately equipped to address these new technologies. Passive adoption of mHealth will not guarantee success in terms of clinical outcomes or value for money. Successful integration of mHealth in health care systems requires a number of adaptations: the performance and clinical utility of mobile applications must be assessed for reliable and efficient use in health care, and financial incentives are needed to encourage take-up of mobile applications that are effective and cost-effective. In addition, exchanges of information must be protected by appropriate levels of cybersecurity.

2.4. *Wearable devices and sensors with digital tools may complement traditional diagnostics*

Traditional medical devices such as implantables (e.g. pacemakers) are employing digital communication tools to deliver and/or receive data, for example via a mobile application on a patient or provider's smartphone. Wearable devices and sensors can continuously transmit a person's vital signs to his provider in real time, permitting more effective and tailored management of health problems. Such technologies combine the existing challenges in regulating medical devices with the emerging regulatory challenges surrounding mHealth described above. In particular, the performance of digital communication tools is paramount, as is adequate training and monitoring of users (providers and/or patients). This is true for any input to clinical decision making, but is amplified as such treatment decisions become automated.

Biosensors facilitate the remote monitoring of biological, physical and lifestyle parameters; devices can be worn anywhere on the body, swallowed (disposable) or implanted. Monitoring sleep is fairly well-established. Wellness/fitness wearables are already available and increasing in popularity and the field is evolving to collect additional data elements using both internal and external sensors, permitting real-time monitoring by patients and/or providers.

The convergence of wireless network technology (e.g. smartphones) and biometric sensors offers patients the opportunity for home-based monitoring of their health status. A well-developed literature exists on the use of biometric sensors for home-based health monitoring as part of a comprehensive eHealth infrastructure. For example, wireless oesophageal pH monitoring was authorised for clinical use in recent years, and a new endoscopic technology that combines wireless telemetry with video is being discussed.

As cited by the European COST foresight exercise, the backbone of life-enhancement technologies will be data, gathered in part from ubiquitous lightweight wearable biosensors (COST, 2009). These tiny devices will provide basic monitoring and measurement data in real time and place, thereby providing advanced, patient-focused health care services. These sensors and cameras will continuously check body functions such as blood pressure, heartbeat, alcohol levels, concentrations of drugs and individuals' emotional state.

The Ninth Japanese Delphi process yielded numerous market access predictions involving biosensor technology between now and 2030, such as: a medical chip embedded in the human body that enables health-condition monitoring, self-powered by bioenergy sources such as body heat or blood flow; nanochamber arrays that enable instantaneous detection of many biological reactions; wireless sensor networks strongly supporting human activities as needed by means of many sensors placed in the living space; and an assistant network robot that predicts risks by summarising life space information detected by sensors and/or various information from networks (NISTEP, 2010).

As far as impact on process of care, RAND noted that in relation to surveillance and public health, a range of technological capabilities will be needed, such as data mining and data fusion, the use of intelligence sensor networks, grid computing, and biosensor and biomarkers. "Big Data" capacity (see Chapter 6) will also be required, particularly in the use of smart analytics and integrating data in surveillance links with informatics and modelling (RAND, 2013).

2.5. *Additive manufacturing to permit "3D printing" of devices and potentially of transplant organs*

3D printing is already in common use in health care, for example in dental care and joint replacement (Tremblay, 2006; COST, 2009). 3D printing enables providers to create a device matched to a patient's anatomy, which may in turn improve patient outcomes. However, this causes disruption in the traditional supply chain of such products, challenging not only the economic business model of the medical device industry, but also the regulation of these devices.

3D bioprinting, currently in development, is even more challenging. 3D bioprinting applications engineer tissue from human cells. The ultimate goal of 3D bioprinting is seen as replacing damaged neurological tissue and entire organs to help meet the growing public health crisis of transplant organ shortages. However, other potential clinical applications of this technology arise – regenerative scaffolds and bones, bridge to transplant, in-situ printing of cells directly onto a wound, or even potential cosmetic applications (Murphy and Atala, 2014).

While currently all bioprinted tissue is still experimental for human implantation, some tissues are beginning to enter clinical trials. A market is growing for bioprinted tissues to aid in R&D – for example, studies of liver toxicity using 3D bioprinted liver tissue could be an eventual replacement for preclinical animal testing. This is seen as potentially saving significant cost in the R&D process by limiting the number of products that fail in clinical trials (Fischer, 2013).

The range of intertwined technical and regulatory questions this technology will raise is vast: for example, in the case of 3D bioprinting, should cells be the patient's own or from a donor? Will tissue be printed into patients within the operating suite, within the health service facility, or off site? Would printed tissue be regulated as a device, tissue therapy, or a medical service? How could policy makers assess the economic benefit of such an intervention (Box 2.3)?

Box 2.3. Analysing potential impacts of 3D bioprinting on health care delivery

3D bioprinting is cited by many across the OECD as having the potential to both create new therapies for unmet medical needs and replace existing standards of care. For example, if tissues can be engineered for transplant using autologous (i.e. the patient's own) cells, the need for antirejection medication will decrease significantly. Furthermore, if the technology does indeed advance to the point where transplantable organs can be printed (a longer-term objective), reduced time on donation lists and costs of interim care (such as dialysis or ventricular assist devices) could truly affect the process of care for many conditions.

To assess the gaps in the existing body of knowledge on the potential impact of 3D bioprinting on health care delivery, in 2015 the OECD analysed key health care delivery impact indicators for 3D bioprinting. Key stakeholders were consulted to elucidate primary concerns for 3D bioprinting dissemination, and identify potential needs for health care system changes stemming from 3D bioprinting. Academic research scientists, product developers, policy/regulatory authorities, legal/ethical specialists and clinicians discussed in-depth their views on the current state of the technology and its potential future impact on health care systems.

A key finding was the lack of consensus on key elements of the process of care that will affect nearly every aspect of the impact this technology has on care delivery. In particular, strong disparities arose among experts interviewed related to the source of the cells for use in 3D bioprinting (the patient's own or from a donor), as well as the dissemination model/process of care to put those cells to clinical use (whether tissue can print directly into a patient versus printing tissue for transplant). Perhaps the biggest question is process of care – i.e. whether printing will take place within the operating suite, within the health service facility, or offsite – as this will affect many aspects of its regulation and reimbursement. Similarly, regulatory considerations largely hinge on the chosen model of dissemination – bioprinter (device), bioprinted tissue (biopharmaceutical cell/tissue therapy) or surgical intervention (medical service).

These decision points demonstrate the large spectrum for applications of this innovation. This is of great interest at this stage, since each decision point regarding the 3D bioprinting delivery model has a series of outcomes, costs and regulatory trade-offs. For example, facilities will need to consider whether volume will be adequate to justify investment in 3D bioprinting equipment or to source the tissue from another facility (or commercial manufacturer), which in turn may limit their ability to pursue any of the in-situ applications of the technology.

Despite the significant research taking place in OECD countries and its high potential to "disrupt" process of care for surgeries and patients awaiting transplant, 3D bioprinting is not yet "on the radar" of many policy makers. Modelling is needed to affirm whether offsets will translate to economic benefits, but it is clear that broader issues beyond cost must be addressed to effectively understand and achieve the promise of this technology.

Therefore, policy makers will need to consider the differential impact on care delivery, and strategies to mitigate potential access barriers, across the various scenarios. Such domains to help drive towards an ideal state could include various elements discussed throughout this report, including a data infrastructure, frameworks for evaluating evidence, evidence communication, and transparency of coverage and payment. While the challenges facing each technology will be different, when placed against one another these themes can be validated and potential sources for a more rigorous quantitative analysis could emerge. This will permit a more thorough analysis on existing impact frameworks, care delivery evaluation indicators, measures of adoption/dissemination success, and processes for adapting regulatory/reimbursement policies to new technologies.

3. Preparation for and promotion of high-value technology in health care systems

Imagining a future health care system that incorporates these technologies can easily enter the realm of science fiction. Therefore, policy makers have to find the right balance between strategic foresight, based on hypothetical future advances for sciences, and horizon scanning, which aims to assess the impact of health technologies about to enter the market.

Health care systems' sustainability depends on intelligent adoption of technologies that enable gains in population-based needs and outcomes. When technologies emerge that provide clear evidence of patient benefits in an affordable manner, they must be integrated into the health care system in a way that can improve that system's performance. This will very much depend on how the technology is used and on associated financing models.

The development of rational, systematic, early and ongoing decision-making processes to adopt value-adding technology could aid health care systems in preparing to reap potential benefits, and overcome barriers to adoption. Therefore, this section describes how proactive thinking about the potential impact of new technologies on care delivery can help OECD member health care systems manage uncertainties to ensure that patients and societies benefit from innovation.

3.1. *Existing early awareness and alert programmes vary in objectives, authority and methods*

As a first step towards priority setting and prudent allocation of scarce health resources, many countries are increasingly thinking proactively about medical technologies that are not yet on the market. Over half of OECD countries now deploy some degree of horizon scanning, most often considering technologies in a short-term time horizon, for example two to three years prior to market entry, although some engage in longer-term technology foresight. Some prominent national experiences within OECD countries that have published their methods and impact are described in Box 2.4.

Box 2.4. **Examples of early awareness and alert activity across OECD countries**

Australia and **New Zealand** conduct joint horizon scanning via HealthPACT, a subcommittee of the Australian Health Ministers' Advisory Council (AHMAC), reporting directly to the Hospitals Principal Committee (HPC) and giving priority to technologies diffusing rapidly in the health care system that do not yet have published assessments (ANZHSN, 2004).

Austria's Ludwig Boltzmann Institute for HTA (LBI-HTA) specifically focuses on horizon scanning in oncology, periodically publishing assessments on novel cancer drugs with a likely therapeutic and/or financial outcome. These assessments (59 published since 2009) serve as decision aids for funding agencies and the HTA in hospitals' decision-making network.

The **Italian** Horizon Scanning Project (IHSP) is developing a forecasting model to allow prediction of impact on the Italian National Health System (NHS) or Regional Health Systems (RHS) of emerging medicines identified via horizon scanning.

Korea's National Evidence-based Healthcare Collaborating Agency (NECA) started to undertake horizon scanning for early detection of developments and trends regarding emerging technologies starting in 2014. NECA H-SIGHT conducts both identification and

Box 2.4. **Examples of early awareness and alert activity across OECD countries** *(cont.)*

filtration, distinguishing between "New Health Technology under Development" at a pre-developmental stage, "Emerging New Health Technology" selected after prioritisation and assessment as worthy of national-level support for a clinical trial, and "New Health Technology" that is reaching launch.

Spain has several horizon-scanning initiatives, owing to the regional nature of its health care system. Assessments are carried out by the Agencia de Evaluacion de Tecnologias (AETS), the Agencia de Evaluación de Technologías Sanitarias de Andalucía (AETSA), as well as the Basque Office for Health Technology Assessment (Osteba).

The **United Kingdom** has a long-established Horizon Scanning Programme Team to co-ordinate strategic horizon-scanning work across departments. Specific to health, its National Institute for Health Research (NIHR) Horizon Scanning Centre (HSC) is set up in the Department of Public Health and Epidemiology at the University of Birmingham.

The Agency for Healthcare Research and Quality (AHRQ) in the **United States** contracts with the non-profit ECRI Institute (formerly the "Emergency Care Research Institute") to publish several Status Update Reports and Potential High Impact Reports per year. In the last updated report, published online in January 2016, ECRI was tracking 661 interventions in 15 priority condition areas (ECRI Institute, 2015). They note, "It is NOT the goal of the AHRQ Healthcare Horizon Scanning System to make predictions on the future use and costs of any health care technology. Rather, the reports will help to inform and guide the planning and prioritisation of research resources" (ECRI Institute, 2015).

International co-operation is common and developing in horizon-scanning activities, most commonly among regional and international HTA networks with an explicit or implicit horizon-scanning function: the Central and Eastern European Society of Technology Assessment in Health Care (CEESTAHC), the European Network for Health Technology Assessment (EUnetHTA), EuroScan, Health Technology Assessment International (HTAi), HTAsiaLink, the International Network of Agencies for Health Technology Assessment (INAHTA), and the HTA Network of the Americas (*Red de Evaluación de Tecnologías en Salud de las Américas*, RedETSA).

Early awareness and alert systems differ widely in their purpose, audience, time horizon, scope of technologies to be reviewed, stakeholder role, and processes for filtration, prioritisation and assessment. Horizon-scanning systems use scoring systems with varying degrees of quantitative rigor to assess expected impact on dimensions such as expected utilisation and financial impact. However, many technologies will not yet have any clinical or economic data publicly available on which to base such a quantitative assessment.

Many of these early awareness and alert systems and international collaborations exhibit good practice by considering the broader governance impact of new technologies along the following dimensions:

- *Expected patient benefits:* expected application and timing, potential use in patient treatment relative to existing standards of care, including endpoints.
- *Expected impact on process of care:* new skills or staffing required to deploy, likely adoption model, and other adjustments needed/desirable to ensure appropriate uptake of the technology.

- *Regulatory considerations:* any changes or adaptations of current regulatory framework required, or will it fit into current regulation.
- *Purchasing/reimbursement/pricing considerations:* anticipated scenarios and potential models for reimbursement authorities regarding financing for related health care activities.
- *Expected utilisation and financial impact:* perceived demand for utilisation; available comparisons to any current alternatives that could demonstrate cost-effectiveness.
- *Legal/ethical considerations:* any necessary/desirable adaptations to patients' rights to adapt to use, additional legal and ethical considerations for policy makers.
- *Dissemination considerations:* perceived acceptance by payers, providers and patients.

Evaluating the potential impact of a medical technology further into the future than existing horizon-scanning capacity presents a key challenge. Technology foresight studies, which adopt a longer-term perspective of 5 to up to 30 years, can help plan for introduction of new technologies into health care systems but seem to be of less relevance for health policy decision makers for day-to-day management of the system (Box 2.5).

Box 2.5. **Technology foresight study use by OECD health care systems**

Technology foresight studies are performed by a variety of different stakeholders within the health care system, ranging from the private sector to regional intergovernmental frameworks such as the European Cooperation in Science and Technology (COST, 2009). Many of these, however, represent one-off projects versus a sustained commitment to long-term forecasting. Foresight studies related to health focus generally on future grand challenges, such as demographic changes and ageing populations, multiple chronic conditions, climate change and changes in infectious disease patterns. Technological foresight studies specifically target technological innovation, and usually include a section on life sciences and health care.

Since 1971, large-scale science and technology foresight surveys have been conducted roughly every five years in Japan, housed since 1992 at the National Institute of Science and Technology Policy (NISTEP). In 2008, the US Food and Drug Administration (FDA) conducted a foresight exercise specifically designed to identify medical devices likely to emerge or develop substantially over the next decade (Herman and Devey, 2011). The OECD has been commissioned to perform foresight activities for member countries in the past, such as the report on "The Ageing Society 2030" commissioned from the OECD International Futures Programme Unit by the Danish Agency for Science, Technology and Innovation (DASTI, 2007).

Most long-term technology foresight studies discuss innovation trends in general terms, although research is emerging on characterising technology developments at the stage of early emerging applications. These methods propose to provide information supporting early decisions in health care systems and in the industry, and can classify the scenarios identified in the prioritisation stage according to their timing and likelihood. Examples include forecasting innovation pathways for emerging technologies (Robinson et al., 2013) or prospective HTA (Kolominsky-Rabas et al., 2014).

Limited evidence exists on the impact of foresight studies on health care systems. While not specific to health, the European Foresight Platform published a brief case study in 2012 measuring foresight impact, in particular noting that, "The challenge was to assess how to effectively measure impacts of foresight for government sponsors, operating in the short to medium term of 1-3 years when ideally these foresight impacts occur over a (mid to long

Box 2.5. **Technology foresight study use by OECD health care systems** *(cont.)*

term) 5- to 15-year time horizon" (Smith, 2012). Still, the question remained as to whether current or adapted technology foresight methods could adequately affect decision-maker awareness of emerging technologies in the mid to long term to influence policy decisions.

Participants in the OECD Workshop on New Health Technologies on 22 March 2016 suggested that perhaps the biggest need lies in "medium-term" technology planning: i.e. longer-term than what is currently captured by horizon scanning but shorter-term than what is often captured in technology foresight studies. Delegates noted that analysis on emerging trends in health technology innovation may be more valuable than attempts to predict the impact of specific technologies in early clinical development, but technology foresight can still play a role in health care systems. Such scenario planning can aid health care systems in anticipating potential reforms needed for regulation, reimbursement or process of care.

In practice, health care systems most often use early awareness and alert systems to focus their immediate priorities for HTA. Such shortened purview is understandable in an era of limited resources, but horizon scanning runs the risk of failing to consider other critical dimensions of a technology's impact on health care delivery. For example, the costs associated with dissemination of new health technology include not only the price of the technology itself, but also associated disruptions to the process of care, ethical debates, and reforms to regulatory and reimbursement systems. Important indirect benefits such as reduced costs in other parts of the health care system should also be considered. A more holistic approach to horizon scanning/technology foresight could aid in taking such elements into account.

3.2. Limited evaluation of horizon scanning in health care systems demonstrates areas for improvement

Conducting a thorough assessment of the impact of such efforts is hampered by a lack of evidence. Only a few studies to date have assessed and published the outcomes of early assessment of health technologies and their utility in affecting decision makers' awareness of and choices for emerging technologies. The National Institute for Health Research (NIHR) Horizon Scanning Centre (HSC) in the United Kingdom explored its ability to inform key policy and decision makers, with a study showing that 40% of pharmaceutical and non-pharmaceutical technologies recommended to the National Institute for Health and Clinical Excellence (NICE) by the HSC were selected by NICE for technology appraisal/HTA (Packer et al., 2012). HSC missed 7.8% of pharmaceuticals that received NICE appraisals.

Packer and colleagues (2006) assessed the impact of horizon-scanning activity on technology diffusion in ten EU countries from 1995 to 2004. This study specifically examined six technologies to explain any differential adoption and diffusion, finding that a positive or negative horizon-scanning recommendation did not have a significant impact on diffusion (defined as daily defined doses per quarter or vials/implants per million people). However, early notice of emerging technologies usually leads to an in-depth HTA, as noted in the study above for NICE in the United Kingdom.

In thinking about the broader international impact of horizon-scanning findings, Packer et al. (2012) noted that, "A major problem [with assessing early awareness and alert systems] is that the value of a technology is not absolute and will be interpreted differently within separate health care systems and between health professionals and patients."

Nachtnebel and colleagues (2016) evaluated the impact of Austria's horizon scanning in an oncology programme at Ludwig Boltzmann Institute for HTA after five years in operation. They found that demand exists for analysis in this domain, and the relevancy and content of reports are adequate, but users are mainly industry and entities outside Austria. In addition, users find some reports come too late (within four months after approval by the European Medicines Agency on average) and there are redundancies with work of other HTA agencies (although the timing of their analyses differed). The Institute has already taken steps to act on suggestions, including an improved dissemination strategy and improved collaboration with groups like EUnetHTA.

A study of the Australian health care system assessed the success of horizon scanning in identifying new and emerging technologies suitable for government-subsidised funding in the private health care sector. Forty-three technologies were subject to full HTA reports from 2004-08, i.e. since the introduction of horizon scanning in Australia (O'Malley and Jordan, 2009). Of the 43 technologies, only 11 had been the subject of either a Prioritising Summary or Horizon Scanning Report. Twelve of the 43 technologies with full HTA received positive recommendations for public funding but had not been the subject of a Prioritising Summary or Horizon Scanning Report. Despite being a preliminary descriptive evaluation, these observations suggested a breakdown in either the horizon-scanning or prioritisation process.

A key element affecting the incorporation of information in policy and decision making is the dissemination of information to users. Horizon-scanning reports vary in depth and dissemination methods depending on their objectives and intended audience. EuroScan conducted a comparative study in 2009 of the horizon-scanning methods employed by its members. According to this study, respondents produce reports of varying lengths, from short one-pagers to comprehensive reports of over 10 pages. Primary dissemination methods include email (70%), websites (50%), paper versions (30%) and medical journals (5%). Some reports are for internal use only and are not disseminated externally (10%). Workshops and conferences are also organised regularly by EuroScan, and the group has ongoing initiatives to explore the impact of such activities on funding, bibliometrics, research gaps, economic impact and health outcomes.

3.3. *Reinforced international co-operation could increase capacity, efficiency and impact*

Opportunities exist to improve collaboration and shared work in this area to improve impact and avoid duplication of efforts. To the extent that these efforts do not already incorporate the process and social considerations for technology dissemination, or foresight scanning for technologies and trends farther into the future, opportunities for strengthened or additional collaboration should be explored.

For example, early awareness and alert activities can be a tool to anticipate disruptions to current care pathways. Making technology a tool that complements decision making and teamwork will require reform in clinical education and models of practice. Infrastructure, work processes and institutions need to be updated as well. For new practices and workflows to have maximum impact and to enable health professionals to embrace the future, investments is required in new technologies, evolving models of practice, and health data. For example, a new medicine or device may disrupt a current process of care, in some instances adding cost/time and in others introducing efficiencies. Anticipating such costs and/or offsets can give policy makers a clearer window into future needs and budgets.

The emergence of new technologies into practice may necessitate reconsideration of payment systems to ensure their appropriate use and to avoid the pitfalls that sometimes occurred in the past. Changes to infrastructure and system design may have to provide incentives for using new technology to allow for systematic adoption that is long-lasting and transformative. Alternatives to financial incentives could include embedding new technology into workflows, providing medical education credits, and fostering closer interactions among health professionals. Deciding among these alternatives is a difficult task prior to knowing final information about a particular technology and its evidence of effectiveness and affordability. However, considering and communicating appropriate scenarios from early awareness and alert activities could ease appropriate uptake when such technologies do come to fruition.

Strategic planning and appraisal of new technologies and health care systems could focus more directly on standards, clinical priorities and outcomes, strategies for investment/procurement and R&D, skill and knowledge issues, and public participation. In addition, it is critical to share information on national innovation policies for member countries and on the feasibility and impact that new technologies will have (on patient outcomes, process of care, regulation, health care system financing, and any evidentiary, legal, or ethical considerations foreseen as potentially affecting their dissemination). These actions could help health care systems characterise the types of innovations that would be most beneficial to both the health sector and patients.

Finally, many early awareness and alert initiatives rely on describing technologies in the pipeline, pushed by industry, providers and other actors. Member countries should be more proactive in defining public health needs and research agendas to help build the right incentives for technology development, especially when the market will not do it. As the old linear model of innovation is replaced by more flexible, responsive and open approaches, additional work is warranted to assess what promotes these ecosystems, and how they can be implemented while preserving proper incentives. Health care systems have an opportunity to use such capacity to define unmet medical needs and propel desired innovation. By clearly identifying research priorities, health care systems can take a more active role in reforming the innovation model to attract new technologies that citizens need.

Conclusion

Informed decisions about new technologies require an understanding of how health technologies diffuse and the dynamic nature of health delivery systems. As noted in the European Commission COST report forecasting technology trends to 2030, "technology itself is rarely the issue; it is about politics as the social and ethical changes in society will be tremendous" (COST, 2009). In the absence of a whole-system approach, individual institutions may fail to optimise their future technology acquisition in terms of wider system requirements and purely think of medical innovation as increasing financial risk (Lakdawalla et al., 2015).

In the past, adoption and diffusion of medical technology across health care systems generally led to considerable gains in longevity and quality of life. However, these advances imparted increasing costs on the health care system, and were a principal driver of health expenditure growth in most developed countries. In contrast to other sectors, health technology had – and continues to have – an expansionary effect on the volume of care and on expenditure. The return on this expenditure appears to have plateaued in recent decades, and the value of continued investment in health technology is beginning to be questioned, particularly when compared to expenditure in other welfare-producing sectors of the economy.

An important lesson from the past is that the value derived from health technologies is primarily a function of how they are used, suggesting that this is amenable to control with the right policy settings. This applies to pure biomedical technology (e.g. drugs and medical devices), to process innovations (e.g. improved care processes and techniques), and to combinations of the two (e.g. same-day surgery). The challenge for policy makers, regulators and payers is to structure incentives across the system to promote appropriate use and discourage inappropriate application of technology.

Horizon scanning, and to a certain degree foresight studies, offer a systematic and information-rich approach to determining technology's capacity to meet the manifest and future population demands, how it is geographically distributed and accessed, and how it is paid for. Better understanding technologies' capabilities, their diffusion patterns and their potential impact in health care systems will help decision making.

At the same time, because innovation in health care is so often incremental, it can be difficult to adequately articulate the expected patient benefits of early emerging technologies without becoming hypothetical. The evidence behind technology in early phases of development is generally not strong enough for adequate health care system intervention. Even at the time of market entry and assessment for reimbursement, information on the absolute effectiveness, comparative effectiveness or cost-effectiveness of new technologies is still incomplete.

Continued work in this area should therefore focus on identifying trends in research and development for health technology, how these technologies affect the health care system, and policy considerations that could help health care systems work through the challenges they present, which will differ depending on the technology.

By reinforcing international co-operation in these areas, the efficiency and impact of such efforts can improve capacity to further analyse the impact of new technologies on care delivery. In so doing, further policy levers become apparent, many of which are specific to a particular technology type. Thus, subsequent chapters of this report contain a more detailed examination of the issues facing pharmaceuticals, medical devices, precision medicine, ICT and electronic health records (EHRs).

Notes

1. Low prices are partly responsible for the concerningly low number of novel antimicrobial agents being developed. A more detailed discussion on the failure of the market-based innovation model to deliver in this context is provided in Chapter 3.
2. These interventions are the application of scientific inquiry to solve the clinical and health problem of IHD, and therefore firmly within the definition of health technology adopted in this report.
3. Higher rates are observed among more affluent geographic regions (ACSQHC, 2015).
4. The impact of these diffuse technologies has been less studied in isolation but they can potentially have a considerable effect. For example, digital information networks that store and archive diagnostic images increase annual hospital costs by 1.8% (Bryan et al., 2000).
5. A "medical arms race" is said to fuel indiscriminate adoption and diffusion of new technology by health insurers fearful of missing out on market share (or political consequences) and health services trying to attract the best clinical talent (Hofman, 2015).

6. Canada, France, Germany, Switzerland and the United States.
7. It is generally assumed that direct development costs are priced into the remuneration for use of the technology. But it is unlikely that this includes the opportunity cost of diverting human capital and investment from R&D in other areas of enquiry (within and outside the health rector).
8. Expenditure was not subjected to sensitivity testing. For impact of medical care on longevity, sensitivity analyses that included a 25% assumption were performed but the headline results used the 50% assumption.
9. The favourable cost-benefit of the medical technologies aimed at combatting infectious diseases is tempered when important externalities and downstream costs such as antimicrobial resistance are considered.
10. The study did not capture other potentially important dimensions of quality such as patient experience, which may explain cost variation to some extent.
11. See note 9. Although the broader "spillover" benefits are not considered here, they can perhaps be assumed to be similar regardless of sector (health, education or other) although this has not been tested empirically.
12. However, not *all* public health intervention represents value compared to clinical treatments (Cohen et al., 2008).
13. Telehealth describes the provision of health care remotely using telecommunication tools such as telephones, smartphones and mobile devices.
14. This process also requires ongoing investment of resources and thus should be periodically evaluated based on the same principles as the technologies and interventions it examines.
15. Telehealth describes the provision of health care remotely using telecommunication tools such as telephones, smartphones and mobile devices.

References

ACSQHC – Australian Commission on Safety and Quality in Health Care (2015), *Australian Atlas of Healthcare Variation*, Australian Commission on Safety and Quality in Health Care, Sydney.

Angelis, A. and P. Kanavos (2014), "Applying Multiple Criteria Decision Analysis in the Context of Health Technology Assessment: An Empirical Case Study", *Value in Health*, Vol. 7, No. 17, A552.

ANZHSN – Australia and New Zealand Horizon Scanning Network (2004), "National Horizon Scanning Unit Horizon Scanning Report Combined CT and PET Scanner", Adelaide, February.

Asacaso, F. and V. Huerva (2013), "The History of Cataract Surgery", in F. Zaidi (ed.), *Cataract Surgery*, InTech, Rijeka, pp. 75-90.

Atella, V. and F. D'Amico (2015), "Who Is Responsible for Your Health: Is It You, Your Doctor or the New Technologies?", *European Journal of Health Economics*, Vol. 16, pp. 835-846.

Atkinson, L. and A. Zacest (2016), "Surgical Management of Low Back Pain", *Medical Journal of Australia*, Vol. 204, No. 8, pp. 299-300.

Baker, L. et al. (2003), "The Relationship Between Technology Availability and Health Care Spending", *Health Affairs*, *http://dx.doi.org/10.1377/hlthaff.W3.537.*

Barnato, A. et al. (2007), "Are Regional Variations in End-of-Life Care Intensity Explained by Patient Preferences?", *Medical Care*, Vol. 45, No. 5, pp. 386-393.

Batsawrous, A. et al. (2015), "Development and Validation of a Smartphone-Based Visual Acuity Test (Peek Acuity) for Clinical Practice and Community-Based Fieldwork", *JAMA Ophthalmology*, Vol. 133, No. 8, pp. 930-937.

Bellan, L. (2008), "The Evolution of Cataract Surgery: The Most Common Eye Procedure in Older Adults", *Geriatrics and Ageing*, Vol. 11, No. 6, pp. 328-332.

Binanay, C. et al. (2005), "Evaluation Study of Congestive Heart Failure and Pulmonary Artery Catheterization Effectiveness: The ESCAPE Trial", *Journal of the American Medical Association*, Vol. 294, No. 13, pp. 1625-1633.

Bochner, B., D. Sjoberg and V. Laudone (2014), "A Randomized Trial of Robot-Assisted Laparoscopic Radical Cystectomy", *New England Journal of Medicine*, Vol. 371, pp. 371-390.

Breeden, J. (2013), "Statement on Robotic Surgery by ACOG President", *www.acog.org/About_ACOG/News_Room/News_Releases/2013/Statement_on_Robotic_Surgery* (accessed 27 June 2016).

Bryan, S., M. Buxton and E. Brenna (2000), "Estimating the Impact of a Diffuse Technology on the Running Costs of a Hospital", *International Journal of Technology Assessment*, Vol. 16, pp. 787-798.

Buchbinder, R. et al. (2009), "A Randomized Trial of Vertebroplasty for Painful Osteoporotic Vertebral Fractures", *New England Journal of Medicine*, Vol. 361, pp. 557-568.

Cardona-Morrell, M. et al. (2016), "Non-beneficial Treatments in Hospital at the End of Life: A Systematic Review on Extent of the Problem", *International Journal for Quality in Health Care*, Vol. 28, No. 3, pp. 1-14.

Chandra A. and D. Goldman (2015), "Understanding Health Care's Short-Termism Problem", *Measuring Costs and Outcomes in Healthcare*, Harvard Business Review and New England Journal of Medicine, pp. 5-6.

Chandra, A. and J. Skinner (2012), "Technology Growth and Expenditure Growth in Health Care", *Journal of Economic Literature*, Vol. 50, No. 3, pp. 645-680.

Chandra, A. and J. Skinner (2008), "Technology and Expenditure Growth in Health Care", *NBER Working Paper Series*, Cambridge, United States.

Chang, W. and M. Shapiro (2016), "Association Between Intensive Care Unit Utilization During Hospitalization and Costs, Use of Invasive Procedures, and Mortality", *JAMA Internal Medicine*, *http://dx.doi.org/10.1001/jamainternmed.2016.4298*.

Chernew, M. and J. Newhouse (2012), "Health Care Spending and Growth", in M. Pauly, T. McGuire and P. Barros (eds.), *Handbook of Health Economics*, Vol. 2, Elsevier.

Chew, D.P. et al. (2016), "Variation in Coronary Angiography Rates in Australia: Correlations with Socio-demographic, Health Service and Disease Burden Indices", *Medical Journal of Australia*, Vol. 205, No. 3, pp. 114-120.

Chhatwal, J. et al. (2015), "Cost-Effectiveness and Budget Impact of Hepatitis C Virus Treatment With Sofosbuvir and Ledipasvir in the United States", *Annals of Internal Medicine*, Vol. 162, No. 6, pp. 397-406.

Cohen, J., P. Neumann and M. Weinstein (2008), "Does Preventive Care Save Money? Health Economics and the Presidential Candidates", *New England Journal of Medicine*, Vol. 358, No. 7, pp. 661-663.

COST – European Cooperation in Science and Technology (2009), "Foresight 2030: Benefitting from the Digital Revolution", Workshop on Life Enhancement, Workshop Report: 30 June-2 July 2009.

Culyer, A.J. (2016), "Cost-effectiveness Thresholds in Health Care: a Bookshelf Guide to their Meaning and Use", *Health Economics, Policy and Law*, Vol. 11, pp. 415-432.

Cutler, D. (2007), "The Lifetime Costs and Benefits of Medical Technology", *NBER Working Paper Series*, No. 13478, Cambridge, United States.

Cutler, D. and M. McClellan (2001), "Is Technological Change in Medicine Worth It?", *Health Affairs*, Vol. 20, No. 5, pp. 11-29.

Cutler, D. and E. Meara (2000), "The Technology of Birth: Is It Worth It?", in A. Garber (ed.), *Frontiers in Health Policy Research*, MIT Press, Cambridge, United States, pp. 33-67.

Cutler, D., A. Rosen and S. Vijan (2006), "The Value of Medical Spending in the United States, 1960-2000", *New England Journal of Medicine*, Vol. 355, No. 9, pp. 920-927.

Dalen, J. (2001), "The Pulmonary Artery Catheter – Friend, Foe, or Accomplice?", *Journal of the American Medical Association*, Vol. 286, No. 3, pp. 348-350.

DASTI – Danish Agency for Science, Technology and Innovation (2007), "OECD-DASTI Horizon Scan", August 2007.

de Meijer, C. et al. (2013), "The Effect of Population Aging on Health Expenditure Growth: A Critical Review", *European Journal of Ageing*, Vol. 10, No. 4.

Dermio (2016), "Dermio" [online], *www.dermio.com/* (accessed 3 March 2016).

Dormont, B., M. Grignon and H. Huber (2006), "Health Expenditure Growth: Reassessing the Threat of Ageing", *Health Economics*, Vol. 15, No. 9, pp. 947-963.

Drummond, M.F. et al. (2005), "Methods for the Economic Evaluation of Health Care Programmes", in Drummond M.F. et al. (eds.), Oxford University Press.

Duffy, J. (2015), "10 Apps that Are Changing Healthcare" [online], *www.pcmag.com/article2/0,2817,2476623,00.asp* (accessed 3 March 2016).

ECRI Institute (2015), "AHRQ Healthcare Horizon Scanning System – Status Update November 2015", Plymouth Meeting.

Eklund, A., T. Nichols and H. Knutsson (2016), "Cluster Failure: Why fMRI Inferences for Spatial Extent Have Inflated False-positive Rates", *Proceedings of the National Academy of Sciences (PNAS)*, *http://dx.doi.org/10.1073/pnas.1602413113*.

Elshaug, A. et al. (2012), "Over 150 Potentially Low-value Health Care Practices: An Australian Study", *Medical Journal of Australia*, Vol. 197, No. 10, pp. 556-560.

Fischer, S. (2013), "The Body Printed", *IEEE Pulse*, November/December, pp. 27-31.

Ford, E. et al. (2007), "Explaining the Decrease in U.S. Deaths from Coronary Disease, 1980-2000", *New England Journal of Medicine*, Vol. 356, pp. 2388-2398.

Garber, A. and J. Skinner (2008), "Is American Health Care Uniquely Inefficient?", *Journal of Economic Perspectives*, Vol. 22, No. 4, pp. 27-50.

Garrison, L.P. and A. Towse (2014), "Personalized Medicine: Pricing and Reimbursement Policies as a Potential Barrier to Development and Adoption", in Anthony J. Culyer (ed.), *Encyclopedia of Health Economics*, Vol. 2, Elsevier, San Diego, pp. 484-490.

Gelijins, A. and N. Rosenberg (1994), "The Dynamics of Technological Change in Medicine", *Health Affairs*, Vol. 13, No. 3, pp. 28-46.

Goldstein, D. et al. (2016), "Global Differences in Cancer Drug Prices: A Comparative Analysis", *Journal of Clinical Oncology* (suppl; abstr LBA6500) *http://meetinglibrary.asco.org/content/164423-176* (accessed 11 October 2016).

Hartwell, D. et al. (2005), "Clinical Effectiveness and Cost Effectiveness of Immediate Angioplasty for Acute Myocardial Infarction: Systematic Review and Economic Evaluation", *Health Technology Assessment*, Vol. 9, No. 17, 1-99, pp. iii-iv.

Harvey, S. et al. (2006), "An Evaluation of the Clinical and Cost-effectiveness of Pulmonary Artery Catheters in Patient Management in Intensive Care: A Systematic Review and a Randomised Controlled Trial", *Health Technology Assessment*, Vol. 10, No. 29, pp. 1-166.

Herman, W.A. and G.B. Devey (2011), *Future Trends in Medical Device Technologies: A Ten-year Forecast*, U.S. Food & Drug Administration, Washington, DC.

Hofman, B.M. (2015), "Too Much Technology", *British Medical Journal*, Vol. 350, h705.

Holahan, J., A. Dor and S. Zuckerman (1990), "Understanding the Recent Growth in Medicare Physician Expenditures", *Journal of the American Medical Association*, Vol. 263, No. 12, pp. 1658-1661.

Howard, D. et al. (2015), "Pricing in the Market for Anticancer Drugs", *Journal of Economic Perspectives*, Vol. 29, No. 1, pp. 139-162.

Hurley J. (2000), "An Overview of the Normative Economics of the Health Sector", in A.J. Culyer and J. Newhouse (eds.), *Handbook of Health Economics*, Vol. 1, pp. 55-117.

Hutton, G. and L. Haller (2004), *Evaluation of the Costs and Benefits of Water and Sanitation Improvements at the Global Level*, WHO, Geneva.

IMS – Institute for Healthcare Informatics (2015), "Patient Adoption of mHealth: Use, Evidence, and Remaining Barriers to Mainstream Acceptance", September, Parsippany.

Jena, A. et al. (2015), "Mortality and Treatment Patterns Among Patients Hospitalized with Acute Cardiovascular Conditions During Dates of National Cardiology Meetings", *JAMA Internal Medicine*, Vol. 175, No. 2, pp. 237-244.

Keeler, E. and S. Cretin (1983), "Discounting of Life-saving and Other Nonmonetary Effects", *Management Science*, *http://dx.doi.org/10.1287/mnsc.29.3.300*, pp. 300-306.

Kolominsky-Rabas, P.L. et al. (2014), "Technology Foresight for Medical Device Development Through Hybrid Simulation: The ProHTA Project", *Technological Forecasting & Social Change*, Vol. 97, pp. 105-114.

Kuo, N., S. Wang and W. Chen (2016), "Using Information and Mobile Technology Improved Elderly Home Care Services", *Health Policy and Technology*, *http://dx.doi.org/10.1016/j.hlpt.2016.02.004*.

Lakdawalla, D. et al. (2015), "The Insurance Value of Medical Innovation", *NBER Working Paper* No. 21015, March.

Lambooij, M., P. Engelfriet and G. Westert (2010), "Diffusion of Innovations in Health Care: Does the Structural Context Determine Its Direction?", *International Journal of Technology Assessment in Health Care*, Vol. 26, No. 4, pp. 415-420.

Lamiraud, K. and S. Lhuillery (2015), "Endogenous Technology Adoption and Medical Costs", ESSEC Business School, Cergy.

Lane, H., N. Blum and E. Fee (2010), "Oliver Wendell Holmes (1809–1894) and Ignaz Philipp Semmelweis (1818-1865): Preventing the Transmission of Puerperal Fever", *American Journal of Public Health*, Vol. 100, No. 6, pp. 1008-1009.

Lee, D. and F. Levy (2012), "The Sharp Slowdown in Growth of Medical Imaging: An Early Analysis Suggests Combination of Policies Was the Cause", *Health Affairs*, Vol. 31, No. 8.

Legorreta, A. et al. (1993), "Increased Cholecystectomy Rate After the Introduction of Laparoscopic Cholecystectomy", *Journal of the American Medical Association*, Vol. 270, No. 12, pp. 1429-1432.

Lichtenberg, F. (2013), "The Effect of Pharmaceutical Innovation on Longevity: Patient-Level Evidence from the 1996-2002 Medical Expenditure Panel Survey and Linked Mortality Public-Use Files", *Forum for Health Economics & Policy*, Vol. 16, No. 1, pp. 1-33.

Morden, N. et al. (2012), "End-Of-Life Care for Medicare Beneficiaries with Cancer Is Highly Intensive Overall and Varies Widely", *Health Affairs*, Vol. 31, No. 4, pp. 786-796.

Murphy, K. and R. Topel (2006), "The Value of Health and Longevity", *Journal of Political Economy*, Vol. 114, No. 5, pp. 871-904.

Murphy, S.V. and A. Atala (2014), "3D Bioprinting of Tissues and Organs", *Nature Biotechnology*, Vol. 32, No. 8, pp. 773-785.

Nachtnebel, A. et al. (2016), "Looking Back on 5 Years of Horizon Scanning in Oncology", *International Journal of Technology Assessment in Health Care*, Vol. 32, No. 1, pp. 1-7.

Newcomer, L. (2012), "Changing Physician Incentives for Cancer Care to Reward Better Patient Outcomes Instead of Use of More Costly Drugs", *Health Affairs (Millwood)*, Vol. 31, No. 4, pp. 780-785.

NISTEP – National Institute of Science and Technology Policy (2010), "The 9th Science and Technology Foresight: Contribution of Science and Technology to Future Society (The 9th Delphi Survey, Summary)", *NISTEP Report* No. 140, March.

Nolte, E. and M. McKee (2004), *Does Health Care Save Lives?*, Nuffield Trust, London.

Nundy, S. et al. (2014), "Mobile Phone Diabetes Project Led to Improved Glycemic Control and Net Savings for Chicago Plan Participants", *Health Affairs (Millwood)*, Vol. 33, pp. 265-272.

OECD (2015a), *Health at a Glance: OECD Indicators*, OECD Publishing, Paris, *http://dx.doi.org/10.1787/health_glance-2015-en*.

OECD (2015b), *Data-driven Innovation: Big Data for Growth and Well-being*, OECD Publishing, Paris, *http://dx.doi.org/10.1787/9789264229358-en*.

OECD (2014), *Geographic Variations in Health Care: What Do We Know and What Can Be Done to Improve Health System Performance?*, OECD Publishing, Paris, *http://dx.doi.org/10.1787/9789264216594-en*.

OECD (2012), *Mortality Risk Valuation in Environment, Health and Transport Policies*, OECD Publishing, Paris, *http://dx.doi.org/10.1787/9789264130807-en*.

O'Malley, S.P. and E. Jordan (2009), "Horizon Scanning of New and Emerging Medical Technology in Australia: Its Relevance to Medical Services Advisory Committee Health Technology Assessments and Public Funding", *International Journal of Technology Assessment in Health Care*, Vol. 25, No. 03, pp. 374-382.

Packer, C. et al. (2012), "Analysing 10 Years of Early Awareness and Alert Activity in the United Kingdom", *International Journal of Technology Assessment in Health Care*, Vol. 28, No. 3, pp. 308-314.

Packer, C. et al. (2006), "International Diffusion of New Health Technologies: A Ten-country Analysis of Six Health Technologies", *International Journal of Technology Assessment in Health Care*, Vol. 22, pp. 419-428.

Porter, M.E. (2010), "What Is Value in Health Care?", *New England Journal of Medicine*, Vol. 363, No. 26, pp. 2477-2481.

Productivity Commission (2005), *Impacts of Advances in Medical Technology in Australia*, Australian Government, Canberra.

Rajaram, S. et al. (2013), "Pulmonary Artery Catheters for Adult Patients in Intensive Care", *Cochrane Database of Systematic Reviews*, Vol. 28, No. 2, CD003408.

RAND (2013), *The Future of Public Health: A Horizon Scan*, RAND Europe, Cambridge, United Kingdom.

Regelado, A. (2016), "For $999, Veritas Genetics Will Put Your Genome on a Smartphone App", *MIT Technology Review*, 4 March, *www.technologyreview.com/s/600950/for-999-veritas-genetics-will-put-your-genome-on-a-smartphone-app/#/set/id/600954/.*

Reinhardt, U. (2012), "Divide et impera: Protecting the Growth of Healthcare Incomes (Costs)", *Health Economics*, Vol. 21, pp. 41-54.

Robinson, D.K.R. et al. (2013), "Forecasting Innovation Pathways (FIP) for New and Emerging Science and Technologies", *Technological Forecasting & Social Change*, Vol. 80, pp. 267-285.

Scitovski, A. (1985), "Changes in the Costs of Treatment of Selected Illnesses, 1971-1981", *Medical Care*, Vol. 23, No. 12, pp. 1315-1357.

Scitovski, A. and N. McCall (1976), "Change in Treatment Costs for Selected Illnesses, 1951-1964-1971", National Center for Health Services Research, Washington, DC.

Sedlis, S. et al. (2015), "Effect of PCI on Long-Term Survival in Patients with Stable Ischemic Heart Disease", *New England Journal of Medicine*, Vol. 373, No. 20, pp. 1937-1946.

Shivonen, R. et al. (2013), "Arthroscopic Partial Meniscectomy versus Sham Surgery for a Degenerative Meniscal Tear", *New England Journal of Medicine*, Vol. 369, pp. 2515-2524.

Showstack, J., S. Schroeder and M. Matsumoto (1982), "Changes in the Use of Medical Technologies, 1972-1977 – A Study of 10 Inpatient Diagnoses", *New England Journal of Medicine*, Vol. 306, pp. 706-712.

Skinner, J., D. Staiger and E. Fisher (2006), "Is Technological Change in Medicine Always Worth It? The Case of Acute Myocardial Infarction", *Health Affairs*, Vol. 25, pp. w35-w47.

Smith, J. (2012), "Measuring Foresight Impact", *European Foresight Platform Brief*, No. 249, July.

Smith, S., J. Newhouse and M. Freeland (2009), "Income, Insurance and Technology: Why Does Health Spending Outpace Economic Growth?", *Health Affairs*, Vol. 28, No. 5, pp. 1276-1284.

Somogyi-Zalud, E., Z. Zhong and J. Lynn (2002), "The Use of Life-sustaining Treatments in Hospitalized Persons Aged 80 and Older", *Journal of the American Geriatric Society*, Vol. 50, No. 5, pp. 930-934.

Sorenson, C., M. Drummond and B. Khan (2013), "Medical Technology As a Key Driver of Rising Health Expenditure: Disentangling the Relationship", *Clinicoeconomics and Outcomes Research*, Vol. 5, pp. 223-234.

Steiner, C. et al. (1994), "Surgical Rates and Operative Mortality for Open and Laparoscopic Cholecystectomy in Maryland", *New England Journal of Medicine*, Vol. 330, No. 6, pp. 403-408.

Swartz, M. (2004), "Bacterial Meningitis: A View of the Past 90 Years", *New England Journal of Medicine*, Vol. 351, No. 18, pp. 1826-1828.

Temel, J. et al. (2010), "Early Palliative Care for Patients with Metastatic Non-Small-Cell Lung Cancer", *New England Journal of Medicine*, Vol. 363, pp. 733-742.

Tremblay, M. (2006), "Horizon Scan of Diagnostic Technologies, Technology Push or Treatment Pull", prepared by Tremblay consulting for the Ontario Diagnostics Services Committee, Rainmaker Publications.

US Department of Health, Education, and Welfare (1976), "Report of the President's Biomedical Research Panel: Appendix B", US Government Publishing Office, Washington, DC.

Vaccarella, S. et al. (2016), "Worldwide Thyroid-Cancer Epidemic? The Increasing Impact of Overdiagnosis", *New England Journal of Medicine*, Vol. 375, No. 7, pp. 614-617.

Van Nuys et al. (2015), "Broad Hepatitis C Treatment Scenarios Return Substantial Health Gains, But Capacity Is A Concern", *Health Affairs*, Vol. 34, No. 10, pp. 1666-1674, *http://dx.doi.org/10.1377/hlthaff.2014.1193.*

Varley, R., J. Tarvid and D. Chao (1998), "A Reassessment of the Cost-effectiveness of Water and Sanitation Interventions in Programmes for Controlling Childhood Diarrhoea", *Bulletin of the WHO*, Vol. 76, No. 6, pp. 617-631.

Weinstein, R., A. Lopez and E. Krupinski (2014), "Telemedicine: News from the Front Line", *American Journal of Medicine*, Vol. 127, No. 3, pp. 172-173.

Weisbrod, B. (1991), "The Health Care Quadrilemma: An Essay on Technological Change, Insurance, Quality of Care, and Cost Containment", *Journal of Economic Literature*, Vol. 29, No. 2, pp. 523-552.

WHO Regional Office for Europe (2013), *Health 2020: A European Policy Framework and Strategy for the 21st Century*, WHO, Geneva.

Wunsch, H. et al. (2009), "Use of Intensive Care Services During Terminal Hospitalizations in England and the United States", *American Journal of Respiratory and Critical Care Medicine*, Vol. 180, No. 9, pp 875-880.

New Health Technologies: Managing Access, Value
and Sustainability

Chapter 3

Innovation, access and value in pharmaceuticals

by
Valérie Paris *and* Allison Colbert

Pharmaceutical markets are changing across the world, raising a number of new questions that need to be addressed. This chapter first examines trends in R&D and in market approvals, highlighting gaps in R&D investments and the focus of new treatments on small population targets. Then, it looks at current challenges faced by policy makers, from pressure to speed market access to worrying trends towards the proliferation of high-cost products, which do not always deliver value. Finally, it reviews policy responses to these challenges and possible options to go further.

We thank Ane Auraaen and Annalisa Belloni for their contributions to this work. We thank country delegates and experts, as well as BIAC members, for their comments on earlier versions of this chapter and during the OECD Health Committee meeting of 28-29 June 2016. We also thank Mark Pearson (OECD) and Michel Grignon (McMaster University) for their detailed comments on earlier drafts.

Introduction

Current trends in pharmaceutical markets arouse both hopes and concerns. Some recent medicines are breakthrough innovations, bringing huge benefits to patients (e.g. new treatments for hepatitis C) and the pipeline shows promise to bring real improvements in areas such as cancer. On the other hand, prices of new medicines have skyrocketed, at times without an apparent systematic link with associated health benefits. Pharmaceutical spending is increasingly skewed towards high-priced "specialty medicines",[1] raising questions about static and dynamic efficiency.

This chapter first examines recent trends in pharmaceutical markets (Section 1). It shows that the pharmaceutical pipeline is rich, but does not adequately address some priority medical needs. The section reviews recent trends in approvals, highlighting the high proportion of targeted and/or orphan medicines. As a result of these trends, many new medicines are priced at very high levels that are not always related to high health benefits. Section 2 describes and assesses policies implemented so far by OECD countries to provide quicker access to new treatments, from faster approval pathways to managed entry agreements (MEAs), used to mitigate budget impact or to get better value-for-money. None of these instruments, however, seems to fully address growing concerns about the affordability of new and future treatments, access for patients, and sustainability of health spending. Section 3 thus suggests a set of policy options, currently experimented or envisaged, that could be explored to respond to these challenges.

1. Current trends in pharmaceutical markets

Current dynamics in the pharmaceutical market stir both hopes and concerns. While thousands of drugs are currently in development, some medical needs, such as treatments for neglected diseases, antimicrobial resistance (AMR) and dementia, are not yet adequately addressed (Section 1.1). The number of new medicines approved each year is on the rise, with an increasing share of therapies targeting small patient groups, reflecting both advances in biomedical science and the attractiveness of some market segments such as oncology and orphan medicines. Some of these new treatments may bring real benefits for patients (Section 1.2). At the same time, pharmaceutical spending is increasingly skewed towards high-cost products; in some market segments, medicines are launched at high prices that do not always coincide with high health benefits for patients (Section 1.3).

1.1. The pharmaceutical industry pipeline is rich but some unmet medical needs require further investment

According to Pharmaprojects (2016), more than 13 700 pharmaceutical products are in the pipeline in 2016, of which nearly 6 900 are in a clinical phase of development. Oncology is by far the most targeted therapeutic area, with almost one-third of medicines in development in 2016, followed by prophylactic vaccines and anti-infectives, and antidiabetics (Pharmaprojects, 2016). To some extent, these developments reflect priority health needs, especially those of high-income countries. Cancer accounts for 16.9% of the burden of disease in high-income countries, ranking second after cardiovascular diseases (21.3%) and before mental and behavioural disorders (12.3%).[2]

Pharmaceutical and biotech companies are the main investors in biomedical research and development (R&D). In 2009, the last year for which consolidated data are available, USD 240 billion were spent in health R&D globally, 90% of which was in high-income countries. Sixty per cent of these investments came from the private sector, 30% from the public sector and the remaining 10% from other sources (including private non-profit organisations) (Røttingen et al., 2013). The proportion of private investment in the pharmaceutical sector is likely much higher than in biomedical research as a whole. Private entities have no natural incentives to invest in development of products with poor market prospects. As a result, pharmaceutical R&D does not yet adequately address some unmet medical needs, such as the development of preventive, diagnostic and curative solutions to treat neglected diseases, fight AMR and address dementia.

Research for neglected diseases needs to be further encouraged

As early as the end of the 1990s, research gaps were identified for so-called "neglected diseases";[3] i.e. diseases mainly affecting populations in low-income countries with low ability to pay. Many initiatives adopted by governments, international organisations such as the World Health Organization (WHO), and non-governmental organisations (NGOs) encourage and fund R&D for these diseases, notably through grants and public-private partnerships (Pugatch et al., 2012). In 2014, USD 3 377 million was invested in neglected disease R&D, of which 68% was for HIV/AIDS, malaria and tuberculosis alone. The public sector contributed 64% of this global investment, the philanthropic sector 20%, and industry the remaining 16% (Policy Cures, 2015). Looking at R&D for about 40 very neglected diseases, Di Procolo and Jommi (2014) noted a growing interest in terms of research. The authors identified 650 clinical studies in 2012, almost 60% of which were sponsored by the public sector, 24% by industry and 9% by NGOs. More than prevalence or unmet medical need, the risk of disease diffusion seems to be one of the most important determinants in determining research targets.

Development of novel antibiotics to fight AMR is essential

AMR is now recognised as a top-order global health problem. Worldwide, AMR results in 700 000 deaths each year and if not addressed could escalate into a full-blown global health and economic crisis (Cecchini et al., 2015). Yet only a few of the products currently in development target resistant bacteria (Butler et al., 2013, Renwick et al., 2016b). In addition, cheap and effective diagnostic devices at the point of care are needed to appropriately target treatment and avoid unnecessary antibiotic use. Some rapid diagnostic tests are available at a cost that makes them cost-effective, but cheaper tests providing quicker results are much needed. The same can be said for effective vaccines.

Investment in R&D to discover new antimicrobials has become unattractive. Incentives for private companies to develop new antibiotics are quite low as the expected profitability is much lower than for other therapeutic categories, such as chronic diseases. The market is clearly not delivering in this important area, and additional measures should be implemented in parallel with policies supporting the reduction of resistance emergence, such as use of antimicrobials both in agriculture and in human health care.

Recent proposals suggest policy options to address this innovation failure (Renwick et al., 2016a; O'Neill et al., 2016; WHO, 2015; Cecchini et al., 2015). These options fall into two categories. Upstream interventions target the early phases of development, including basic research, which typically requires public funding due to the uncertainty of success, the time lags involved and the difficulties to get appropriate returns. Examples include public grants and partnerships between the public and private sector, and seed funding. Downstream mechanisms aim to reward successful companies at the end of the development process and at market entry. They take the form of milestone or end prizes,[4] patent buyouts[5] or advance market commitments,[6] and can potentially delink the reward from sales volume. These "pull mechanisms" reduce the risk to funders but may inflate the amount required to make investments attractive for developers. An ideal approach would combine up- and downstream mechanisms to encourage global innovation by lowering early development costs and boosting the reward at the end of the development process. Global research platforms will make research spending more cost-effective (Cecchini et al., 2015).

Given the global concern and cross-border nature of AMR, a number of regional and international initiatives are under way to combat this issue. AMR was a key topic of the recent G20 and G7 meetings – the latter resulting in the Global Union for Antibiotics Research and Development (GUARD) Initiative – and the UN General Assembly in 2016 included a high-level meeting on AMR. International initiatives aim to co-ordinate efforts and/or to secure funding. These initiatives include, for instance, the European Joint Programming Initiative on Antimicrobial Resistance (JPIAMR),[7] which aims to co-ordinate research efforts through joint calls for proposals to maximise the impact of dedicated funds and avoid duplication of research. This initiative brings together funding and research organisations in 22 countries. Other initiatives are the Transatlantic Task Force on Antimicrobial Resistance (TATFAR), the European and Developing Countries Clinical Trials Partnership, and the Global Action Plan on Antimicrobial Resistance. The European Commission also invested in public-private partnerships with the pharmaceutical industry through the Innovative Medicines Initiative (IMI) (see Renwick et al., 2016b for a full review and assessment of these initiatives). Work has been commissioned by stakeholders such as WHO (Renwick et al., 2016a) and the governments of Germany (Chorzelski et al., 2015) and the United Kingdom (O'Neill et al., 2016) on recommendations to enhance antibiotic R&D (Box 3.1 summarises the recommendations of the UK AMR review).

Box 3.1. **Recommendations of the United Kingdom AMR Review to encourage innovation and development of new technologies**

In 2014, the UK Government and the Wellcome Trust commissioned a Review on AMR, chaired by economist Lord Jim O'Neill. The review consisted of broad consultation and a research project assessing the strategies and costs of combatting AMR. In May 2016, the review released its final report and recommendations. It sets out specific interventions aimed at minimising the spread of infectious disease, promoting more judicious use of antimicrobial agents (which includes promoting the development of rapid diagnostics and vaccines), and stimulating development of new antimicrobials to combat resistance.

To stimulate innovation to combat AMR, the review first calls for better incentives for continued investment in new and improved antimicrobial agents, diagnostics and vaccines. Although annual antibiotic sales are worth about USD 40 billion per year, just over 10% of these are on patented products – about the same as the annual sales of one top-selling

Box 3.1. **Recommendations of the United Kingdom AMR Review to encourage innovation and development of new technologies** *(cont.)*

cancer drug. The review urges aligning commercial incentives with public health needs through policy intervention in the purchase and distribution of antimicrobials. This needs to ensure that innovation is adequately rewarded, but also decoupled from sales volumes and overuse. Downstream mechanisms – or "payments for success" – are proposed. These include market entry rewards – prizes of around USD 1 billion for each effective treatment of resistant infection – and harmonised regulatory frameworks and clinical trial networks are also suggested – which can significantly lower development costs.

The second recommendation is to establish a Global Innovation Fund for early-stage and non-commercial research. This fund will support "blue sky" research as well as work focused on neglected areas such as vaccines and diagnostics to overcome barriers to entry, and will ensure relevant organisations have sufficient funds to do this important upstream work, which does not always carry commercial or scientific appeal. The proposed worth of the fund is USD 2 billion over five years. An overarching objective of the fund is to link up and increase the size of existing initiatives such as the United Kingdom and China's Innovation Fund focused on AMR, the US Biomedical Advanced Research and Development Authority (BARDA), the Innovative Medicines Initiative (IMI) and European Joint Programming Initiative on Antimicrobial Resistance (JPIAMR). In this way it is hoped that the collective output can be increased.

The review estimates that all initiatives, including the ones described here, will cost USD 3-4 billion per year, or up to USD 40 billion over ten years. This assumes 15 new antimicrobial agents to be produced over the decade, of which 4 would be breakthrough products targeting areas of greatest concern, as well as the development and roll-out of rapid diagnostics. The review calls on governments to contribute funding and proposes several methods to cover this cost. These include creating new funding streams – such as taxes on antibiotics or transferable vouchers to reward new antimicrobials – all of which have advantages and disadvantages in terms of their impact on health care systems and health care. Another is an antibiotic investment charge imposed widely across the pharmaceutical sector and applied on a "pay or play" basis. This model shifts supply-side resources towards research. Relevant companies would have the option of paying a charge or investing in R&D in an area of need with regard to AMR. Money raised by the charge would fund the commercial, downstream incentives outlined above.

The review urges international co-operation and establishment of a global coalition through the G20 and the United Nations. While the proposals raised by the UK AMR Review merit ongoing assessment and consideration in the context of additional existing and emerging initiatives outlined above, such proposals hold promise in encouraging innovation and development of new technologies to combat AMR.

Source: O'Neill, J. et al. (2016), "Tackling Drug-resistant Infections Globally: Final Report and Recommendations – The Review on Antimicrobial Resistance Chaired by Jim O'Neill", Wellcome Trust and HM Government, London.

Development of dementia treatments needs to be boosted

Dementia is emerging as another leading health priority across the world, with a number of national and international initiatives taking shape in the last decade. Of all causes of early death in 2013, Alzheimer's caused the fifth-most years of life lost in developed countries (GBD, 2014). Here the innovation problem is largely due to the complexity of the disease and the difficulty in understanding its underlying mechanisms of action.

This complexity results in high rates of research failure, and alternative innovation models that reduce these risks are needed. These include shared public-private funding and a higher public investment in basic, upstream research (dementia comprises less than 0.5% of R&D budgets). Permitting early-phase clinical studies involving people with pre-symptomatic dementia must also be examined. As with AMR, global sharing of research data is crucial (OECD, 2015a, 2015b).

Regulatory and reimbursement reform is another way to stimulate investment. Costs can be reduced by simplifying processes and harmonising them across countries. Clear reimbursement policies that ensure sufferers have access to effective interventions can reduce investor uncertainty. Industry, academia, regulators, payers and patients' organisations each play important roles at various stages, and stronger collaboration between these groups is needed (OECD, 2015a, 2015b).

1.2. *Many new medicines approved are therapies targeting small populations*

The number of new products approved every year is on the rise. While experts noted a decline in pharmaceutical R&D productivity and output in the first decade of the 2000s (Scannell et al., 2012), the number of new active substances approved has been increasing since 2010 (Figure 3.1). Due to both advances in science and economic incentives, new medicines increasingly target small populations. The paragraphs below illustrate these trends in three areas: rare diseases, oncology and gene and cell therapies.

Figure 3.1. **Number of new active substances approved by six regulatory authorities, approval years 2006-15**

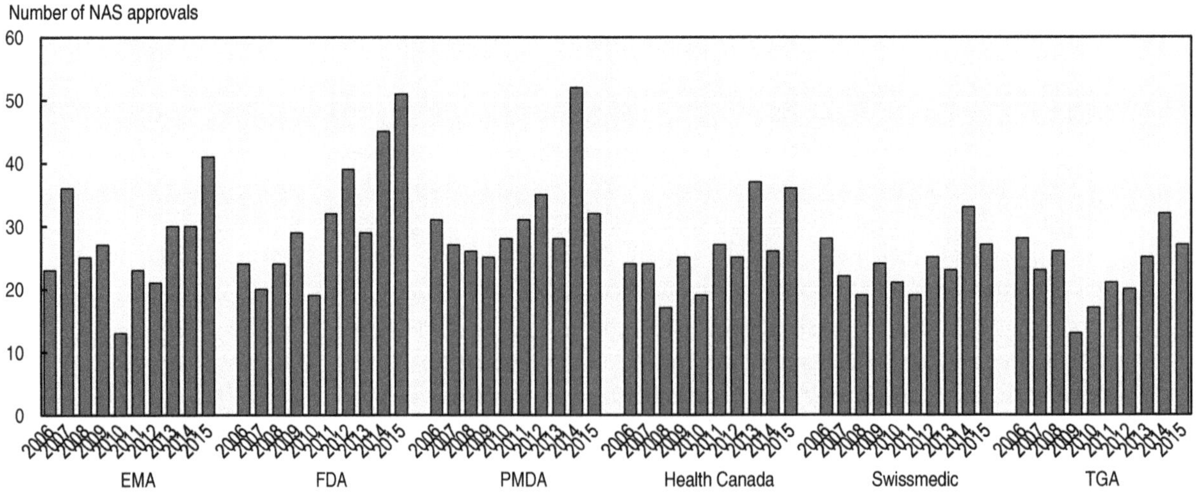

Note: EMA: European Medicines Agency, FDA: US Food and Drug Administration, PMDA: Regulatory authority in Japan, TGA: Australian Therapeutic Goods Administration.
Source: Based on Bujar, M., N. McAuslane and L. Liberti (2016), "R&D Briefing 59: The Impact of the Evolving Regulatory Environment on the Approval of New Medicines Across Six Major Authorities 2006-2015", Centre for Innovation in Regulatory Science.
StatLink http://dx.doi.org/10.1787/888933442896

Orphan drugs have become attractive for pharmaceutical companies

Policies adopted by OECD countries to encourage development of treatments for orphan diseases (see Annex 3.A1) undoubtedly contributed to the proliferation of orphan medicines (Figure 3.2). Following the United States in 1983, OECD countries such as Japan, Australia and the European Union introduced incentives for R&D investment in the treatment of rare

Figure 3.2. **Number of orphan drug designations/approvals in the United States and the European Union, 2000-15**

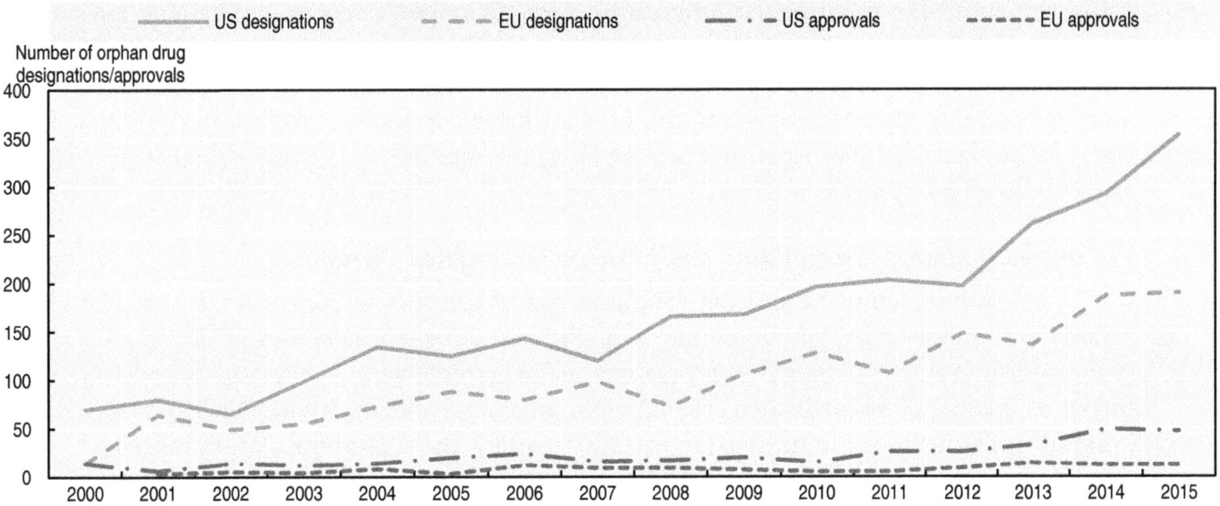

Source: Based on FDA Office of Orphan Drug Products; European Commission.

StatLink http://dx.doi.org/10.1787/888933442905

diseases. Though eligibility criteria and related advantages of getting an orphan drug status differ across countries, these incentives generally consist of subsidised R&D spending, expedited or facilitated regulatory approval and extended market exclusivity. During the first 25 years of the United States Orphan Drug Act, 326 new drugs were approved by the US Food and Drug Administration (FDA) and marketed. Orphan medicines now account for up to half of new molecular entities approved by the FDA every year. This trend is generally considered proof of success, though it is important to stress that treatments are available for less than 5 per cent of the approximately 7 000 rare diseases.

The recent surge in the number of orphan designations and orphan medicines proves that the industry has an interest to develop them. The probability for an orphan drug to be approved is 25.3% in Phase I, 33.3% in Phase II and 65.7% in Phase III, far higher than for other diseases such as oncology (respectively, 5.1%, 8.1% and 33.0%), although treatments with biomarkers fare better (25.9%, 33.8% and 72.3%, respectively) (Thomas et al., 2016). The expected return on investment of Phase III/Filed orphan drugs is estimated to be 1.14 times greater than that of non-orphan drugs (EvaluatePharma, 2015).

Orphan drug legislation is increasingly suspected to incentivise pharmaceutical companies, through the practice of "salami slicing". While the majority of orphan drugs are marketed only for their original orphan indication, several are subsequently marketed for additional orphan or non-orphan indications. For instance, the drug rituximab, originally approved to treat follicular B-cell non-Hodgkin's lymphoma, a disease that affects about 14 000 patients a year, is now used to treat several other types of cancer, organ rejection following kidney transplantation and auto-immune diseases, including rheumatoid arthritis, which affects 1.3 million Americans. Rituximab is the 12th-all-time drug best seller in the United States and generated USD 3.7 billion in domestic sales in 2014. Seven of the top ten best-selling drugs worldwide in 2015 have an orphan designation in the United States (Daniel et al., 2016). By 2020, the 20 top-selling orphan drugs will all be blockbusters (EvaluatePharma, 2015).

It is important to note, however, that the "actual benefits" attached to orphan drug status may differ across products. Orphan status is not granted to a medicine but to the combination of "one product-one indication". A medicine with several indications may have orphan and non-orphan indications. If a product has no competition in any of its indications, an orphan status extending market exclusivity can result in a long period of monopoly pricing. By contrast, when the product faces competitors from other original "me-too" products, price competition is more likely to occur and to become strong as soon as competitors go off-patent.[8]

The oncology market is expanding and focusing on targeted therapies

Oncology medicines accounted for about one-third of new approvals in the past decade and increasingly targeted small populations. Between 2006 and 2015, the FDA granted approval for 154 original or supplemental indications for oncology medicines. Over the whole period, of all medicines granted an original approval, 49 out of 75 (65%) had an indication linked to a biomarker (Figure 3.3). Among the 154 original/supplemental indications for oncology approved in 2006-15, 84 (55%) had received an orphan designation (Figure 3.4). The proportion of targeted therapies may increase in the future. According to the Pharmaceutical Research and Manufacturers of America (PhRMA) and the American Association for Cancer Research (AACR), three-quarters of the 836 medicines and vaccines in development for cancer in the United States in 2015 had the potential to be personalised medicines (PhRMA and AACR, 2015).

Figure 3.3. **Original FDA approval for oncology, stratified by personalised medicine status, 2006-15**

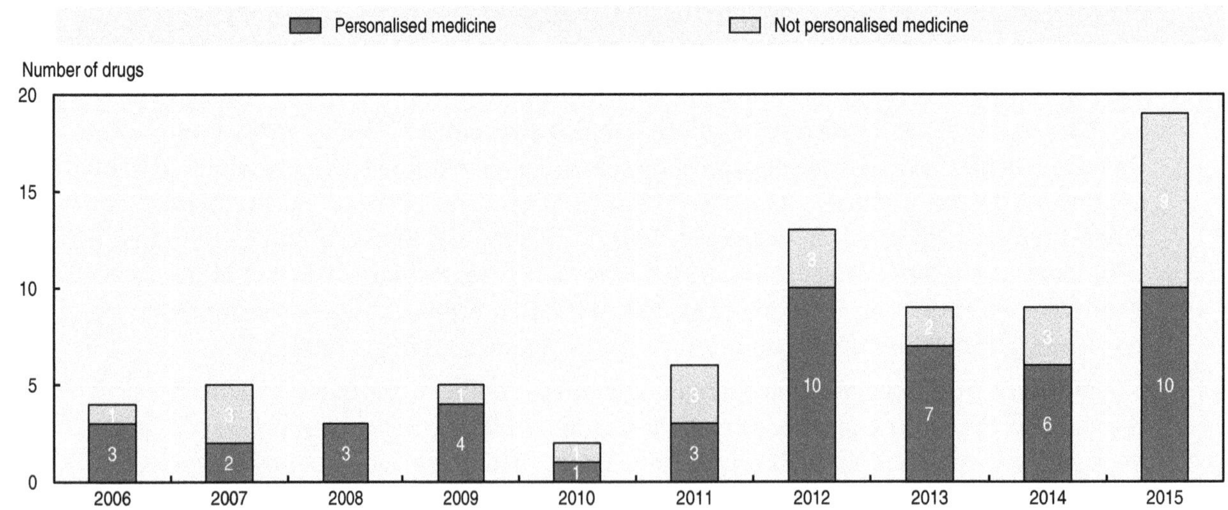

Note: Personalised medicines were defined as medicines associated with a biomarker.
Source: Authors' estimates, based on FDA.

StatLink http://dx.doi.org/10.1787/888933442916

Cell and gene therapy development is under way

Cell and gene therapies are being developed for a number of indications. According to the Alliance for Regenerative Medicines, nearly 700 gene therapy trials are under way by both industry and charitable foundations, with 70 in Phase III. Many of these drugs are expected to be one-off treatments curing one of about 5 000 rare diseases caused by errors

Figure 3.4. **Original FDA approval for oncology, stratified by orphan status, 2006-15**

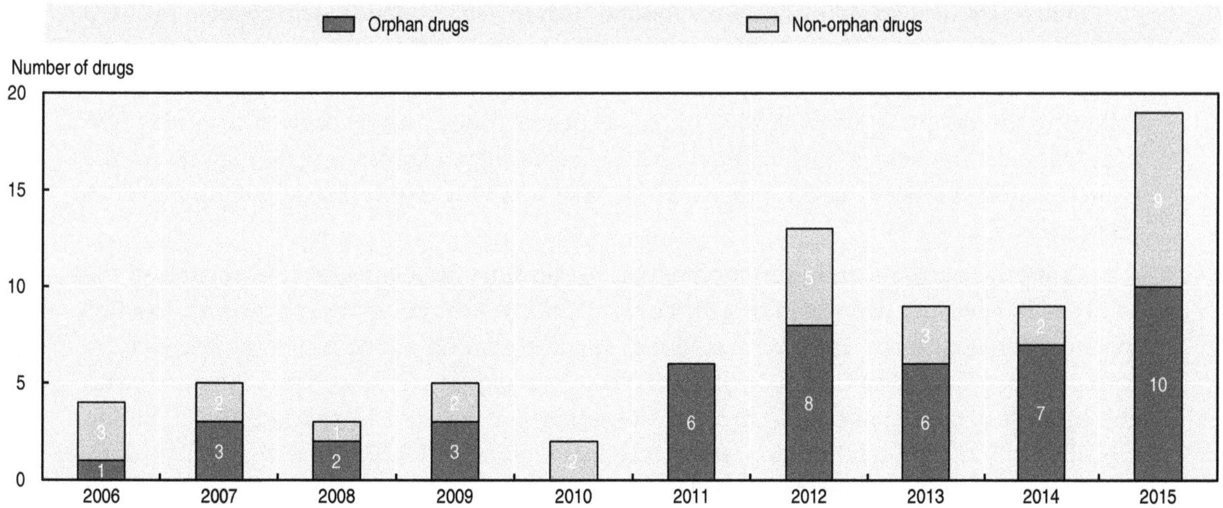

Note: Medicines were considered "orphan" when their initial approval was for an indication with an orphan designation.
Source: Authors' estimates, based on FDA.

StatLink http://dx.doi.org/10.1787/888933442922

in a single gene (Regalado, 2015, 2016a, 2016b). These medicines combine all the characteristics leading to high prices: high development and production costs, often very small target populations, and potentially high effectiveness and even potential cures. The first gene therapy to obtain European Medicines Agency (EMA) approval (Glybera®, used to treat an ultra-rare disease) struggles to reach patients due to the rarity of the condition and difficulties in obtaining health care system funding for its price tag (~EUR 1 million per cure). A new gene therapy treatment for the "bubble-boy" disease (severe combined immunodeficiency) targets only about 14 cases a year in Europe and 12 in the United States (Regalado, 2015, 2016a, 2016b).

Cell therapies are also being developed in oncology. More than 30 companies have started tests or intend to do so. The idea is to remove cells from a patient's immune system (T cells), engineer them genetically to target their cancer and then drip them back into the patient's blood. Such so-called chimeric antigen receptor T cell (CAR-T) therapies are currently being tested for diseases such as acute lymphoblastic leukaemia. At the time of writing, most stakeholders are optimistic regarding the promise of this method though others, such as the Recombinant DNA Advisory Committee, the federal body in the United States overseeing gene therapy (within the National Institutes of Health), point to the urgency for researchers to ensure that expected benefits outweigh the potential risks of damaging vital organs (Regalado, 2015, 2016a, 2016b).

The development of cell and gene therapy perhaps holds some of the greatest promise of the precision medicine movement. However, in addition to price concerns noted above, such therapies will have difficulty demonstrating effectiveness using traditional trial models, particularly when the treatment is by definition tailored to the individual patient. If such treatments indeed become the rule rather than the exception, there will be an urgent need to reassess current development, regulatory, coverage and pricing models to ensure sustainable access to innovative therapies.

1.3. Pharmaceutical spending is increasingly skewed towards expensive medicines

Pharmaceutical spending accounts for one-fifth of health spending on average in OECD countries, taking into account medicines used in outpatient and inpatient care (Belloni et al., 2016).[9] While overall spending for medicines did not increase or even decreased in the years following the economic crisis of 2008-09, it has become increasingly skewed towards high-cost "specialty medicines" (Belloni et al., 2016). According to Express Scripts analyses, in the United States, specialty drugs represented 37.7% of total prescription drug spending in 2015 (Express Scripts, 2016).

Oral cancer agents and immunomodulators account for a considerable portion of the increase in specialty drug spending (Trish et al., 2014). According to reports from the IMS Institute for Healthcare Informatics, global spending on oncology drugs increased from USD 84 billion in 2010 to USD 107 billion in 2015. Oncology is also the therapeutic area with the highest expected spending growth: spending is predicted to reach USD 150 billion globally by 2020 (IMS Institute for Healthcare Informatics, 2016). While these trends partly reflect an increase in the incidence and burden of cancer in OECD countries, they also result from commercial strategies of pharmaceutical companies and high prices.

New treatments tend to be priced at high levels

Specialty drugs' prices increased considerably over the years. In the United States, companies' median revenue per patient for the top 100 selling drugs saw a seven-fold increase in just four years, from USD 1 260 in 2010 to USD 9 400 in 2014 (EvaluatePharma, 2014). In the United States again, a treatment for multiple sclerosis now costs USD 60 000 per year, about ten times what it cost ten years ago (Hartung et al., 2015). In oncology, the median monthly price of cancer treatment for Medicare patients has dramatically increased, especially since 2000 (Figure 3.5): 12 out of 13 cancer drugs approved in 2012 cost more than

Figure 3.5. **Median monthly costs of cancer drugs at FDA approval in the United States, 1965-2015**

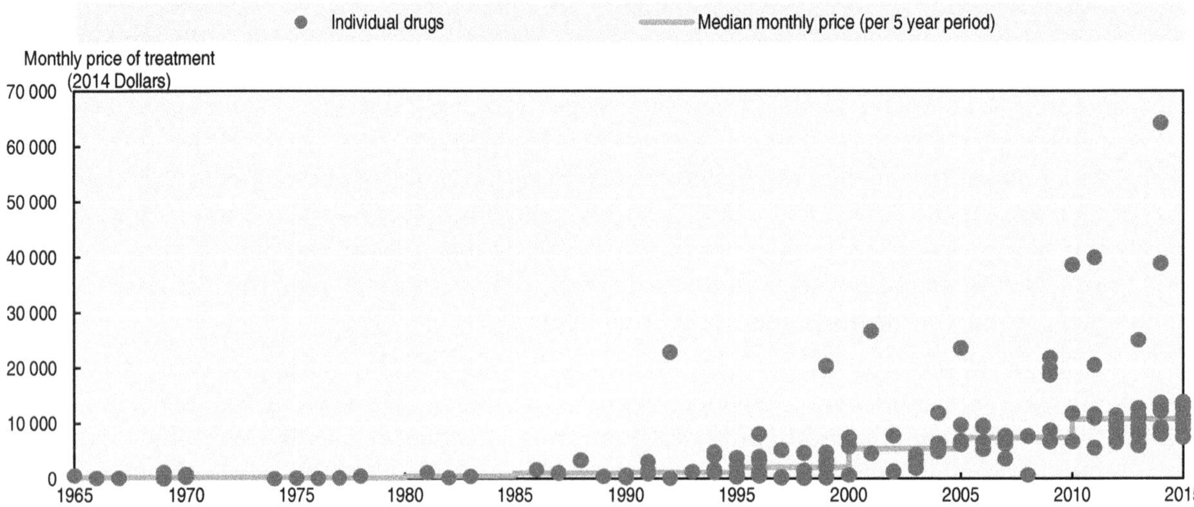

Note: The price of a monthly treatment refers to the treatment of a person who weighs 70 kg or has a body-surface area of 1.7 m^2. The gray line indicates median prices during a five-year period. Prices were adjusted to 2014 dollars and reflect the price for the drug at the time of approval, including both the amount of Medicare reimbursement and the amount paid by the patient or by a secondary payer.
Source: Based on Peter B. Bach, Memorial Sloan-Kettering Cancer Center, available at: *www.mskcc.org/research-areas/programs-centers/health-policy-outcomes/cost-drugs.*

StatLink http://dx.doi.org/10.1787/888933442936

USD 100 000 per year (Light and Kantarjian, 2013). Although prices vary widely, price increases are observed across many OECD countries (Box 3.2). In Australia, the average reimbursement price per anticancer prescription drug increased by 133% in real terms over the period 1999-2000 to 2011-12, while the price of all other prescription drugs only increased by 37% in the same period (Karikios et al., 2014).

Box 3.2. **Cross-country variations in list prices of expensive medicines**

Actual prices paid by payers for expensive therapies are generally not known, due to the development of managed entry agreements (MEAs), which disconnect list prices from actual prices paid (Section 2.3). That said, important variations in list prices are observed across OECD countries.

A recent study by Vogler et al. (2016) compared list prices of 31 originator cancer drugs in 16 European countries, Australia and New Zealand.[1] This study found that price differences between the highest- and lowest-priced country for each drug surveyed varied between 28% and 388%. The difference between the prices of a drug in the highest- and lowest-priced country was between 28% and 50% for ten drugs (one-third of the drugs sampled), between 50% and 100% for half of the sample, and between 100% and 200% for three medicines. Prices reported in Sweden, Switzerland and Germany were generally high while prices in Mediterranean countries such as Portugal, Spain and especially Greece and in the United Kingdom tended to be lower. However, as mentioned later in the chapter, oncology medicines are increasingly subject to all sorts of MEAs, which disconnect their list prices from the actual price paid. This practice represents a clear limitation, both for price comparisons in this class and for the use of international price benchmarking in price regulation.

List prices of hepatitis C treatments vary two-fold between OECD countries. In 2015, the ex-factory list price of a 12-week course of sofosbuvir across 26 OECD countries ranged from USD 48 999 in Japan to USD 84 000 in the United States. When adjusted for purchasing power parity, list prices appeared to be particularly high in Poland, Turkey, the United States and the Slovak Republic. By contrast, the lowest list prices were observed in Nordic European countries, Switzerland and the United Kingdom. Treating the entire population in these countries – assuming a 23% rebate in all of them – would cost from 10.6% of total pharmaceutical spending in the Netherlands to more than 150.0% of total pharmaceutical spending in New Zealand or Poland (Iyengar et al., 2016).

Price variations across countries are not all bad. Cross-country differential pricing is commonly envisaged as an appropriate policy to widen access to medicines in lower-income countries while allowing companies to derive profits from markets in higher-income countries and continue to invest in R&D. However, in the current situation, there is no guarantee that poorer countries pay lower prices than richer ones. List prices, which are used as a benchmark for further negotiations at a local level, suggest this is not the case.

1. In Austria, Denmark, Finland, Germany, Italy, Norway, Sweden and the United Kingdom, price information was available for all or all but one drug surveyed whereas the availability of price data was restricted for some drugs in other countries, especially New Zealand and Portugal.

In addition, the duration of treatment with new cancer drugs has increased, partly due to their ability to prolong life. In the United Kingdom, the average median duration of treatment with a new drug rose from 181 days in 1995-99 to 263 days in 2010-14. In parallel, the average cost of treatment increased from GBP 3 037 (20.6% of gross domestic product [GDP] per capita) in 1995-99 to GBP 35 383 (141.7% of GDP per capita) in 2010-14 (Savage and Mahmoud, 2015).

Medicine prices are not always commensurate with health benefits

High prices of new medicines are not always associated with high benefits (Howard et al., 2015; Light and Kantarjian, 2013). Typically, the prices of medicines used for very severe conditions and/or diseases with no alternative treatment are too often disconnected from the health benefits they bring to patients. Many of these drugs are not cost-effective according to standard thresholds.[10]

In oncology, many new cancer drugs provide small added benefits over existing ones. Among the 12 new anticancer drugs approved by the FDA in 2012, only one provides survival gains that exceed two months. The launch price of 58 cancer drugs approved during this period increased regardless of the drug's impact on survival. "In 1995 patients and their insurers paid USD 54 100 for an additional year of life. A decade later, in 2005, they paid USD 139 100 for the same benefit. By 2013, they paid USD 207 000" (Howard et al., 2015). This represents a 10% annual increase over the period, even when adjusted for inflation (Figure 3.6). And these costs do not include the costs of other medicines or treatments used in combination nor the costs of dealing with adverse effects (Howard et al., 2015).

Figure 3.6. **Price per life year gained versus FDA approval date for oncology products, 1995-2013**

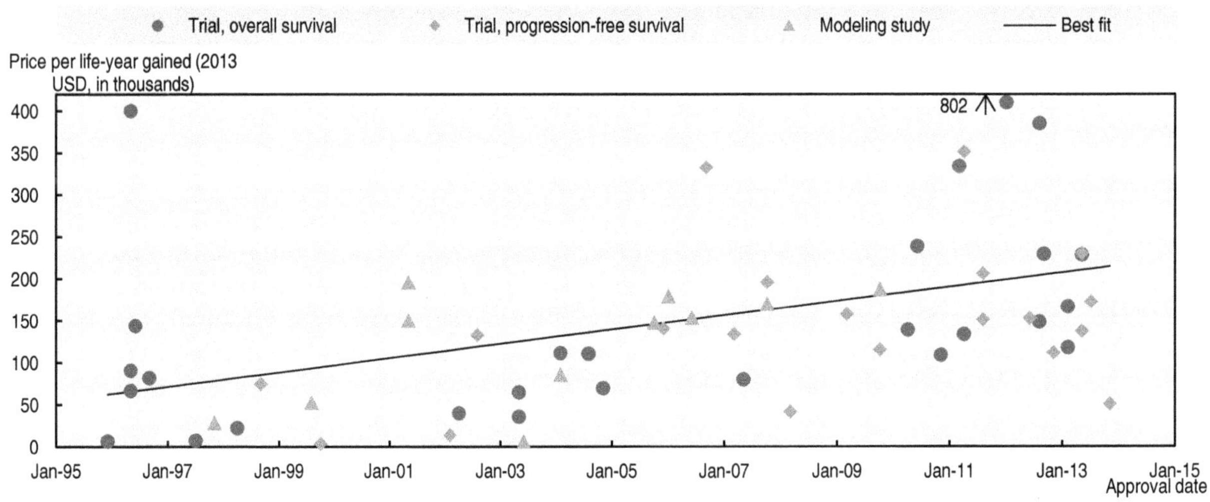

Source: Adapted from Howard, D. et al. (2015), "Pricing in the Market for Anticancer Drugs", *Journal of Economic Perspectives*, Vol. 29, No. 1, pp. 139-162.

StatLink http://dx.doi.org/10.1787/888933442948

New products targeting severe diseases often do not meet standard cost-effectiveness thresholds. The proportion of oncology drugs not recommended by the National Institute for Health and Care Excellence (NICE) has increased over the years. While it is 31% for the whole period between 2000 to 2016, nearly 60% of new indications approved after 2007 were not recommended, despite an increase in the threshold for products used at the end of life (NICE, 2016; Polton et al., 2015).

Orphan drugs often do not meet standard ICER thresholds. Incremental costs per quality-adjusted life year (QALY) gained often exceed USD 100 000 and even EUR 1 million in extreme cases (Schuller et al., 2015). A systematic review of economic evaluations of ultra-orphan[11] medicines showed that high-quality studies are scarce and that results differ substantially depending on assumptions on clinical benefits, models used and perspectives adopted. For instance, ICERs of treatments ranged from EUR 351 622 to EUR 3 282 252 per

QALY for Fabry disease, from EUR 153 405 to EUR 1 043 868 per QALY for Pompe disease, and from EUR 43 532 to EUR 432 540 for Gaucher disease (Schuller et al., 2015). As it stands, prices of orphan drugs seem to be mainly justified by the market power of sellers and by the size of the target population (the smaller the population, the higher the price), independent of the "quantity" of clinical benefits, let alone cost-effectiveness or cost-utility considerations (Lancet Haematology, 2015; EvaluatePharma, 2015).

Even cost-effective medicines can potentially raise significant challenges for health budgets

The approval of new treatments for hepatitis C in 2013 and 2014 raised a novel type of challenge in all OECD countries. These medicines represent a great medical advancement for patients: sofosbuvir-based regimens achieve a sustained virological response of more than 90% in several patient groups, and are far less toxic than the former standard of care. Despite high prices, these treatments are cost-effective in most patients in comparison with the old standard of care (Luhnen et al., 2016). Some experts assessed the societal benefits of using these new treatments in the United States over 50 years, for several scenarios depending on the initial population target, ranging from treating only the most severely affected patients to treating the whole population diagnosed with hepatitis C (Van Nuys et al., 2015). According to these estimates, societal benefits are always positive due to savings in avoided health care and monetised benefits due to health gains.[12] They are greater in the scenario where all diagnosed patients are treated. Yet the authors acknowledge that such a scenario is unaffordable for US payers. Indeed, in most OECD countries, payers decided to limit access to the most severely affected patients (CNAMTS, 2015, pp. 82-84).

The pricing strategy of Gilead, the US biopharmaceutical company distributing sofosbuvir, raised legitimate questions. It led to an investigation by the US Senate. Sofosbuvir (Solvadi®) was initially priced at USD 84 000 for a standard 12-week course of therapy and sofosbuvir/ledipasvir (Harvoni®) at USD 94 500. In the United States, these two products contributed to a 12.2% increase in US prescription drug spending in 2014, despite access restrictions imposed by all payers. The US Senate report estimates the outlay for R&D for sofosbuvir at between USD 125.6 million and USD 942.4 million (respective estimates provided by Pharmasset – the initial developer of sofosbuvir – and by Gilead) (Kapczynski and Kesselheim, 2016). In 2011, Gilead purchased Pharmasset for USD 11.2 billion to complete the development of sofosbuvir and sofosbuvir/ledipasvir and bring the two products to market. By the first quarter of 2016, Gilead had earned over USD 35 billion in global revenue from hepatitis C medicines since their launch – three times the initial acquisition of Pharmasset and nearly 40 times Gilead and Pharmasset's combined reported outlays for developing sofosbuvir-based medicines (Roy and King, 2016).

Many stakeholders condemn Gilead and believe that the company could reduce its price to widen access while keeping a sufficient return on investment. Though this reasoning seems at odds with the logic of value-based pricing (the medicine is cost-effective by usual standards at the proposed price), it holds if one considers that the drug would be even more cost-effective at a lower price and that the total value created would be better shared between the company and society. Gilead's returns have been exceptional and do not reflect the average return on investments of pharmaceutical companies. Nevertheless, such returns raise the question of the relevance of the business model and policy responses.

Spending dynamics raise concerns about compromised access for patients

High prices clearly compromise access to orphan medicines in some countries. Eurordis analysed the availability of 60 orphan medicines in several EU countries in 2010 and found that almost all of them were available in France, the Netherlands and Denmark, two-thirds of them were available in Belgium, Hungary and Italy but only one-third were available in Spain and Greece (Eurordis, 2010).

The high prices of hepatitis C treatments compromised access in several OECD countries. In the United States, only 2.4% of infected Medicaid beneficiaries got access to these treatments and the situation is even worse in prisons, where only 222 infected patients got access to these treatments in 2015, despite the high prevalence in this subpopulation (Kapczynski and Kesselheim, 2016). Though Gilead made notable efforts to make these treatments available in low-income countries at highly discounted prices, affordability in high- and middle-income countries has also proven a real issue. Even though countries may not want to treat all patients with a drug whose long-term effects are not yet known, current access appears too restrictive in a number of countries.

Such potential for compromised access to treatments is among the key concerns raised by policy makers when considering current pharmaceutical market trends. While the pipeline is robust, the trend towards expensive specialty medicines has sparked debates as to whether current conditions produce the "right" innovations that patients need. The following section analyses policies implemented in OECD countries to speed approval and to make coverage and pricing decisions.

2. Recent policy initiatives to provide faster access to pharmaceutical treatments

In the pharmaceutical sector, regulation of market entry is often perceived as too stringent by pharmaceutical and biotech companies and by some patients' associations. New drug approvals rely on demanding standards for producing evidence on safety and efficacy, based on randomised controlled trials (RCTs), which take several years to conduct and are costly. The regulatory process itself takes several months, including review time by the competent authority and time used by the applicant to answer questions and update documentation. This sometimes delays access to promising medicines that treat unmet medical needs.

From another perspective, public health experts consider that current regulation is not entirely satisfactory. Several studies show that information communicated by companies responsible for conducting clinical trials is incomplete and biased towards good results. Too often, RCTs compare new products to a placebo, while in reality they will compete with existing treatments. In addition, patients recruited for RCTs are often not representative of the entire patient population, who for example may be affected by more than one disease, which affects their response rate to the medicine (AHRQ, 2011; House of Commons, 2013).

2.1. *Regulators are under pressure to speed up the regulatory process*

The approval time for New Active Substances (NASs) by leading regulatory agencies has reduced and converged over the past decade. In 2006, the median approval time of six regulatory authorities[13] was 565 days. In 2016 it was 374 days. The difference in the median approval time between the fastest and slowest agencies reduced from 530 days to 180 days over that time. The greatest reduction in median approval times was achieved by the

Japanese authority, the PMDA. Others remained relatively stable (Figure 3.7). Meanwhile, the total number of NASs approved by these agencies annually increased over 2011-15 compared to 2006-10. Agencies have tried to implement initiatives that improve the quality and timeliness of review. These include pre-submission activity with companies to ensure adequate levels of quality, and expedited priority systems for promising NASs. The changes are likely to reflect improvements in the quality of companies' submissions (Bujar et al., 2016).

Figure 3.7. **New Active Substance median approval time for six regulatory authorities, 2006-15**

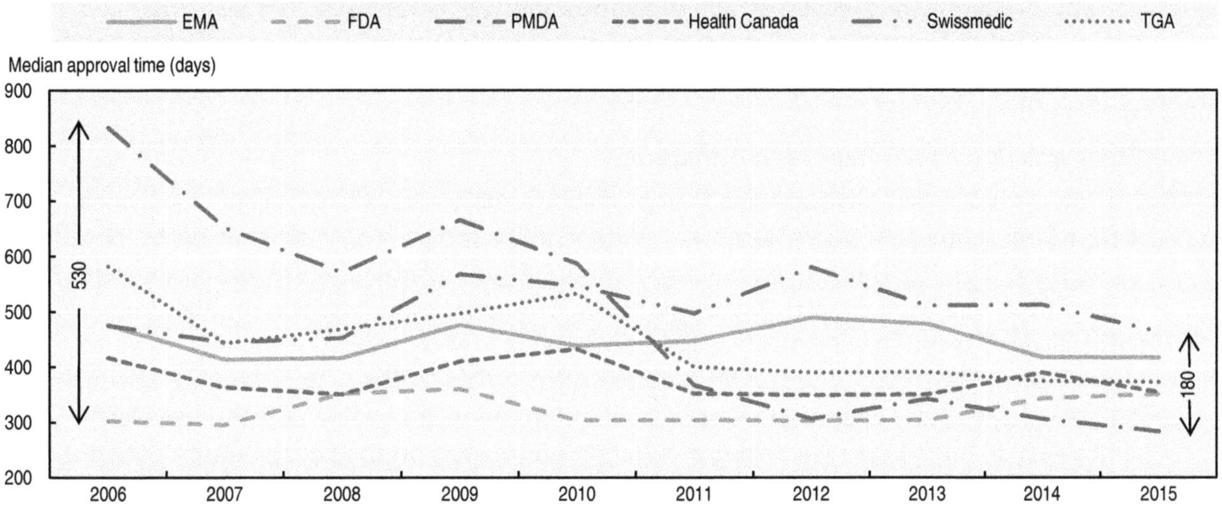

Note: EMA: European Medicines Agency, FDA: US Food and Drug Administration, PMDA: Regulatory authority in Japan, TGA: Australian Therapeutic Goods Administration. EMA approval time includes EU Commission time.

Source: Adapted from Bujar, M., N. McAuslane and L. Liberti (2016), "R&D Briefing 59: The Impact of the Evolving Regulatory Environment on the Approval of New Medicines Across Six Major Authorities 2006-2015", Centre for Innovation in Regulatory Science.

StatLink http://dx.doi.org/10.1787/888933442950

Several countries have already implemented accelerated pathways

Since the end of the 1980s and following pressure from the HIV patient community to expedite access to new treatments, regulatory agencies have implemented accelerated pathways to approve promising treatments for high unmet medical needs earlier and more quickly (i.e. for severe diseases without any available treatments). Such treatments can be approved earlier in their development phase, with lower levels of evidence requirements, based on surrogate markers[14] instead of survival, for instance. In the United States, the European Union and Switzerland, conditional approval[15] can be granted on the condition that the company provides further evidence on the medicine's benefits in real life. In Australia, work has commenced for implementation of a provisional approval pathway to allow earlier access to new treatments.

Different types of accelerated pathways contributed to the reduction of approval time. In 2015, 53% of FDA approvals were through an expedited pathway. This figure was 47% for the Japanese PMDA. The remaining agencies approve a considerably lower proportion of NASs through expedited pathways. The proportion of applications that qualified for an accelerated review increased for all five agencies that use them between 2011 and 2015, most notably for Swissmedic, the EMA and PMDA. Furthermore, in 2016 the EMA launched the PRIME (PRIority MEdicines) scheme, specifically designed to promote accelerated assessment for medicines to address unmet medical needs (Bujar et al., 2016). It is unclear if these recent changes reflect a longer-term trend.

The approval of orphan medicines raises a number of issues that some regulatory agencies have partially addressed. Agencies tend to approve medicines with lower standards of evidence, balancing licensing requirements with high patient needs and the obvious difficulty to recruit patients for clinical trials. For instance, the number of patients in Phase III trials is lower than for non-orphan medicines (median 538 patients versus 1 558) and FDA approval time is shorter than for non-orphan medicines (EvaluatePharma, 2015). Bujar et al. (2016) calculate that median approval times are generally shorter for orphan than for non-orphan medicines, especially in Switzerland (126 fewer days; 35% less time) and Japan (44 fewer days; 15% less time). Of the six regulatory agencies examined, only the EMA took longer to approve medicines with orphan status (median 37 more days; 9% more time).

Early access schemes have been introduced

Several countries have systems to grant patients early access to promising medicines before final approval. France's "temporary authorisation for use" (ATU) scheme has been in place since 1994. It grants exceptional and temporary authorisation for use and coverage to a specific patient or a cohort of patients with a serious or rare disease with high unmet clinical need before market authorisation. ATU approval requires the manufacturer to submit an application to the French National Agency for Medicines and Health Products Safety (ANSM). The application must include: information from clinical trials on efficacy and safety to infer a positive benefit-risk ratio; information on the patient or the patient group to which the treatment will be provided; a justification for the treatment's use and proof of the absence of a suitable therapeutic alternative. ATU drug prices are freely set by the manufacturer and are 100% reimbursed by the National Health Insurance.

The United Kingdom's Early Access to Medicines Scheme (EAMS) was established in April 2014 with the aim of giving patients with life-threatening or seriously debilitating conditions access to drugs that are yet to receive market authorisation in situations where clear unmet clinical need is established. As of December 2015, early access was approved for four products (targeting melanoma, lung cancer and heart failure) from 18 applications under the EAMS. It is estimated that early access to medicines has been provided to over 500 patients since the scheme's launch. The drugs are not reimbursed by National Health Service (NHS) England. The longest period that a drug has remained on the EAMS before market authorisation is 131 days (MHRA, 2016).

The United States also conducts an expanded access scheme, commonly referred to as "compassionate use", for drugs, biologics and medical devices. Although primarily intended for patients ineligible to participate in a clinical trial for a given product, in 2009 the FDA regulations were revised to provide three categories of expanded access: individual patient, intermediate-size patient population, and widespread treatment use – submitted either via a treatment protocol amending an existing investigational new drug (IND) application or via a distinct "treatment IND" (Federal Register, 2009).

Stakeholders urge faster access to promising treatments

Experts and regulators are exploring innovative pathways to speed market access (Eichler et al., 2012; OECD, 2013). Such pathways consist of early approval, based on incomplete clinical trial results, followed by post-marketing studies to be performed by companies. For instance, in Europe, the EMA launched a pilot project in 2014 to explore the feasibility of "adaptive pathways". Adaptive licensing refers to one of the following strategies: approval in stages, beginning with a restricted patient population then expanding to wider patient populations; or confirming the benefit-risk balance of a product, following a conditional approval based on early data (using surrogate endpoints) considered predictive of important clinical outcomes. Adaptive licensing requires 1) gathering evidence through real-world use to supplement clinical trial data, and 2) early involvement of patients and Health Technology Assessment (HTA) bodies in discussions on a medicine's development.

Similarly, Canada is developing a progressive licensing framework under the assumption that knowledge and experience about a therapeutic product can be gained at every stage of its lifecycle. Continuous re-evaluation of the risks and benefits of medications is expected to allow identification of any serious safety issues earlier and to improve the targeting of drug therapy through pro-active risk management. This lifecycle approach aims to better inform decisions of patients, consumers and health care professionals and to better address health needs, including those of patients with rare diseases (OECD, 2013).

While it is reasonable to respond to patients with desperate needs for treatment, countries should consider several conditions to make the system work. First, patients must be adequately informed of the quasi-experimental status of products approved through such pathways. Second, regulatory agencies must be provided with the means to ensure that companies comply with their commitment to produce further evidence within the agreed delay. The threat of withdrawal in case of non-compliance might be more effective than current systems of fines, which do not seem high enough to encourage compliance. Such an option would also clearly put the responsibility on firms in case of withdrawal. Finally, since adaptive pathways have the potential to significantly reduce the cost of producing evidence before market entry and provide companies with earlier returns on investments, payers and patients should also benefit from these financial gains though lower prices and greater affordability.

A convergence of evidence requirements of regulatory agencies (approval) and HTA agencies seems desirable to the extent feasible. Stronger synergies between developers of health technologies, regulators, HTA bodies and decision makers can improve patient access to new treatments, especially innovative medicines. It could reduce development time and costs and accelerate access to treatment. A multistakeholder dialogue was engaged in Europe to move in this direction. While international work on this issue must continue to ensure objectivity and avoid duplication of efforts, such future work must also consider the minimum requirements justifying the grounds of reimbursement decisions in particular countries. There should be collaborative discussion in evaluating the safety and needed resources for early access tools such as adaptive pathways and the EMA launch of the PRIME scheme in 2016, specifically designed to promote expedited assessment of medicines for unmet medical needs. An appropriate balance is needed between incentives for pharmaceutical research, HTA, patients' access to innovative medicines and their safety.

2.2. Payers struggle to assess benefits and pay for value

Many countries aim to pay for medicines in relation to the benefits they bring to patients and/or society. Value-based pricing is envisaged as a promising option to ensure static and dynamic efficiency of pharmaceutical spending (see, for instance, Paris and Belloni, 2013).

Many countries use HTA to inform coverage and pricing decisions

In many OECD countries, marketing authorisation is followed by an assessment of the added therapeutic value of new treatments over standards of care and/or of economic aspects, whose aim is to inform coverage and/or pricing decisions. OECD countries use HTA either systematically, for each new indication or medicine (e.g. Australia, France), or occasionally, only for medicines raising particular concerns related to high prices and/or uncertain benefits (Table 3.1).

Table 3.1. **Use of HTA to make coverage and pricing decisions for pharmaceuticals in OECD countries**

	Countries
Systematically used to inform coverage decisions	Australia, Belgium, Canada, Chile,[1] Finland, France, Hungary, Ireland, Israel, Italy, Korea, Luxembourg, Netherlands, New Zealand, Norway, Poland, Slovenia, Sweden, Switzerland
Used in some circumstances to inform coverage decisions	Austria, Denmark, Mexico, Portugal, Spain, United Kingdom
Used to help determine reimbursement level or price	France, Hungary, Ireland, Japan, New Zealand, Norway, Poland, Sweden

1. Only for products and services to be included in GES (i.e. explicit guarantees expected to be covered by all plans).
Source: Auraaen et al. (2016).

HTA does not always provide an answer to decision makers

The trend towards earlier approval, based on lower levels of evidence, complicates HTA. For a number of recently approved medicines, HTA agencies have struggled to assess clinical benefits, let alone cost-effectiveness, and have been unable to provide conclusive assessments to decision makers. In such cases, payers face a dilemma: they can either delay decisions to reimburse a product or base their decisions on incomplete evidence. Such decisions are increasingly accompanied with requirements for manufacturers to produce further evidence (see Section 2.3).

Cost-effectiveness of medicines in oncology is more complex to assess than in other therapeutic areas since medicines are assessed in isolation but increasingly used in combination. OECD analysis indicates that of the 124 drugs with an original or supplemental indication in oncology approved in 2006-15 by the FDA, 56 (45%) were approved for use in combination as part of a multi-agent treatment regimen or with specific diagnostic tests. In addition, treatment for cancer nearly always involves a combination approach with surgery, chemotherapy, radiation therapy and/or supportive care.

Oncology products are often funded even when not cost-effective

In oncology, many products are funded at incremental cost-effectiveness ratios (ICERs) that do not meet standard thresholds (Paris and Belloni, 2013). In all countries, governments and payers perceive a high public pressure to pay for oncology drugs, even when they are not cost-effective, although public preferences are not always clearly assessed (Aggarwal et al., 2014). Patients generally want access to these treatments, either because they value the small benefits they bring or because they overestimate potential benefits. In a study of more than 1 000 patients with incurable cancer in the United States, for example, 69% of those with lung cancer and 81% of those with colorectal cancer responded in a way that showed they did not understand that chemotherapy was "not at all likely" to cure their cancer; chemotherapy in such cases can prolong life by weeks or months and may provide palliation, but it is not curative (Weeks et al., 2012). To respond to this public pressure, several OECD countries created special access schemes.

In Australia, access to medicines with a high ICER can be granted through a special access process called "Section 100", reserved for medicines treating chronic and severe disease, highly specialised treatments and expensive medicines (small target populations). Access to medicines listed in Section 100 is limited to authorised centres with allocated budgets. The number of doses and quantities administered to patients are often limited. In Italy, patients can also access specific treatments on individual request (Act 648/96) but funding is only continued if the medicine is effective.

In England, oncology medicines often did not meet the ICER threshold adopted by NICE. Since negative decisions were difficult to accept for English patients, the ICER threshold was first increased for "end-of-life treatments" in 2008. Yet the scheme was quite restrictive and did not guarantee access to all new cancer medicines, a very unpopular situation. A report showed that English patients' access lagged behind their counterparts in other European countries (Richards, 2010). In 2010, the Cancer Drug Fund (CDF) was established for medicines used outside their licensed indication, or for medicines NICE has not appraised or recommended. The CDF began with GBP 50 million interim funding, increased in 2011 to GBP 200 million per year for three years. The fund overspent due to more patients requesting access, and to virtually no constraint on prices. In 2014 and again in 2015, the CDF went through a re-evaluation process and delisted some products. Following a public consultation, NHS England outlined a new process for appraisal and funding of cancer drugs effective July 2016, under which the CDF became a managed access scheme (NHS, 2016).

Orphan drugs may be exempt from economic evaluation

The fact that orphan medicines often target severe diseases and unmet medical needs results in high pressure on decision makers to fund them, especially from associations advocating for patients affected by rare diseases. The extent to which the general public supports such decisions – reflecting a higher willingness to pay for patients with rare diseases – has been explored, providing contradictory results and no definitive conclusion (Drummond and Towse, 2014). Countries tend to fund orphan medicines even when they are not cost-effective.

A few countries explicitly exempt orphan medicines from economic evaluation. For instance, in France, medicines whose budget impact during the first two years of commercialisation does not exceed EUR 20 million are not subject to economic evaluation (HAS, 2014). In Germany, an orphan medicine has to undergo regular assessment only if spending of statutory health insurance funds (at pharmacy prices including VAT) exceeded EUR 50 million within the last 12 months. Innovative medicines whose annual turnover is below EUR 1 million are excluded from the evaluation process.

Experts and stakeholders are considering alternative ways to define "value"

In several OECD countries, "value" in pharmaceutical policies has most often been defined by the ratio of incremental costs to incremental QALYs, adopting an extra-welfarist approach according to which health policy aims to maximise health gains from a given budget. This approach is sometimes assessed as too restrictive and some countries are adopting a wider "societal" approach in economic evaluation, where benefits are extended, for instance, to account for productivity gains. Such approaches do not really respond to challenges raised by the very high prices of medicines in therapeutic areas such as oncology and rare diseases, however. Experts and stakeholders are now considering alternative ways to define value.

In Europe, a specific "value framework" was proposed to help European payers and other stakeholders assess the value of orphan medicines for reimbursement and pricing purposes (MoCA-OMP, 2014). This framework considers four criteria: 1) the availability (or not) of therapeutic alternatives; 2) the clinical effect; 3) the response rate; and 4) the degree of uncertainty attached to evaluation. It suggests qualitative and quantitative benchmarks to assess the value of orphan medicines (Table 3.2). It would be interesting to see whether this framework can be used in practice to inform decisions or negotiate the prices of new medicines.

Table 3.2. **Transparent value framework proposed for orphan drugs in European countries**

Criterion	Lower degree	Medium degree	High degree
Available alternatives/ unmet need, including non-pharmaceutical treatment options	Yes, new medicine does not address unmet need	Yes, but major unmet need still remains	No alternatives except best supportive care – New drug addresses major unmet need
(Relative) effectiveness, degree of net benefit (clinical imporvement, QoL, etc. vs. side effects, societal impact, etc.) relative to alternatives, including no treatment	Incremental	Major	Curative
Response rate (based on best available clinically relevant criteria)	< 30%	30-60%	> 60%
Degree of certainty (documentation)	Promising but not well-documented	Plausible	Unequivocal

Source: MoCA-OMP Working Group on Mechanism of Coordinated Access to Orphan Medicinal Products (2014), "Transparent Value Framework, Process on Corporate Social Responsibility in the Field of Pharmaceuticals Platform on Access to Medicines in Europe".

More recent research, not specific to orphan medicines, also explores the possibility of using multi-criteria decision analysis (MCDA) to make reimbursement and pricing decisions, in order to go beyond "cost-effectiveness" when considering value and to incorporate preferences and values in the equation (Angelis and Kanavos, 2014).

These approaches may provide arguments for paying higher prices for some medicines, to reflect population preferences (albeit, noting the lack of a clear evidence base around such preferences). They will not, however, solve issues related to the affordability of medicines.

2.3. *Managed entry agreements are used to address uncertainty on effectiveness or contain costs*

To respond to challenges raised by new medicines, many countries increasingly use MEAs. According to a taxonomy proposed by Garrison et al. (2013), these agreements can be classified in two main categories:

- financial agreements, which seek to obtain discounts on list prices based on confidential discounts, price-volume agreements or caps per patient or for the whole population
- performance-based agreements, which link coverage conditions or prices to health outcomes observed in real life, either on each patient or on the whole patient population; these are further split into:
  - coverage with evidence development (CED), where the product/indication is covered under the condition that the company will provide further evidence

- performance-linked reimbursement, where the price finally paid by the payer depends on health outcomes observed in real life (for each patient or for the whole population); they can take the form of rebates paid *ex post* by the company or of provision of free stock, for instance.

Countries often use a mix of MEAs, depending on circumstances. Interestingly, the type of MEA for a single product/indication may vary across countries (Ferrario and Kanavos, 2015). While some countries (e.g. Italy, the United Kingdom) publish the content of MEAs, other countries keep the content of the agreement confidential (e.g. Belgium) or even the mere existence of an agreement (e.g. France). In all cases, the financial outcomes of MEAs are kept confidential for individual products, even though countries sometimes publish, at the aggregate level, the total amount of spending recouped through these agreements. According to a survey conducted in EU countries in 2011-12, the majority of agreements aim to control budget impact (75%) either in isolation (42%) or combined with cost-effectiveness (16%) or use (15%).

By therapeutic focus, antineoplastic and immunomodulating agents account for nearly 40% of MEAs in Europe (Vitry and Roughead, 2014; van de Vooren et al., 2014; Ferrario and Kanavos, 2013). They represented 89% and 74% of MEAs in England and the Netherlands, respectively, in 2012 (Ferrario and Kanavos, 2015) and 84% in Italy (van de Vooren et al., 2015). Morel and colleagues examined MEAs for orphan medicinal products in seven European countries between 2006 and 2012. Here again, antineoplastic agents were the primary target of the 42 MEAs identified. Just over half of these were performance-based risk-sharing arrangements; the rest were budget-based (Morel et al., 2013).

Financial arrangements are common practice in many OECD countries

Financial agreements aim to mitigate budget impact. They take the form of simple discounts or rebates, for the whole spending or beyond an agreed cap. In Europe, price-volume agreements are the most common feature of MEAs (40%), just before data collection requirements (30%) (Ferrario and Kanavos, 2013). In England, MEAs are mainly discounts and dose-capping and aim to influence prices and cost-effectiveness. Belgium developed a price-volume agreement for orphan drugs whereby manufacturers' "payback" rises incrementally as the actual volume dispensed exceeds pre-agreed budget caps (Morel et al., 2013). France imposed a budget cap in 2014 for several medications, including sofosbuvir (CEPS, 2015:55). In Australia, 71 MEAs were active in 2013. The majority were non-outcome based agreements; either price-volume agreements or dose-capping arrangements (Vitry and Roughead, 2014).

Financial agreements are relatively easy to manage, as long as data to monitor them are available. All things being equal, manufacturers prefer confidential discounts over reductions in list prices, since the latter are used by other payers using international benchmarking to determine their own reimbursement prices.

CED schemes deliver mixed results

CED, which conditions positive coverage decisions on further development of evidence, is used in several countries as an option for select medicines, devices and procedures. At the end of a specified period of evidence development, payers are expected to get more information from the company on the technology's effectiveness and sometimes cost-effectiveness. Payers then decide whether to continue or stop coverage or to restrict coverage to subgroups of indications or populations. The Netherlands, Sweden and Portugal, for instance, use such an approach (Ferrario and Kanavos, 2013). In the Netherlands and

Sweden, CED schemes aim to assess effectiveness and/or cost-effectiveness of new medicines (Ferrario and Kanavos, 2015).

In some cases, CED schemes are effective. For instance, in Sweden, the CED arrangement on Ropinirole (for idiopathic restless leg syndrome) showed that the drug was not cost-effective, which led to a price reduction (Ferrario and Kanavos, 2015). By contrast, the experience with CED on orphan drugs in the Netherlands is less positive. In spite of clear evidence that some drugs were not even close to cost-effective, it was impossible to stop coverage due to public pressure (Franken, 2014).

Finally, results of experiences with CED are mixed but enough experience has been accumulated to draw some lessons. First, it is very difficult to stop coverage on economic grounds, whatever the results of the assessment, especially when the treatment targets severe diseases with no alternative treatments. Second, in some cases, compliance with CED requirements is poor, suggesting that incentives for companies to respect their commitments are insufficient.

Performance-based agreements should be used with parsimony

To deal with uncertainty and lack of evidence, payers increasingly use performance-based MEAs for pharmaceuticals, linking the final price paid for a medicine to its performance in real life. In such arrangements, the effectiveness of the medicine observed in real life is compared with benefits claimed by the manufacturer. If observed outcomes are lower than expected, the company must refund a share of the costs incurred. Most often, financial arrangements take the form of *ex post* rebates, but they can also consist of provision of free stocks, for instance. These agreements are widely used in Italy and England, mainly for oncology medicines.

In England, Patient Access Schemes (PAS), often established to ensure that the medicine becomes cost-effective, seem to achieve this objective, at least in certain cases (Ferrario and Kanavos, 2015). In Italy, financial results of MEAs were published for the first time in 2013. The amounts recouped by the government from manufacturers through performance-based arrangements are modest, representing 5% of total expenditure for the relevant indications (Garattini et al., 2015; Navarria et al., 2015; van de Vooren et al., 2014). This outcome does not reflect high therapeutic success. It results from high management and administrative costs, disputes with pharmaceutical companies and late requests from hospitals (in charge of collecting refunds) (Navarria et al., 2015; van de Vooren et al., 2015).

Performance-based agreements do not increase knowledge on therapeutic benefits of new drugs. In Italy, registries were established for 78 therapeutic indications related to 66 compounds (Garrison et al., 2013). Despite a stated objective of contributing to the evidence base, no published data exist on the drugs subject to MEA in Italy that can contribute to further assessment of effectiveness (van de Vooren et al., 2014). MEAs do not seem to contribute to clinical evaluation of new drugs in a meaningful way (Garattini et al., 2015). More generally, clinical results of performance-based MEAs – 40% of which concern oncology medicines in Europe – are generally not made available beyond involved parties due to confidentiality provisions. While information collected through these agreements might be difficult to aggregate to derive meaningful information on products' performance, if decision makers and payers continue to rely on MEAs, they should make sure that clinical data and final value assessments are made available to the scientific community and their international counterparts.

The potential consequences of the failure of performance-based MEAs would mean that not only are health care systems potentially paying prices that are not justified by a new drug's proven benefits, but they are also incurring extra costs to administer schemes that add no therapeutic value. Wider consequences may also arise, for example if a product that is reimbursed only because of an MEA is used as a comparator to assess a new treatment on the basis of the original, unproven assumptions.

Nevertheless, some of these challenges can be overcome through better planning and innovative process design. The digitisation of health data and improved data infrastructure are likely to improve the availability and quality of information outcomes, potentially making performance-based MEA more viable. MEA may yet become a useful instrument for decision makers. Drummond (2015) made recommendations to increase appropriateness, design and implementation of MEAs. First, decision makers must make sure that the uncertainty surrounding clinical and economic benefits or new drugs can be reduced by further evidence and that relevant clinical or economic outcomes can be clearly defined and measured. The timeline of MEAs must be reasonable; data collection and analysis must be easy to implement and affordable; and, importantly, the consequences of the results of the analysis must be clearly defined. Yet unless and until the substantial challenges associated with MEAs are demonstrably overcome, it would be sensible to limit usage of such arrangements, or to use them only in exceptional circumstances where it is certain that clinically valuable information can be generated and published.

In addition, Section 2 identified several accelerated pathways that result in health care systems paying for pharmaceuticals with less information about safety, effectiveness or cost-effectiveness. These pathways in effect shift aspects of drug development risk onto health care systems, and it is important to identify the appropriate situations for health care systems to accept such a role. This should be limited to cases where the expected benefits are really promising and can only be verified post-market and should be reflected in price determination.

3. Exploring new policy options to ensure sustainable access to innovation

Health policy makers, other stakeholders and analysts are increasingly worried about current trends in pharmaceutical prices and their affordability (Council of the European Union, 2016), with many now questioning industry pricing strategies. In addition, some researchers point out that paying high prices for low benefits may generate duplication of R&D efforts and redundant pipelines (Fojo et al., 2014). There is an apparent need to rebalance the negotiation powers of buyers and sellers in some therapeutic areas. Beyond this, incentives created for orphan medicines several decades ago might be worth re-examining to take into account recent trends in medicine development. Finally, some stakeholders are imagining new ways to steer and finance R&D in the pharmaceutical sector to ensure they address priority needs and produce effective and affordable treatments.

3.1. In some market segments, negotiation powers of purchasers and sellers need to be rebalanced

In some pharmaceutical markets, negotiation powers of purchasers and sellers need to be rebalanced. Several options are emerging on the international scene to revamp pharmaceutical pricing mechanisms, based on very different rationales. Cost-plus pricing has been suggested to set prices in relation to disclosed R&D development costs to allow a reasonable profit to companies, capable of incentivising further investments in research.

However, this option does not encourage efficient R&D processes, since any cost incurred could be covered. In addition, it is very difficult to implement in a global market.

Another, more promising option to increase purchasers' power in negotiations with global companies is multicountry joint procurement. More traditionally used in exceptional circumstances such as epidemics or complex supply chains such as vaccines,[16] joint procurement is expected to facilitate access to essential medicines. Several countries in Europe and Latin America are now working on such initiatives. The ability of international joint procurement to lead to lower prices and broadened access to medicine is not known yet. At a minimum, countries and payers should increase transparency and exchange of information to reduce the information asymmetry between them and global companies.

Payers are also seeking opportunities to foster competition in some therapeutic areas, such as oncology. One option envisaged is to offer bundled payments for a specific oncologic indication. Competition could occur at the level of providers or at the level of purchasers, through calls for tender for instance, provided that several medicines have the same indication and comparable effects on patients. This is not an easy task as providers and patients generally value choice and like having access to a wide range of therapeutic options. This is complicated by the fact that treatments are increasingly tailored to patient categories (e.g. precision medicine, as discussed in Chapter 5), reducing opportunities for competition.

Finally, more radical options are proposed, such as compulsory licensing where affordability of essential treatments is impaired by pricing strategies. OECD countries have been reluctant so far to use this option, even where it could be used (Kapczynski and Kesselheim, 2016), for fear of sending a too negative signal to investors that may result in disincentivising research and affecting the pharmaceutical industry's financial sustainability.

3.2. *A re-assessment of orphan legislation would be welcome*

The costs and benefits of incentives for the development of orphan medicines, in particular, need to be re-examined. Incentives to invest in the development of treatments for rare diseases have been successful: the number of orphan medicines has continuously increased. The industry now envisages the development of orphan medicines as a good business opportunity, since all incentives are now combined with exceptionally high prices (EvaluatePharma, 2015).

From payers' point of view, however, this is becoming a bitter pill to swallow. In spite of public support, including funding of basic research in addition to incentives described above and in Annex 3.A1, orphan medicines are not available and affordable to all patients who need them. In addition, companies are suspected of adopting "salami-slicing strategies", marketing new medicines with narrow indications to claim an orphan status and a high price, and then developing other indications or promoting off-label use (Daniel et al., 2016).

Finally, some orphan medicines perform very well – two of them are in the 50 top-selling medicines worldwide – which suggests that they may not need additional public subsidies to be commercially viable. It might be worth launching a global assessment of the costs of public incentives for orphan medicines and associated benefits, in terms of access to treatment and health benefits brought to patients. For instance, concerned by the high price and low benefits of medicines for Fabry and Pompe's diseases, van den Brink (2014) asks "Why are these enzyme therapies so expensive? Why are they so mediocre? Is it true that the industry lacks incentives to come up with a better product since the limited one generates such a substantial amount of money?"

In Australia, the regulation of orphan drugs is currently being reviewed to consider whether the existing orphan drug scheme is fit for purpose as the global trend for increasing numbers of orphan designations continues.

3.3. Imagining new ways to steer and finance pharmaceutical R&D

Policy makers increasingly question the appropriateness of the current model of financing pharmaceutical innovation. The Dutch Health Care Institute and the Belgian Health Care Knowledge Centre convened a group of experts and stakeholders to imagine new and disruptive ways to finance pharmaceutical development and to pay for medicines. They proposed four scenarios (Box 3.3). All four aim to give a greater role to public authorities in the definition of priorities for pharmaceutical R&D, and to ensure affordable access to new medicines to all patients who need them.

Box 3.3. **Future scenarios about drug development and drug pricing**

These disruptive scenarios result from an expert consultation led by ShiftN and commissioned by the Belgian Health Care Knowledge Centre of Expertise and the Dutch Health Care Institute. The aim of the consultation was to imagine disruptive ways to finance R&D that could potentially better respond to public health needs.

Scenario 1: Needs-oriented Public-Private Partnerships

Public actors and drug developers are tackling public health priorities in vigorous and pragmatic partnerships. The public actor identifies indications representing high public health needs; specifies criteria for the performance levels of drugs to be developed for those indications; and indicates his willingness to pay. Through procurements with enforceable contractual commitments, the public actor enters into a partnership with drug developers to find solutions for these needs. Developers are prepared to enter into the partnership and to give price concessions for a pre-negotiated fixed agreement on price and volume, and speedier access to market, which reduces their development risk. This drug development and pricing model is close to existing governmental procurement practices in research-intensive areas such as public transport, defence and space exploration.

Scenario 2: Parallel Drug Development Track

EU member states set up a parallel, not-for-profit drug development track that exists alongside, but independent of, the pharmaceutical and biotechnological industry. The aim of the parallel track is to develop cheaper drugs without compromising safety and effectiveness. After having made up an inventory of the public health gaps and priorities in health care, EU member state authorities ask leading public research institutes which discoveries, assets, tools and capabilities they possess to develop solutions addressing (some of) the needs that were identified. Starting from the match between demand and available expertise, coalitions are built between these (not-for-profit) research institutes, payers, authorities and patients' organisations. All these partners make the commitment to participate in an open and transparent way in clinical research projects. Intellectual property (IP) rights are acquired early on in the development process by the partners of the consortium, and ownership is shared. Alternatively, the parallel research infrastructure can completely deprioritise ownership; i.e. inventions and developments in the parallel track are not protected and are in the public domain.

Box 3.3. **Future scenarios about drug development and drug pricing** *(cont.)*

Scenario 3: Pay for Patents

A consortium of European countries join forces and establish a "Public Fund for Affordable Drugs". Each of the participating countries deposits a fixed annual percentage of what it currently spends on drugs into the Fund. Private payers (including insurance companies) can also join the Fund. The Fund continuously screens the research market for "interesting" drugs that are being developed in Phase II or in Phase III for indications with clear health priorities. The Fund buys the patent from developers, conducts or commissions the last phases of research in public research institutes or subcontracts to private partners (with strict public oversight), and guides the submission process for market authorisation. Because the drug is then put on the market at a relatively low price, substantial savings are generated for the public payer. Once the system is functioning "at cruising speed", these savings can (partly) serve to replenish the Fund. The "Pay for Patents" model delinks R&D from manufacturing and sales. The prices decrease because the partners in the Fund consider medicines as public goods that should not be financed through monopoly prices. Hence, once the patent is owned by the public sector, after a successful development and authorisation trajectory, the rights to produce, distribute and sell the drug can be licenced to manufacturers and distributors that provide the best deal in terms of quality, safety and accessibility for the lowest cost. As a rule, various private partners compete with each other, with the result that "new drugs enter the market at generic prices".

Scenario 4: Public Good from A to Z

Drug development is essentially a public enterprise, and is radically re-oriented from serving private profits towards serving the public interest and patients' needs. In a drug development system that is essentially a public enterprise, private drug companies still have a role, albeit with a completely different business model. They mainly manufacture drugs and deliver services to the public provider on a competitive basis. With drugs and other health technologies essentially public goods, patents and monopolistic prices have no role. Patients and public health providers, not corporations, choose which unmet needs research should address. Public authorities regularly publish lists of research priorities, based on objectively established and patient-informed unmet medical needs. Governments organise and fund that research through a variety of mechanisms, including requests for proposals based on well-defined targets that any research team, public or private, can compete for, or milestone compensation, and active management of the innovation process. By paying directly for R&D and active management of the drug development pipeline, nations and health care systems pay much less than the patent-protected prices of the past. Ultimately, drug prices are set on the basis of the real costs of manufacturing, quality control and distribution, which are decoupled from R&D.

Source: Vandenbroeck, Ph. et al. (2016), "Future Scenarios About Drug Development and Drug Pricing", *Health Care Knowledge Centre (KCE) Report* 271, D/2016/10.273/59, Health Services Research (HSR), Brussels.

Conclusion

Current trends in pharmaceutical markets are simultaneously viewed with optimism and concern. The wealth of the pipeline and the increasing number of new drugs approved every year, boosted by the development of targeted therapies, sound promising. Targeted therapies are expected to provide better outcomes and less toxic treatments to populations identified by a biomarker. On the other hand, a new business model seems to be emerging where companies claim high prices for medicines targeting small populations affected by severe diseases.

These new trends have several policy implications. Regulatory agencies are pressured to accelerate approval and give faster access to patients, sometimes with less available evidence. HTA agencies struggle to assess health benefits and cost-effectiveness of new treatments, while payers are urged to provide access to these treatments and bypass standard rules to determine coverage and reimbursement prices.

In response to these trends, OECD countries are exploring a number of policy instruments, including MEAs, to contain budget impact or increase value-for-money. But these tools do not really address current concerns about accessibility and affordability of new and future treatments or the sustainability of health spending. A number of stakeholders feel the need to explore new policy options to respond to these challenges and make sure that incentives in pharmaceutical markets encourage innovations that bring real benefits to patients at an affordable price.

Notes

1. Specialty medicines do not have a unique definition. They usually include injectable and biologic agents used to treat complex conditions such as rheumatoid arthritis, multiple sclerosis and cancer and often require special handling or delivery mechanisms.
2. In these statistics, the burden of disease is estimated by the number of disability-adjusted life years (DALYs) lost by cause in 2012. See *www.who.int/healthinfo/global_burden_disease/estimates/en/index2.html*, DALY estimates, 2000-12, DALYs by cause and by World Bank income category and WHO region, consulted on 22 October 2016.
3. No single definition of "neglected diseases" exists. The WHO experts working group on Public Health, Innovation and Intellectual Property identifies two groups. Neglected diseases refer to diseases that "are incident in both rich and poor countries, but with a substantial proportion of the cases in the poor countries...HIV/AIDS and tuberculosis are examples: both diseases are present in both rich and poor countries, but more than 90 per cent of cases are in the poor countries". Very neglected diseases are "those that are overwhelmingly or exclusively incident in the developing countries, such as African sleeping sickness (trypanosomiasis) and African river blindness (onchocerciasis)". Such diseases receive extremely little R&D, and essentially no commercially based R&D in the rich countries (WHO, 2006).
4. A prize is a payment made to a research entity that is conditional on the achievement of a particular outcome. It can reward the accomplishment of certain research milestones, such as discovery and isolation of a lead compound or be proposed for the development of an entire treatment with a significant health impact (Pugatch et al., 2012).
5. A patent buyout consists of purchasing a patent or patents from the patent holder to place the object of the patent(s) in the public domain or ensure the development and distribution of the related product at an affordable price. The purchaser could be the government or an NGO, for instance.
6. An Advanced Market Commitment is a legally binding agreement for an amount of funds to subsidise the purchase, at a given price, of an as yet unavailable product.
7. See *www.jpiamr.eu/* (accessed 16 October 2016).
8. For instance, Humira®, the top-selling prescription drug in the United States for the 12-month period before March 15, obtained in 2015 an orphan designation for the treatment of moderate to severe hidradenitis suppurativa (a chronic skin condition that features pea-sized to marble-sized lumps under the skin). This status provides Humira® with an extended period of exclusivity up to 2022 in the US market for this indication. However, Humira® is indicated in several other conditions, among which rheumatoid arthritis. In this indication, price competition already exists and will likely increase when competing products lose patent protection. Although Humira®'s orphan indication may not be exposed to biosimilars competition before 2022, the marketing authorisation holder might not be able to keep a monopoly price (*www.fda.gov*, *www.medscape.com/viewarticle/844317#vp_2*,).
9. This estimate aggregates pharmaceutical expenditure in the inpatient and outpatient sectors for eight OECD countries for which data are available in 2013 (or most recent available year).

10. In practice, economic evaluation most often consists of cost-utility analysis via estimation of an ICER; i.e. the ratio of incremental costs to incremental benefits (measured in QALYs). In principle, this should go along with the definition of an ICER threshold, beyond which the assessed technology will not be funded through health coverage schemes. Countries are often reluctant to set ICER thresholds. According to an OECD survey conducted in 2014-15, only five member countries (Hungary, Korea, Poland, the Slovak Republic and the United Kingdom) have published such a threshold.

11. Ultra-orphan drugs target diseases with a prevalence of less than one in 50 000. Among the 124 orphan drugs approved by the EMA between 2000 and 2015, 32 were ultra-orphan drugs (Schuller et al., 2015).

12. Authors propose to derive the societal value of a QALY from estimates of the value of statistical life (VSL) and produce estimates of overall societal benefits of using new hepatitis C treatments for three different values of a QALY (USD 100 000, USD 150 000 and USD 200 000).

13. European Medicines Agency (EMA), US Food and Drug Administration (FDA), Japanese Pharmaceuticals and Medical Devices Agency (PMDA), Health Canada, Swissmedic and Australian Therapeutic Goods Administration (TGA).

14. A "surrogate marker" is a laboratory measurement or physical sign used in therapeutic trials as a substitute for a clinically meaningful endpoint that is a direct measure of how a patient feels, functions or survives. It is expected to predict the effect of the therapy.

15. Conditional approval consists of temporary approval of a medical product for a given period during which the company is required to provide further evidence of its safety and effectiveness.

16. See *http://ec.europa.eu/health/preparedness_response/joint_procurement/jpa_signature_en.htm* (accessed 22 October 2016).

References

Aggarwal, A., O. Ginsburg and T. Fojoc (2014), "Cancer Economics, Policy and Politics: What Informs the Debate? Perspectives from the EU, Canada and US", *Journal of Cancer Policy*, Vol. 2, pp. 1-11.

AHRQ – Agency for Healthcare Research and Quality (2011), "Correcting for Publication Bias in the Presence of Covariates", *Methods Research Report*, AHRQ Publication No. 11-EHC041-EF, United States, September.

Auraaen, A. et al. (2016), "How OECD Health Systems Define the Range of Good and Services to be Financed Collectively?", *OECD Health Working Paper*, No. 90, OECD Publishing, Paris, *http://dx.doi.org/10.1787/5jlnb59ll80x-en.*

Angelis, A. and P. Kanavos (2014), "Applying Multiple Criteria Decision Analysis in the Context of Health Technology Assessment: An Empirical Case Study", *Value in Health*, Vol. 7, No. 17, A552.

Belloni, A., D. Morgan and V. Paris (2016), "Pharmaceutical Expenditure and Policies: Past Trends and Future Challenges", *OECD Health Working Papers*, No. 87, OECD Publishing, Paris, *http://dx.doi.org/10.1787/5jm0q1f4cdq7-en.*

Bujar, M., N. McAuslane and L. Liberti (2016), "R&D Briefing 59: The Impact of the Evolving Regulatory Environment on the Approval of New Medicines Across Six Major Authorities 2006-2015", Centre for Innovation in Regulatory Science.

Butler, M.S. et al. (2013), "Antibiotics in the Clinical Pipeline in 2013", *Journal of Antibiotics*, Vol. 66, pp. 571-591.

Cecchini, M., J. Langer and L. Slawomirski (2015), "Antimicrobial Resistance in G7 Countries and Beyond: Economic Issues, Policies and Options for Action", OECD, Paris, *www.oecd.org/els/health-systems/Antimicrobial-Resistance-in-G7-Countries-and-Beyond.pdf.*

CEPS – Comité Economique des Produits de Santé (2015), *Rapport d'activité 2014/2015*, Comité Économique des Produits de Santé, Paris.

Chorzelski, S. et al. (2015), "Breaking through the Wall: Enhancing Research and Development of Antibiotics in Science and Industry", Report for the Global Union for Antibiotics Research and Development (GUARD) Initiative Commissioned by the German Federal Ministry of Health, October 2015.

CNAMTS – Caisse Nationale de l'Assurance Maladie des Travailleurs Salariés (2015), *Améliorer la qualité du système de santé et maîtriser les dépenses – Propositions de l'Assurance Maladie pour 2016*, Caisse Nationale d'Assurance Maladie des Travailleurs Salariés, Paris.

Council of the European Union (2016), "Council Conclusions on Strengthening the Balance in the Pharmaceutical Systems in the EU and its Member States", *Press release 350/16*, 17 June.

Daniel, M.G. et al. (2016), "The Orphan Drug Act: Restoring the Mission to Rare Diseases", *American Journal of Clinical Oncology*, Vol. 39, No. 2, pp. 210-213.

Di Procolo, P. and C. Jommi (2014), "Current Pipelines for Neglected Diseases", *PLoS Neglected Tropical Diseases*, Vol. 8, No. 9, e3092, *http://doi.org/10.1371/journal.pntd.0003092*.

Drummond, M. (2015), "When Do Performance-based Risk-sharing Arrangements Make Sense?", *European Journal of Health Economics*, Vol. 16, No. 6, pp. 569-571.

Drummond, M. and A. Towse (2014), "Orphan Drugs Policies: A Suitable Case for Treatment", *European Journal of Health Economics*, Vol. 15, pp. 335-340.

Eichler, H.G. et al. (2012), "Adaptive Licensing: Taking the Next Step in the Evolution of Drug Approval", *Nature Clinical Pharmacology & Therapeutics*, Vol. 91, No. 3, pp. 426-437 (advance online publication 15 February 2012).

Eurordis (2010), "Inventory of Access and Prices of Orphan Drugs across Europe", Paris.

EvaluatePharma (2015), *Orphan Drug Report 2015*, EvaluatePharma, London.

EvaluatePharma (2014), *Budget-busters: The Shift to High-priced Innovator Drugs in the USA*, EvaluatePharma, London.

Express Scripts (2016), "Express Scripts 2015 Drug Trend Report", The Express Scripts Lab, St. Louis, March.

Federal Register (United States) (2009), "Expanded Access to Investigational Drugs for Treatment Use", Federal Register 74 FR 40900, 13 August.

Ferrario, A. and P. Kanavos (2015), "Dealing with Uncertainty and High Prices of New Medicines: A Comparative Analysis of the Use of Managed Entry Agreements in Belgium, England, the Netherlands and Sweden", *Social Science and Medicine*, Vol. 124, pp. 39-47.

Ferrario, A. and P. Kanavos (2013), *Managed Entry Agreements for Pharmaceuticals: The European Experience*, London School of Economics and Political Science, London.

Fojo, T. et al. (2014), "Unintended Consequences of Expensive Cancer Therapeutics – The Pursuit of Marginal Indications and a Me-Too Mentality That Stifles Innovation and Creativity", *JAMA Otolaryngology*, E1-E11, 28 July 2014.

Franken, M. (2014), "Decision Making in Drug Reimbursement", Erasmus University, Rotterdam.

Gammie, T., C.Y. Lu and Z.U-D. Babar (2015), "Access to Orphan Drugs: A Comprehensive Review of Legislations, Regulations and Policies in 35 Countries", *PLoS ONE*, Vol. 10, No. 10, e0140002.

Garattini, L., A. Curto and K. van de Vooren (2015), "Italian Risk-sharing Agreements on Drugs: Are They Worthwhile?", *European Journal of Health Economics*, Vol. 16, pp. 1-3.

Garrison, L. et al. (2013), "Performance-based Risk-sharing Arrangements – Good Practices for Design, Implementation and Evaluation", *Value in Health*, Vol. 16, pp. 703-719.

GBD 2013 Mortality and Causes of Death Collaborators (2014), "Global, Regional, and National Age-sex Specific All-cause and Cause-specific Mortality for 240 Causes of Death, 1990-2013: A Systematic Analysis for the Global Burden of Disease Study 2013", *The Lancet*, Vol. 385, No. 9963, pp. 117-171, 10 January 2015 (published online 17 December 2014).

Hartung, D. et al. (2015), "The Cost of Multiple Sclerosis Drugs in the US and the Pharmaceutical Industry – Too Big to Fail?", *Neurology*, Vol. 84, pp. 1-8.

HAS – Haute Autorité de Santé (2014), "L'évaluation micro-économique des médicaments et dispositifs médicaux", Haute Autorité de Santé, Paris.

House of Commons, Science and Technology Committee (2013), "Clinical Trials: Third Report of Session 2013-2014", HC104, United Kingdom, 17 September.

Howard, D.H. et al. (2015), "Pricing in the Market for Anticancer Drugs", *Journal of Economic Perspectives*, Vol. 29, No. 1, pp. 139-162.

IMS Institute for Healthcare Informatics (2016), "Global Oncology Trend Report: A Review of 2015 and Outlook to 2020", June, Danbury.

Iyengar, S. et al. (2016), "Prices, Costs, and Affordability of New Medicines for Hepatitis C in 30 Countries: An Economic Analysis", *PLoS Medicine*, Vol. 13, No. 5, e1002032.

Kapczynski, A. and A.S. Kesselheim (2016), "Government Patent Use: A Legal Approach To Reducing Drug Spending", *Health Affairs*, Vol. 35, No.5, pp. 791-797.

Karikios, D.J. et al. (2014), "Rising Cost of Anticancer Drugs in Australia", *Internal Medicine Journal*, Vol. 44, No. 5, pp. 458-463.

Lancet Haematology (2015), "The Rising Cost of Orphan Drugs – Editorial", *Lancet Haematology*, Vol. 2, November.

Light, D.W. and H. Kantarjian (2013), "Market Spiral Pricing of Cancer Drugs", *Cancer*, Vol. 119, No. 22, pp. 3900-3902, 15 November.

Luhnen, M. et al. (2016), "Health Economic Evaluations of Sofosbuvir for Treatment of Chronic Hepatitis C: A Systematic Review", *Applied Health Economics and Health Policy*, Vol. 14, No. 5, pp. 527-543.

Mathieu, A. (2016), "EU Regulatory Framework on Orphan Medicinal Products", Presentation at the OECD closed workshop on pharmaceutical reimbursement and pricing policies, 25 January, Paris.

MHRA – Medicines and Healthcare Products Regulatory Agency (2016), *Independent review of Early Access to Medicines Scheme (EAMS)*, Medicines and Healthcare Products Regulatory Agency, London.

MoCA-OMP Working Group on Mechanism of Coordinated Access to Orphan Medicinal Products (2014), "Transparent Value Framework, Process on Corporate Social Responsibility in the Field of Pharmaceuticals Platform on Access to Medicines in Europe", Brussels.

Morel, T. et al. (2013), "Reconciling Uncertainty of Costs and Outcomes with the Need for Access to Orphan Medicinal Products: A Comparative Study of Managed Entry Agreements Across Seven European Countries", *Orphanet Journal of Rare Diseases*, Vol. 8, No. 198, *www.ojrd.com/content/8/1/198*.

Navarria, A. et al. (2015), "Do the Current Performance-based Schemes in Italy Really Work? 'Success Fee': A Novel Measure for Cost-containment of Drug Expenditure", *Value in Health*, Vol. 18, pp. 131-136.

NHS – National Health Service (2016), "Appraisal and Funding of Cancer Drugs from July 2016 (including the new Cancer Drugs Fund): A New Deal for Patients, Taxpayers and Industry", NHS, United Kingdom, 8 July.

NICE – National Institute for Health and Care Excellence (2016), "NICE and Cancer Drugs – The Facts", *www.nice.org.uk/news/nice-statistics* (accessed 24 October 2016).

OECD (2015a), *Addressing Dementia: The OECD Response*, OECD Publishing, Paris, *http://dx.doi.org/10.1787/9789264231726-en*.

OECD (2015b), *Dementia Research and Care: Can Big Data Help?*, OECD Publishing, Paris, *http://dx.doi.org/10.1787/9789264228429-en*.

OECD (2013), *Strengthening Health Information Infrastructure for Health Care Quality Governance:* Good Practices, New Opportunities and Data Privacy Protection Challenges, OECD Publishing, Paris, *http://dx.doi.org/10.1787/9789264193505-en*.

O'Neill, J. et al. (2016), "Tackling Drug-resistant Infections Globally: Final Report and Recommendations – The Review on Antimicrobial Resistance Chaired by Jim O'Neill", Wellcome Trust and HM Government, London.

Paris, V. and A. Belloni (2013), "Value in Pharmaceutical Pricing", *OECD Health Working Papers*, No. 63, OECD Publishing, Paris, *http://dx.doi.org/10.1787/5k43jc9v6knx-en*.

Pharmaprojects (2016), "Blockbuster Trends and Rising Stars of Global R&D", Pharmaprojects annual report 2016, Pharmaprojects, London.

PhRMA – Pharmaceutical Research and Manufacturers of America (PhRMA) and AACR – American Association for Cancer Research (2015), "Medicines in Development for Cancer", *http://phrma.org/sites/default/files/pdf/oncology-report-2015.pdf*.

Policy Cures (2015), "G-FINDER Report 2015 – Neglected Disease Research and Development: The Ebola Effect", *www.policycures.org/downloads/Y8%20GFINDER%20full%20report%20web.pdf*.

Polton, D. et al. (2015), "Rapport sur la réforme des modalités d'évaluation des médicaments" (in French), *http://social-sante.gouv.fr/IMG/pdf/rapport_polton_-_evaluation_medicaments.pdf*.

Prater, D. (2016), "Orphan Drug Designations and Approvals: A U.S. Perspective", Presentation at the OECD closed workshop on pharmaceutical reimbursement and pricing policies, Paris, 25 January.

Pugatch M.P., R. Chu and D. Torstensson (2012), "Assembling the Pharmaceutical R&D Puzzle for Needs in the Developing World", Pugatch Consilium, Geneva.

Regalado, A. (2016a), "Gene Therapy's First Out-and-Out Cure Is Here – A Gene Therapy for an Inherited Immune Disease Completes a 27-year Journey", *MIT Technology Review*, May 6, *www.technologyreview.com/s/601390/gene-therapys-first-out-and-out-cure-is-here/#/set/id/601407/*.

Regalado, A. (2016b), "The World's Most Expensive Medicine Is a Bust", *MIT Technology Review*, 6 May, *www.technologyreview.com/s/601165/the-worlds-most-expensive-medicine-is-a-bust/*.

Regalado, A. (2015), "Biotech's Coming Cancer Cure – Supercharge Your Immune Cells to Defeat Cancer? Juno Therapeutics Believes Its Treatments Can Do Exactly That", *MIT Technology Review*, June 18, *www.technologyreview.com/s/538441/biotechs-coming-cancer-cure/*.

Renwick, M.J., D.M. Brogan and E. Mossialos (2016a), "A Systematic Review and Critical Assessment of Incentive Strategies for Discovery and Development of Novel Antibiotics", *Journal of Antibiotics*, Vol. 69, No. 2, pp. 73-88, *http://doi.org/10.1038/ja.2015.98*.

Renwick, M.J., D.M. Brogan and E. Mossialos (2016b), "Targeting Innovation in Antibiotic Drug Discovery and Development: The Need for a One Health – One Europe – One World Framework", *Health Policy Series Study* No. 45, European Observatory on Health Systems and Policies, Brussels.

Richards, M. (2010), "Extent and Causes of International Variations in Drug Usage", A report for the Secretary of State for Health, July, London.

Røttingen, J.A. et al. (2013), "Mapping of Available Health Research and Development Data: What's There, What's Missing, and What Role Is There for a Global Observatory?", *The Lancet*, Vol. 382, pp. 1286-307, 12 October.

Roy, V. and L. King (2016), "Betting on Hepatitis C: How Financial Speculation in Drug Development Influences Access to Medicines", *British Medical Journal*, Vol. 354, i3718.

Savage, P. and S. Mahmoud (2015), "Development and Economic Trends in Cancer Therapeutic Drugs: A 5-year Update 2010-2014", *British Journal of Cancer*, Vol. 112, pp. 1037-1041.

Scannell, J. et al. (2012), "Diagnosing the Decline in Pharmaceutical R&D Efficiency", *Nature Reviews Drug Discovery*, pp. 191-200.

Schuller, Y., C.E.M. Hollak and M. Biegstraaten (2015), "The Quality of Economic Evaluation of Ultra-orphan Drugs in Europe – A Systematic Review", *Orphanet Journal of Rare Diseases*, Vol. 10, p. 92.

Thomas, D.W. et al. (2016), "Clinical Development Success Rates 2006-2015", BIO, Biomedtracker, Amplion.

Trish, E., G. Joyce and D.P. Goldman (2014), "Specialty Drug Spending Trends Among Medicare and Medicare Advantage Enrollees, 2007-11", *Health Affairs (Millwood)*, Vol. 33, No. 11, pp. 2018-2024.

van den Brink, R. (2014), "Reimbursement of Orphan Drugs: The Pompe and Fabry Case in the Netherlands", *Orphanet Journal of Rare Diseases*, Vol. 9, Suppl. 1, O17.

Vandenbroeck, Ph. et al. (2016), "Future Scenarios About Drug Development and Drug Pricing", *Health Care Knowledge Centre (KCE) Report 271*, D/2016/10.273/59, Health Services Research (HSR), Brussels.

van de Vooren, K. et al. (2015), "Market-access Agreements for Anti-cancer Drugs", *Journal of the Royal Society of Medicine*, Vol. 108, No. 5, pp. 166-170.

van de Vooren, K. et al. (2014), "Market Access Agreements for Anti-cancer Drugs", *Journal of the Royal Society of Medicine*, Vol. 108, No. 5, pp. 1-5.

Van Nuys et al. (2015), "Broad Hepatitis C Treatment Scenarios Return Substantial Health Gains, But Capacity Is A Concern", *Health Affairs*, Vol. 34, No. 10, pp. 1666-1674, *http://dx.doi.org/10.1377/hlthaff.2014.1193*.

Vitry, A. and E. Roughead (2014), "Managed Entry Agreements for Pharmaceuticals in Australia", *Health Policy*, Vol. 117, pp. 345-352.

Vogler, S., A. Vitry and Z.U.-D. Babar (2016), "Cancer Drugs in 16 European Countries, Australia, and New Zealand: A Cross-country Price Comparison Study", *Lancet Oncology*, Vol. 17, pp. 39-47, January.

Weeks, J.C. et al. (2012), "Patients' Expectations about Effects of Chemotherapy for Advanced Cancer", *New England Journal of Medicine*, Vol. 367, pp. 1616-1625.

WHO – World Health Organization (2015), "Antimicrobial Resistance: Global Report on Surveillance", World Health Organization, Geneva.

WHO (2006), "Public Health, Innovation and Intellectual Property Rights", Commission on Intellectual Property Rights, Innovation and Public Health, World Health Organization, Geneva.

ANNEX 3.A1

OECD country policies to boost innovation for orphan diseases

Many OECD countries implemented specific policies to encourage the development of orphan medicines. Though eligibility criteria and related advantages differ across countries (Table 3.A1.1), these incentives generally consist of subsidised R&D spending, expedited or facilitated regulatory approval and extended market exclusivity. Since many orphan medicines target diseases with high unmet medical need, they often also benefit from other provisions, among which is pre-licensing access through different schemes (e.g. temporary use, compassionate use). While compassionate use is often financed by companies themselves, other schemes may be financed by payers (e.g. as in France).

Table 3.A1.1. **Policies to encourage development of orphan drugs in OECD countries**

	Eligibility criteria	Provisions
Australia (1997-)	Medicines targeting a disease affecting less than 2 000 patients	• Waiver of fees for MA evaluation • Use of FDA's evaluation where available • Five-years data protection
European Union (2000-)	• The medicine must be intended for the treatment, prevention or diagnosis of a disease that is life-threatening or chronically debilitating. • The prevalence of the condition in the European Union must not be more than 5 in 10 000 or it must be unlikely that marketing of the medicine would generate sufficient returns to justify the investment needed for its development. • No satisfactory method of diagnosis, prevention or treatment of the condition concerned can be authorised, or, if such a method exists, the medicine must be of significant benefit to those affected by the condition.	• Assessment by a separate Committee of Orphan Medicinal Products of the EMA, but with similar rules as for other products • Ten years market exclusivity during which similar medicines for the same indication cannot be placed on the market • Small and medium enterprises can get further incentives (waiver of registration fees)
Japan (1993-)	• The medicine must target an incurable disease. There must be no possible alternative treatment or the efficacy and expected safety of the drug must be excellent in comparison with other available drugs. • The number of patients affected by this disease in Japan must be less than 50 000 on the Japanese territory, which corresponds to a maximal incidence of 4/10 000.	• Reimbursement of 50% of development costs (some of which must be paid back if the drug is profitable) in addition to the 6% tax credit for R&D spending • Technical assistance with application for marketing authorisation • Eligible for fast-track procedure • Ten years exclusivity
United States (1983-)	• Targeted disease affects less than 200 000 individuals in the United States or affects more than 200 000 individuals in the United States without it being possible to cover the cost of development and distribution by sales on national territory. • If the drug is not the first in this indication, it must show superiority to existing ones to get an orphan designation.	• Tax credit equal to 50% of the costs of clinical trials undertaken in the United States • Technical assistance with application for MA • Eligible for fast-track procedure • + seven-years exclusivity • FDA grants to stimulate product development for rare diseases

MA : Market authorisation.

Source: *www.orpha.net*, *www.fda.gov* ; *www.ema.eu*. Gammie, T., C.Y. Lu and Z.U.-D. Babar (2015), "Access to Orphan Drugs: A Comprehensive Review of Legislations, Regulations and Policies in 35 Countries", *PLoS ONE*, Vol. 10, No. 10, e0140002.

ANNEX 3.A2

Coverage and funding of medicines in OECD countries

	General rule for coverage and funding of medicines	Specific rules for high-cost medicines
Australia	Medicines used in **ambulatory settings** or in private hospitals can be funded by the federal government when listed in the Pharmaceutical Benefit Schedule (PBS). To be listed in the PBS, medicines must be assessed by the Pharmaceutical Benefits Advisory Committee (PBAC) and considered cost-effective. Pharmaceuticals **delivered in hospitals** are funded by states. Hospitals have their own budgets and can purchase any medicine. Most hospitals follow PBAC recommendations even though they are not obliged to do so.	Managed entry agreements (MEAs) can be signed for medicines with a high ICER (volume-price or performance-based). Access to medicines with a high ICER can be granted through a **special access process** called "Section 100", reserved for medicines treating chronic and severe disease, highly specialised treatments and expensive medicines (small target populations). Access to medicines listed in Section 100 is limited to authorised centres with allocated budgets. The number of doses and quantities administered to patients are often limited.
Canada	Medicines used in **ambulatory care** are covered by private insurers (for 2/3 of the population) and public drugs plans. The Common Drug Review (CDR) or the pan Canadian Oncology Drug Review (pCODR) are in charge of assessing new medicines to provide recommendations to public plans, based on HTA results, including cost-effectiveness. Final decisions on funding and pricing are made at the level of public drug plans (provincial or federal). Medicines used **in hospitals** are covered by provinces and territories. Their prices are negotiated between hospitals (or groups of hospitals) and pharmaceutical companies. The maximum price of all patented drugs is subject to regulation at the federal level.	Pharmacy and therapeutic funding policies can include MEAs.
France	Medicines used **in ambulatory care** and **hospitals** are funded by social health insurance when listed in the positive list. The Transparency Commission, part of the national health technology agency (HAS), assesses the therapeutic benefit of the medicines (to recommend funding) and the added therapeutic benefit over standard therapy (to inform price negotiation). In addition, the HAS performs an economic evaluation if the medicine has a significant impact on the health insurance budget (i.e. the medicine generates more than EUR 20 million annual sales during the first two years of commercialisation) or if the manufacturer claims an added therapeutic value (rating I to III). The price is then negotiated by the Pricing Committee (CEPS) for reimbursed medicines used in outpatient care and for medicines used in inpatient care and paid on top of DRG tariffs. Medicines used in **hospitals** are normally included in DRG tariffs with prices negotiated directly with the company, with calls for tender when the price is higher than EUR 4 000. Product-specific agreements (mainly volume-based) may be concluded at the time of price negotiation but are confidential.	In cases of severe diseases and unmet medical need, patients can get access to promising treatments that are not yet approved through temporary authorisation for use (ATU), on request. In this case, health insurance funds pay for these treatments at the price set by the company. The National Institute for Cancer (INCa) facilitates access to diagnostic tests and oncology products. For innovative high-cost medicines, the HAS performs an economic evaluation (cost-effectiveness study, budgetary impact). To facilitate access to expensive treatments, some products are paid on top of diagnosis-related group (DRG), at a price negotiated at the national level by the pricing committee.

	General rule for coverage and funding of medicines	Specific rules for high-cost medicines
Germany	New medicines are reimbursed by health insurance funds unless they belong to one category excluded from reimbursement (e.g. over-the-counter medicines). Within six months after market entry, the Federal Joint Committee (G-BA) evaluates the added benefit of the new medicine. That benefit assessment and appraisal are then used as a basis for negotiations between the statutory health insurance fund and industry to agree on the price. In cases of no additional benefit, the new medicine is clustered into a "reference price group" if possible. The prices of medicines used **in hospitals** are directly negotiated between hospitals and pharmaceutical companies and their cost is included in DRG tariffs.	Innovative medicines whose annual turnover is below EUR 1 million are excluded from the evaluation process. An orphan medicine has to undergo regular assessment if the turnover with the statutory health insurance fund exceeds EUR 50 million (pharmacy prices including VAT) within the last 12 months. Hospitals can obtain extra funding from federal authorities on individual request for medicines and some diagnostic tests whose costs have not been factored in DRG tariffs (NUB).
Italy	The national medicine agency (AIFA) is charge of assessing new medicines, making funding decisions, and negotiating prices. The AIFA rates the innovativeness of the treatment in three categories: minor, modest or major. Medicines of the last category are always reimbursed and their price is negotiated based on the ICER, budget impact and prices abroad. Funding and pricing decisions are made at the national level but regions can negotiate further rebates. Medicines used **in hospitals** are funded through hospital budgets and purchased through calls for tender.	To speed access to treatment, AIFA sometimes agrees to pay for innovative treatments pending the results of the evaluation. Patients can also access specific treatments on individual request (Act 648/96) but funding is only continued if the medicine is effective. Expensive treatments can be partially covered by the regional budget. MEAs may be signed between companies and payers, where the price is linked to performance of the product in real life.
Spain	Every new medicine is assessed by the committee in charge of recommendations for funding, which is part of the Ministry of Health. The committee assesses the clinical benefits, innovativeness and cost-effectiveness of new products, as well as their impact on health care organisation. Regional agencies may also perform assessments. To be reimbursed, medicines have to be included in a positive list and the price is negotiated. Medicines with low therapeutic benefit are excluded from reimbursement. Medicines used **in hospitals** are paid under hospital budgets. Calls for tender are launched at hospital or regional level.	
Sweden	All new products have to be assessed by the TLV (pharmaceutical and dental board) to be included in the positive list. TLV assessment takes the following criteria into account: cost-effectiveness, medical need, national solidarity and the human value principle. Sweden adopts a societal perspective in economic evaluation. There is no explicit ICER threshold. Prices are not negotiated but the company can resubmit an application with a lower price when the TLV issues a negative recommendation because the medicine is not cost-effective. Medicines used **in hospitals** are purchased through calls for tender at the local level.	Price-volume agreements may be negotiated, as well as risk-sharing agreements in some circumstances (uncertain benefits).
Switzerland	Medicines used in ambulatory settings are covered by compulsory health insurance according to the prices and terms and conditions in the positive list, which is determined by the Federal Office of Public Health. Medicines and other services used **in hospitals** are covered by compulsory health insurance and regions (cantons). Generally, the medicines' costs are included in DRG tariffs. The purchase prices of hospital medicines are negotiated between hospitals and pharmaceutical companies.	In general high-cost medicines are only reimbursed when specific terms and conditions are fulfilled and the reimbursement is limited in time before re-evaluation. In specific cases (e.g. combination therapies of oncologic medicines), transparent MEAs with paybacks are implemented. The criteria for pricing high-costs medicines are the same as for low-cost medicines: external price comparison and comparison of the price of medicines with a similar indication.

	General rule for coverage and funding of medicines	Specific rules for high-cost medicines
United Kingdom (England)	New medicines can be funded by National Health Service (NHS) England immediately after market entry, unless they belong to a category excluded from funding (e.g. over-the counter). Prices at market entry are set by manufacturers but regulated through the Pharmaceutical Price Regulation Scheme which caps the annual return on NHS sales. The National Institute for Health and Care Excellence (NICE) assesses many new medicines where national guidance is expected to add value (uncertain effectiveness, high price or budget impact, etc.) through its technology appraisal programme. NICE performs cost-utility analysis and has an explicit ICER threshold of between GBP 20 000 and GBP 30 000 per QALY to recommend new technologies, with flexibility to recommend drugs for patients at the end of their lives at a higher ICER. NICE can take into account Patient Access Scheme proposals. These are schemes offered by companies and agreed with the Department of Health to improve a medicine's cost-effectiveness in the context of a NICE appraisal. Medicines used **in hospitals** are paid on the hospital budgets and purchased with calls for tender.	A small number of very high-cost drugs for very small numbers of patients are evaluated for national specialised commissioning through NICE's Highly Specialised Technologies Programme. Since 2012, the Cancer Drugs Fund provides funding for promising, new cancer drugs where there is uncertainty about their clinical effectiveness and cost-effectiveness.

New Health Technologies: Managing Access, Value
and Sustainability

Chapter 4

Ensuring timely and affordable access to medical devices

by
Valérie Paris, Luke Slawomirski *and* Allison Colbert

Medical devices cover a wide range of products of varying complexity and clinical risk. Practitioners' aptitude in using medical devices in clinical settings also varies. Regulation, coverage and funding of devices thus present a considerable challenge for policy makers who need to balance the often competing objectives of safety, effectiveness, equity and timely access. Regulatory requirements for medical devices were historically less stringent than those for pharmaceutical products. This chapter examines the current state of play for medical device regulation (determining the safety, performance and effectiveness for initial market authorisation and post-market evaluation) and coverage and funding (determining their inclusion in payment schedules and the reimbursement level for their use). It provides a series of recommendations to improve these aspects of regulatory regimes in OECD countries and other health care systems. The chapter also describes the institutional requirements and policy framework needed to enable sound regulatory, coverage and funding decisions. These include governance, information infrastructure and stakeholder involvement.

We thank country delegates and experts, as well as BIAC members, for their comments on earlier versions of this chapter and during the expert meeting of 22 March 2016 and the OECD Health Committee meeting of 28-29 June 2016. We acknowledge in particular suggestions and material provided by Ruth Lopert (George Washington University) Stefano Bonacina (Karolinska Institutet) and Iñaki Gutiérrez Ibarluzea (Osteba).

Introduction

Medical devices comprise a very broad range of health technologies, from tongue depressors, splints, cannulas and endoscopes, to artificial organs and other implantable devices, to complex radiological equipment (Box 4.1). More recent examples include mobile applications (apps) and wearables, web-enabled products and biosensors, and *in vitro* diagnostics (IVD) permitting clinical intervention based on molecular biomarkers. As a category, devices thus cover a uniquely wide spectrum of applications, risks and benefits. They are ubiquitous, embedded in clinical activity in a range of ways, and this interaction is constantly evolving as providers find new uses and applications for existing products. The total number of registered products in the United States and Europe alone exceeds 200 000 (Kirisits and Redekop, 2013).

Box 4.1. **Definition of medical device**

A medical device can be defined as "any instrument, apparatus, appliance, software, implant, reagent, material or other article, intended by the manufacturer to be used, alone or in combination, for human beings for one or more of the specific medical purposes of:

- Diagnosis, prevention, monitoring, prediction, prognosis, treatment or alleviation of disease;
- Diagnosis, monitoring, treatment, alleviation of or compensation for an injury or disability;
- Investigation, replacement or modification of the anatomy or of a physiological or pathological process or state;
- Providing information by means of in vitro examination of specimens derived from the human body, including organ, blood and tissue donations;
- And which does not achieve its principal intended action by pharmacological, immunological or metabolic means, in or on the human body, but which may be assisted in its function by such means.

Products specifically intended for the cleaning, disinfection or sterilisation of medical devices and devices for the purpose of control or support of conception shall be considered medical devices."

Source: Council of the European Union (2016), "Proposal for a Regulation of the European Parliament and of the Council on Medical Devices, and Amending Directive 2001/83/EC, Regulation (EC) No. 178/2002 and Regulation (EC) No. 1223/2009", p. 42, *http://data.consilium.europa.eu/doc/document/ST-9364-2016-REV-3/en/pdf* (accessed 18 July 2016).

Policy governing device regulation, coverage and funding is fundamental in a well-functioning and sustainable health care system. Such policy can determine clinical behaviour and influence health outcomes. As discussed in Chapter 2, diffusion and use of medical technology is an important driver of health care expenditure growth (Chernew and Newhouse, 2012; Chandra and Skinner, 2012), and regulatory and reimbursement policy is an important part of health care system sustainability.

In general terms, a framework for regulating and funding medical devices should aim to balance three core primary objectives:

- ensuring that devices are clinically safe, performant, and effective where relevant;
- facilitating timely and equitable patient access to beneficial health technology; and
- ensuring that expenditure on devices produces value to patients and health care systems.

Tension can arise between these objectives. Expediency must be balanced against adequate rigour, affordability with access. Aligning regulatory objectives with broader economic and industrial policy (e.g. to promote innovation, employment, growth, export and trade) may result in tension with goals of managing costs. In addition, each objective will be prioritised differently by stakeholder groups, adding a political dimension to the process. Finally, concepts such as equity are not easily defined empirically.

These difficulties, as well as the breadth and inherent complexities of medical devices as a class of health technology, present a unique challenge for policy makers. Yet the requirements for approval and clinical use of devices are often less strict than those for pharmaceutical products. The current shift towards hybrid biopharmaceutical products, the convergence of medical information and information and communication technology (ICT), and the increasing complexity of medical product supply chains bring this incongruity into focus and are likely to intensify the challenges associated with device regulation and reimbursement in the near future. At the 67th World Health Assembly, delegates agreed that regulatory systems for medical products, including devices, need to be strengthened and periodically evaluated (WHO, 2014), and recent literature called for medical device regulation to be bolstered (Sorenson and Drummond, 2014; Kirisits and Redekop, 2013; Campillo-Artero, 2013). The WHO subsequently developed a global model for regulatory frameworks for medical devices. This model builds on the 2014 resolution to strengthen regulatory capabilities worldwide, and was open for consultation at the time of writing (WHO, 2016).

This chapter examines current systems of regulation and funding of medical devices in OECD countries, as well as their advantages and weaknesses, and proposes ways to improve value in the management of medical devices. Section 1 discusses *regulation*, which includes marketing authorisation, monitoring, review and post-market evaluation of devices in terms of their safety, effectiveness and performance.

Section 2 focuses on *coverage and funding*. Coverage entails decisions by payers on whether the use of a product should be funded. Funding determines how, and how much of, the use of a device should be paid for. Dedicating separate sections to regulation and funding does not imply that these are completely disconnected processes. Rather, scope exists for recognising alignment between the two. Both face similar conceptual and evidentiary challenges. Considerable overlap often arises in the evidence, expertise and deliberations required to make regulatory, coverage and funding decisions, particularly if established as a cycle of periodic review. Although a critical approach is needed, resource or information sharing could reduce costs and potential delays associated with medical device regulation and market entry.

Section 3 discusses the *institutional and contextual requirements* necessary for regulatory and reimbursement practices to be implemented and to ensure the objectives of a regulatory framework are met. The main focus is the importance of an integrated information infrastructure and of sound public policy fundamentals such as transparency, stakeholder engagement and consultation.

1. Regulating medical devices

Regulation concerns the laws and policies for assessing medical devices for safety and performance, and consequent approval for their clinical use. Regulation comprises two key phases:

- *Market approval*[1] is granted based on detailed evaluation of the product's safety, effectiveness and/or performance for use in clinical settings.
- *Post-market evaluation* comprises the monitoring of safety, effectiveness and/or performance of the product once in routine clinical use.

1.1. Safety, performance and effectiveness are key concepts for medical device regulation

Two fundamental dimensions need to be considered in the regulation of devices: safety and effectiveness or performance. A medical device is considered *safe* if the risk associated with its intended use is deemed acceptably low compared to the expected benefits. *Performance* describes whether the device functions as intended. *Effectiveness* assesses whether the use of a device in usual clinical circumstances does more good than harm and achieves a desired clinical result (Baeyens et al., 2015).

This distinction is illustrated using the example of linear accelerators (linac devices) used in radiation oncology. A linac device would be proven *performant* by demonstrating that it can generate and accurately aim a concentrated stream of high energy particles with a specified intensity at a designated target. This can feasibly be tested in an experimental setting using apparatus only. Establishing its *effectiveness* involves demonstrating that the device actually achieves its desired clinical result – to diminish the size of a tumour by a specified amount. This can only be demonstrated in a clinical setting, and is more challenging than the demonstration of performance. The question of *clinical utility* – does the medical device add any value to the care pathway for a specific diagnosis or disease? – is usually not addressed in regulation of market entry. Rather, this is addressed in Health Technology Assessments (HTAs) used to determine coverage or clinical guidelines.

Market entry regulation varies across device categories and countries

Regulation requirements for medical device marketing authorisation vary widely across countries, but also across device categories. Countries generally categorise devices in three to four classes, according to the level of risk for patients. Requirements for market access are more stringent for devices with higher potential risks for patients (Table 4.1).

In the United States, the Food and Drug Administration (FDA), the body responsible for device approval, examines the *safety* and *effectiveness* of medical devices. Safety standards involve the risk to the patient but also to the provider, for example a laboratory handling blood to perform an IVD procedure. The most stringent requirements apply to Class III products (e.g. implantables), for which applicants need to submit evidence obtained from clinical studies to get market access (pre-market authorisation or PMA). Class II products also require the submission of clinical evidence unless they can demonstrate substantial equivalence with an existing device [the 510(k) regulatory pathway]. In fact, 90% of medical devices in the United States are approved through this pathway (Cohen and Billingsley, 2011).

In Europe, regulation of market access focuses on safety and performance.[2] "CE Marking" provides market access to medical devices in the 28 member states of the European Union plus Iceland, Liechtenstein, Norway and Switzerland. National competent

Table 4.1. **Risk categories and evidentiary requirements for medical devices in the United States and Europe**

Region/Country	Risk stratification	Evidence required
United States	Class I: No to negligible risk (e.g. tongue depressors)	No evidence required; approval concerns registration and labelling requirements (the latter is not required for medical devices that are equivalent to existing ones).
	Class II: Low risk (e.g. endoscopes, infusion pumps)	Most require formal agency notification but no clinical evidence required if "substantial equivalence" demonstrated with existing device [510(k) exemption]. A device seeking classification as low-risk without an existing predicate must submit a scientific evaluation of risks and benefits [510(k) de novo process].
	Class III: Medium to high risk (e.g. coronary stents, defibrillators) includes novel devices with no predicates	Requires approval with evidence of safety and effectiveness from clinical trials, with some exceptions.[1]
Europe	Class I: No to negligible risk (e.g. thermometers)	No approval (self-certification) with clinical evaluation required.
	Class IIa: Low risk (e.g. infusion pumps) Class IIb: Medium risk (e.g. dialysis machines, artificial joints)	Dossier of supporting literature to substantiate *safety* and *performance* comprising clinical and non-clinical data. Assessment by a Notified Body, which involves an audit of the Quality Management System of the manufacturer's production processes.
	Class III: High risk (e.g. pacemakers)	Clinical studies required, can be non-randomised and single arm, focused on demonstrating *safety*. Assessment of the study design and of clinical evidence by a Notified Body is required.

1. Class III devices require PMA to demonstrate "evidence of safety and effectiveness" but there are some exceptions. For instance, devices that were marketed before 1976 or after 1976 but which are substantially equivalent to a device marketed before that date and for which FDA has not established a PMA requirement can go through the 510(k) process (see "Class III Certification and Summary" at *www.fda.gov/MedicalDevices/DeviceRegulationandGuidance/HowtoMarketYourDevice/PremarketSubmissions/PremarketNotification510k/ucm134578.htm*). A GAO report from 2009 found that, despite the goal of discontinuing it, 510(k) approval was still quite common for Class III devices in 2007 (GAO, 2009). Class III devices for a small patient population need to go through PMA but do not need to demonstrate effectiveness under the "Humanitarian Device Exemption" (see *www.fda.gov/medicaldevices/deviceregulationandguidance/howtomarketyourdevice/premarketsubmissions/humanitariandeviceexemption/default.htm*). This lowers entry barriers for devices used to treat rare diseases. Lastly, devices that result from a design change to an existing PMA-approved device can go through a PMA "Supplement" process, with varying requirements regarding new clinical data (see *www.fda.gov/RegulatoryInformation/Guidances/ucm089274.htm#3*). It's difficult to compare the stringency of the various types of supplemental decisions to original PMA process but given that devices follow a process of incremental innovation, supplemental PMA decisions are common (see GAO, 2009, Figure 3, p. 20).

Source: Authors' compilation from various sources.

authorities in each country identify one or several "Notified Bodies" accredited to conduct "conformity [to EU Directive requirements] assessments". This assessment usually involves an audit of the manufacturer's quality system and, depending upon the particular classification of the device, a review of the relevant technical documentation provided by the manufacturer in support of the safety and performance claims for the device. Manufacturers can choose from the many Notified Bodies (59 at the time of writing) in existence across the European common market to file their application.

Weaknesses in current regulations are being addressed by authorities

Problems with the United States regulatory process, as well as its enforcement and application, have been documented. PMA is often granted based on single clinical studies, which are rarely randomised (IOM, 2011) and many medical devices enter the market based on a demonstration of equivalence. This has resulted in frequent and increasing safety recalls (Chen et al., 2012; Sweet et al., 2011; Zuckerman et al., 2011; Ardaugh et al., 2013; Campillo-Artero, 2013). An evaluation of the 113 Class III devices recalled between 2005 and 2009 showed that only 19% were approved through the PMA process, 71% through the

510(k) process, and 7% were exempt from evaluation (Zuckerman et al., 2011). Between 2003 and 2012, the number of annual recalls nearly doubled to 1 190, in part due to efforts to improve the quality and safety of medical devices. In 2012, nearly 88% of recalls were for Class II products, the main contributor to the increase, while recalls for Class III products (7.5%) declined over the period (FDA, 2012).

The FDA is reforming the manner in which it addresses laboratory-developed tests (LDTs), i.e. IVDs designed, manufactured and used within a single laboratory. The FDA did not typically seek oversight of such tests, as they were considered relatively simple and safe, and therefore fell more under the purview of laboratory accreditation. However, as IVDs became increasingly important to the development of precision medicine, concerns arose regarding the apparent evidentiary inequities between LDTs and their commercially developed counterparts. In some cases, laboratories effectively acted as commercial testing operations, a concern in light of a systematic review demonstrating that test results may vary among laboratories (AHRQ, 2010). In 2014, the FDA released a proposed LDT regulatory oversight framework.

The current European system also shows some signs of weakness (Campillo-Artero, 2013; Sorenson and Drummond, 2014), as illustrated by differences in outcomes of regulatory decisions across agencies. The FDA, for instance, reported 12 examples of high-risk medical devices approved in Europe but not in the United States, most of which were later withdrawn from the EU market (FDA, 2012). In addition, the quality of assessment can vary between Notified Bodies, which compete for user fees since manufacturers have to pay for the assessment of their applications for CE marking. Investigations have shown that some of them were ready to grant CE marking to products presented as raising safety problems for patients internationally (Cohen, 2012). Post-marketing surveillance can be improved, and it has sometimes taken several years to withdraw problematic medical devices from the market (Cohen and Billingsley, 2011; Cohen, 2011).[3]

In 2012 the European Commission proposed new regulations to, among others: heighten requirements for clinical evidence; strengthen the supervision of assessment bodies; improve data on device performance and traceability of products through the supply chain; and strengthen co-ordination between national surveillance authorities (European Commission, 2012). The European Parliament and the Council of the European Union recently noted that "Key elements of the existing regulatory approach, such as the supervision of notified bodies, conformity assessment procedures, clinical investigations and clinical evaluation, vigilance and market surveillance should be significantly reinforced, whilst provisions ensuring transparency and traceability regarding devices should be introduced, to improve health and safety" (Council of the European Union, 2016, p. 4).

Revisions to the relevant EU legislation to strengthen the regulatory process were finally agreed upon and were in the process of adoption at the time of writing (Council of the European Union, 2016). These revisions include: a more comprehensive description of risk classification and management; reinforcement of rules concerning clinical data; stricter pre-market control of high-risk devices; reinforced requirements for manufacturers to collect data on real-life performance of their device; and introduction of EU-wide standardised information for patients receiving implants (Hansson, 2016). These changes will increase transparency and improve safety, notably through systematic reporting of clinical investigations, improved oversight of notified bodies by competent authorities, and compliance of rules for clinical investigations with international standards to facilitate use of their results by other jurisdictions. Post-market vigilance will be improved through: an electronic system and a central database of incident reporting; requirements for manufacturers to establish a risk management system; introduction of a unique device identification (UDI) system; and better access to information for all stakeholders.

In the past, post-market evaluation focused almost exclusively on surveillance of a device's safety. Therefore, it is most frequently termed "post-market surveillance". Medical devices' performance or effectiveness in real life was only rarely assessed using data collected after marketing authorisation. Overall, health care system performance would certainly benefit from routine consideration of performance and/or effectiveness. This is reflected in a recently announced policy shift in the United States, where the FDA is strengthening its post-market surveillance system for medical devices (Evans et al., 2015). This will "support optimal patient care by leveraging the experiences of patients to inform decisions about medical device safety, *effectiveness, and quality* in order to promote the public health" (Engelberg Center for Health Care Reform, 2015, p. 23, authors' emphasis). The new EU regulation on medical devices clarifies that post-market surveillance must focus on products' safety *and* performance.

Certain medical devices are, in addition, subject to other types of regulation – radioprotection for imaging and radiology, and certification for laboratories performing diagnostic tests, for example – and more recently, privacy and cyber-security for health data flowing from mobile applications, biosensors and wearable devices. This is discussed in a later section of this chapter.

1.2. *Managing uncertainty may require viewing regulation as a cycle*

Managing uncertainty is a key challenge for regulators. Evidence of the safety of any new medical technology may be incomplete at the market authorisation stage, while, by definition, evidence of effectiveness or clinical utility in real-world settings is lacking. Indeed, this limitation is greater for medical devices than for medicines due to the practical and ethical difficulties of performing robust randomised controlled trials, as well as to other factors such as clinician skill and experience.

Another feature of medical devices that distinguishes them from other health technologies is their multiple determinants of performance, which can include: 1) the intrinsic effectiveness of the device; 2) the skill of the practitioner that operates it; 3) patient-related factors; 4) performance of ancillary technology; and 5) organisational context. Regulation (and funding) should take this into account. Conditions and guidelines for a device or product's use should be stipulated and reviewed periodically based on evidence.

The increasing sophistication and specialised nature of medical technology raises the levels of uncertainty, and highlights the need for more adaptive and flexible approaches that follow a technology through its entire lifecycle. Devices are starting to combine mechanical and pharmaceutical methods of action, and are increasingly converging with ICT. Precision medicine, for example, relies on stratification of patients based on specific biomarkers. This often entails a limited number of potential subjects for clinical trials and results in even greater uncertainty, highlighting the growing need for a more dynamic regulatory framework (Husereau et al., 2014). This is particularly the case when a test for a particular biomarker has not been commercially developed, but rather performed directly by a laboratory.

Regulation can be best conceptualised as a cycle as opposed to a one-off, all-or-nothing decision (Figure 4.1). In this fashion, regulatory decisions can be periodically revisited, taking into account new information about a product's real-world performance and effectiveness. The ideal timeframe for review depends on factors unique to the device, such as level of uncertainty, strength of the initial evidence, level of clinical risk, and how quickly real-world evidence (RWE) can be generated and analysed (partly a function of the device's frequency of use). In this sense, once a product enters routine clinical use, it never actually leaves the regulatory process.

Figure 4.1. **Illustration of the regulatory cycle**

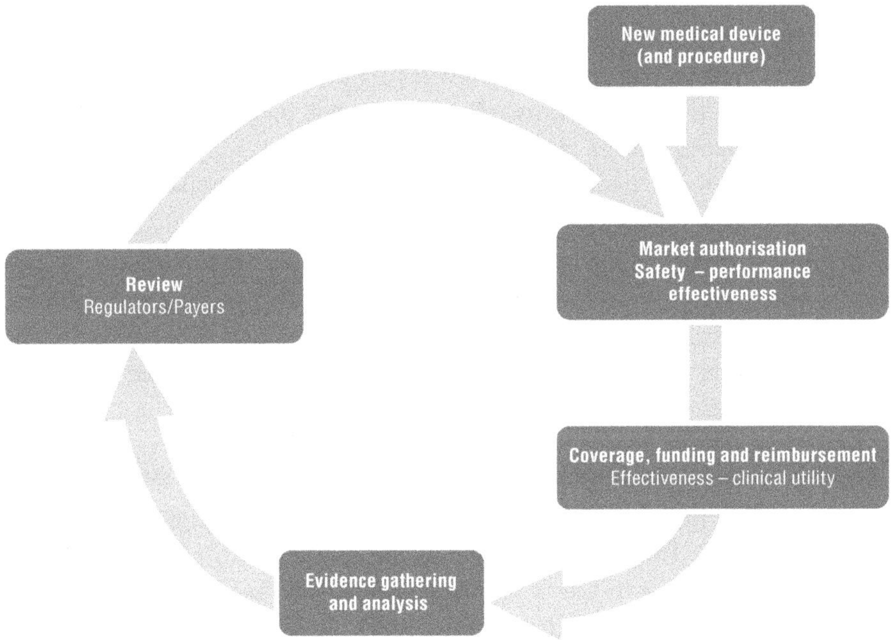

A minority of countries have instituted such a cyclical and dynamic approach to device regulation.[4] While products are monitored and frequently recalled due to safety concerns, routine review and adjustment based on evidence of clinical utility gathered once a product is in widespread clinical use have not been instituted. Indeed, difficulty in re-evaluating and delisting of products based on poor real-world performance is documented in most OECD countries, as explored in Section 2 on coverage and funding (Auraaen et al., 2016). More recently, regulators (and payers) in some jurisdictions are beginning to institute a cyclical approach and are adjusting policy and legislative settings accordingly.

The performance of some devices depends on use and user

Adding to the uncertainty about medical devices is that their real-world clinical utility may change over time as improved ways of using them are discovered by innovative providers, extending their application to a broader patient population. This can manifest in both positive and negative terms for patients and the health care system more broadly. For example, endoscopes were appropriated by gastroenterologists for exploratory colonoscopy after being used by the gynaecological profession for some time (Gelijins and Rosenberg, 1994).[5] Colonoscopy is frequently used as an example of a procedure that, while highly beneficial for some patients, can be used inappropriately with little benefit and considerable risk (ACSQHC, 2015; The Age, 2015). By more precisely and explicitly stipulating the indications for the use of a product, conditional approval can perhaps limit the expansion of use, while ongoing collection and analysis of evidence can inform regulators about the effectiveness of a product's new uses. This can then transfer into the development of guidelines for use, and inform coverage and funding decisions for the product in question.

1.3. *Health care systems should explore opportunities for streamlining the regulatory cycle*

Instituting regulation in a cyclical manner as proposed herein requires better co-ordination, a sound information infrastructure and, therefore, more resources. But not all medical devices need to be subjected to the same level of scrutiny. As described earlier, most systems stratify approval requirements according to the level of clinical risk associated with the product's use.

No right or wrong way prevails to streamline regulation; rather, the local context, regulatory system objectives and available resources should determine this. Given the rapid transformation in this health technology category, regulators may consider additional stratification criteria. These could include, for example, the extra-clinical risks concerning data accuracy and security of portable devices such as biosensors. In fact, it is arguably more important that any such requirements are articulated explicitly and enacted consistently. Stakeholder priorities will differ, challenging regulators to balance expediency, public health and value for money. Manufacturers will be interested in bringing their products to market and deriving an acceptable return on their investment. Patients too will be interested in rapidity but also in ensuring that clinical risks are managed, and citizens expect these imperatives to be balanced.

This highlights the importance of governance (discussed in Section 3). A clearly articulated, explicit set of objectives and principles for the regulatory system can set appropriate expectations and avoid unnecessary confusion among stakeholders. Proactive stakeholder communication and transparent regulatory processes are also required (OECD, 2013b).

Efforts to improve regulation should aim to minimise costs

Current efforts to strengthen regulation should try to minimise associated costs. The benefits of any regulation must always be assessed relative to its costs, in terms of delays in patient access to innovative products, but also in terms of costs for innovators (which are most often ultimately borne by health care payers) and administrative costs.

When advocating against the strengthening of regulation, industry representatives often stress that most companies producing medical devices are small and medium-sized enterprises (SMEs) that do not have the means to conduct high-cost trials, and that medical devices have a short lifecycle,[6] which shortens the period during which inventors can get returns from their investment (WHO, WIPO and WTO, 2012). Indeed, in Europe, 95% of the 25 000 medical technology companies are SMEs (MedTech Europe, 2015). However, not all companies are SMEs: the top five companies account for 28% of global sales and the top 15 for 48% (Gravelle and Lowry, 2015). The market can even be more concentrated in some market segments: the top 4 manufacturers of coronary stents represent 99% of total sales in the United States (Grennan, 2013). In any case, while these considerations are important, they do not justify compromising patient safety and health care system performance.

Some reduction of regulatory costs could be sought through harmonisation of regulatory standards at the international level. The International Medical Device Regulators Forum (IMDRF), formed as a voluntary organisation comprising regulators and industry from Australia, Brazil, Canada, China, the European Union, Japan, Russia, Singapore and the United States, and WHO as an official observer, is working on recommendations to achieve this goal.[7] The IMDRF undertakes wide-ranging activities to strengthen, harmonise and streamline medical device regulation. For example, under its previous incarnation as the Global Harmonization Task Force (GHTF), a study group focused on aligning definitions and concepts around clinical evidence for IVD devices (GHTF, 2012).

As regulation of medical devices is very demanding in terms of volume,[8] efficiencies and economies can be generated by combining efforts and pooling resources with other countries. The WHO urged member states to "engage in global, regional and sub-regional networks of national regulatory authorities... recognizing the importance of collaboration to pool regulatory capacities to promote greater access to quality, safe, efficacious and affordable medical products" and to "promote international co-operation, as appropriate, for collaboration and information sharing, including through electronic platforms" (WHO, 2014, p. 3). Several jurisdictions, such as Australia and Mexico, envisage relying more heavily on market approval by trusted foreign authorities to streamline the process in their own country (Sansom et al., 2015). Indeed, there are sound arguments to reduce the burden of evaluation for any single country by joining forces to assess medical devices at a regional level and by cross-referencing to assessments in other countries.

1.4. *mHealth presents an emerging challenge to regulators*

The emergence of mHealth – mobile apps and portable devices using digital technology and ICT – was briefly outlined in Chapter 2. While these technologies hold considerable potential to advance human health and welfare, their proliferation is generating new and additional regulatory challenges.

A torrent of products is appearing on the market and, as can be expected, their quality and utility vary considerably. Indeed, the emerging evidence on the utility of these products is quite mixed (Bloss et al., 2016; Steinhubl et al., 2015; Free et al., 2013a, 2013b; Hamine et al., 2015; Karhula et al., 2015). The bewildering array of mHealth products can create confusion for providers and consumers. The sheer volume of apps being developed and marketed, the rapidly changing technological landscape, and the entry of stakeholders who are not accustomed to the regulatory processes and institutions unique to health care create a challenging environment for payers and policy makers, who need to manage risks appropriately without stifling potentially useful innovation.

Three types of risks are associated with mHealth products. First, clinical risks and consequences of failure and of poor performance can be as significant for mHealth as for any health technology. Inaccurate results of mobile diagnostics can have grave consequences – for example, insulin doses based on inaccurate blood glucose readings can be fatal.

Second, there are extra-clinical risks concerning privacy and security of individuals' health information that are completely new territory for regulators. A recent study examining 211 diabetes management apps found that 80% did not have privacy policies, and 86% of a randomly selected subset of 65 used tracking cookies that permit information about the user to be sent to other corporations. According to the fine-print permissions users have to accept before downloading the apps, 17% requested to track the user's location, 11% sought to switch on the smartphone's camera, and 64% requested the ability to delete or modify information anywhere on the user's phone.

Third are meta-clinical risks – for example, inaccurate population-wide datasets or flawed research results resulting in harm through erroneous therapeutic algorithms and clinical decision aids. The European Commission is establishing a working group to develop guidelines for assessing the validity and reliability of the data collected and processed through mHealth applications that are not also classified as medical devices, to make these more useful for public health purposes (Brennan, 2016).

An additional challenge is the truly global reach of many mHealth products, especially apps, and their heavy reliance on digital infrastructure. Because these exist in cyberspace, they can be accessed by anyone, anywhere. Traditional borders are not as relevant, and jurisdictions may find it more difficult to administer and enforce regulatory requirements without requisite technical and legal expertise and international co-operation. Another unique feature of mHealth is its heavy reliance on telecommunications infrastructure. The majority of these products rely on Internet connectivity, and only work as intended in areas with access to reliable broadband Internet. Some geographic regions in many middle- as well as high-income countries currently lack reliable connections.

Regulatory systems and institutions for devices are not equipped to deal with the unique requirements and challenges of mHealth, especially software and software/hardware composites. Shoehorning these into current regimes can be problematic. While catastrophic adverse events stemming from these risks have not been reported, cases of product withdrawal have occurred due to concerns over accuracy and performance compromising patient safety (Cortez et al., 2014). As a starting point, three categories of mHealth products are proposed to stratify the level of increasing risk: 1) administrative products (for billing, scheduling of appointments and basic communication); 2) health management products (medication management, reminder apps, activity trackers); and 3) products that perform complex functions (capturing and using variables to calculate therapeutic dosage and other clinical decision support tools).

The regulatory challenge is to create a framework that ensures safety in terms of clinical and privacy/security risks and encourages high-value innovation, while preventing ineffective, unsafe and low-value products from flooding the market and crowding out more effective and beneficial ones. A unique regulatory pathway for approval and ongoing surveillance – separate from that for conventional medical technology and with requisite expertise and oversight – is likely required. The necessary expertise to enable sound judgement and decision making in this regard includes coding, privacy and security, data science and bioethics specialising in this area. Current approaches vary between jurisdictions.

The European Commission developed a draft Code of Conduct for mobile applications in response to consumers' concerns regarding the security and privacy of data collected by mHealth products. This Code of Conduct is targeted at developers, providing specific guidance on how European data protection legislation should be applied in relation to apps. It accounts for both the requirements under the current EU Data Protection Directive as well as the provisions of the new EU General Data Protection Regulation, which will apply from 25 May 2018. The Code of Conduct contains guidance on a number of issues of likely interest to app developers: obtaining consent; information provision requirements; privacy by design and default; data retention and security measures; advertising; processing data for secondary purposes; sharing data with third parties, and the requirement for, and content of, data processing agreements; restrictions on and methods for transferring data outside of the European Economic Area; and steps to be followed in the event of data breaches. The Code of Conduct will not be binding but developers who comply voluntarily will be identified in a centralised register and periodically audited. At the time of writing, the Code of Conduct was in the process of ratification by the Article 29 Working Party, an independent advisory body comprising representatives from all EU data protection authorities (European Commission, 2016a).

In terms of safety and performance, the European Commission established an mHealth Working Group to develop guidelines for assessing the *validity* and *reliability of data* that are collected and processed by apps aimed at lifestyle and well-being (i.e. not apps classified as medical devices). The first draft of the guidelines was published in April 2016 for consultation. They describe a set of criteria relating to quality, safety, reliability and effectiveness to underpin the methodologies that can be used for assessing these apps. They divide the evaluation of an mHealth app into three phases: 1) initial validation and assessment of the app platform; 2) risk assessment to determine the level of scrutiny required, and 3) scrutiny, which sets out a series of questions, taking account of the technology platform and the medical aspects of the app to consider. The draft guidelines focus on the safety and utility evaluation. An assessment of the performance or effectiveness of such apps is being considered separately, along with details of the risk assessment. Like the Code of Conduct, the guidelines will be voluntary (European Commission, 2016b). While not legally binding, guidelines are developed in consultation with member states and interested parties and therefore reflect the experience and positions of key stakeholder groups. For example, one such guideline (MEDDEV 2.1/6) helps software and app designers assess if their product falls into the category of a medical device and, if so, how it should be classified (European Commission, 2016c).

The US FDA focuses regulation on the small subset of mHealth products that meet the regulatory definition of a medical device (FDA, 2015b). These tend to be approved predominantly through the 510(k) pathway, which requires evidence of equivalence to pre-existing, similar technology and thus exonerates developers from more rigorous empirical demonstration of clinical safety and product performance (Cortez et al., 2014). The US Department of Health and Human Services (HHS) and the Office of the National Coordinator for Health Information Technology are partnering in a three-part strategy to spur development of market-ready, user-friendly apps. Two prizes worth USD 350 000 plus additional funding of up to USD 275 000 were established. One prize is for a consumer app that aggregates patient data in one place that is under their control. The other is for an app that can improve providers' experience with electronic health records (EHRs) by making clinical workflows more intuitive and actionable. Importantly, the agencies will supply funding to support development of an open platform for developers to publish their apps, and for providers to discover and compare them (HHS, 2016).

In 2013, in response to concerns voiced by health professionals, the English National Health Service (NHS) launched a system for certifying and curating health apps as clinically safe, trustworthy and compliant with data protection laws. Approved products are listed on the NHS Health Apps Library. The process relies on developer self-certification. However, a recent review found systematic gaps in compliance with data protection principles (Huckvale et al., 2015). In 2014, the UK Medicines and Healthcare Products Regulatory Agency (MHRA) issued a general guidance document for developers of "standalone software" to comply with existing regulatory requirements (MHRA, 2014).

2. Coverage and funding of medical devices

Payers and policy makers need to balance often competing objectives: equitable access to health care; affordability and value; and fostering of medical innovation that helps achieve policy goals (getting the "right" kind of technology developed). Coverage and funding of medical devices – and the clinical procedures or interventions they enable – are important considerations in terms of these aims. They are among the factors that influence adoption and diffusion of products as well as their use in accordance with evidence and clinical guidelines (appropriateness). These are important determinants of therapeutic outcomes, and health benefits to patients and populations. Funding also influences expenditure growth, an important consideration given that adoption of medical technology is a key driver of incremental rises in health spending and costs (Chapter 2).

Determining coverage and funding for medical devices is challenging. As with regulation, payers grapple with the same peculiarities of medical devices as a branch of health technology (e.g. dependence on practitioner skill of the clinical utility of a device; virtual absence of evidence at market approval). More germane to funding is that virtually all medical devices are embedded in some kind of clinical activity. In contrast to drugs, where the medicine is the treatment, the utility of most medical devices is partly a function of how it is applied. Funding and reimbursing the use of medical devices must therefore also incorporate other, often variable, inputs such as labour, supplies and facility costs.

The entwining of technology, devices and practice means that any discussion of coverage and funding will inevitably seek to answer broader questions about health care financing and provider payment. Such a discussion is outside the scope of this document. This chapter does draw on health care financing approaches and models where necessary, using relevant examples to illustrate, but for more detailed description and exploration of provider payments, readers are referred to other literature (OECD, 2016). In practical terms, devices and their application need to be incorporated into the relevant financing instruments – among others, episode (such as diagnosis-related group, DRG) tariffs, fee-for-service (FFS), global budgets and bundled payments. This requires not only frequent updating of reimbursement schedules, but also collection of evidence on cost, utilisation and utility in clinical settings – information that can only be obtained once a device is in routine use.

Coverage and funding decisions differ according to the type of the device and its application. It is useful to distinguish between three types of devices in this regard:

- *Implantable devices* used in medical procedures (hip prosthesis, cardiac stent, pacemaker): coverage decisions are made for individual products or categories of generic products, at the level of each coverage scheme or at regional or national level. Funding for such devices can be included in the payment for the procedure or paid on top of the fee or tariffs for the procedure.
- Devices used to perform a *diagnostic or therapeutic* procedure (imaging scanner, dialyser, IVD): coverage and funding decisions most often relate to individual diagnostic or therapeutic procedures. The cost of using the device is included in the procedure's fee or in bundled payments (DRG tariffs, capitation, global budget, etc.).
- Devices for *individual use* acquired directly by patients[9] (glucose monitor, wheelchair): coverage decisions are made for individual products or categories of generic products at the level of each coverage scheme (insurer or plan) or at a regional or national level. When the device is covered, payers often define a reimbursement price. These devices generally fall into the low clinical risk category.

The following sections first examine coverage, where payers determine whether to include the product in their list or schedule of approved clinical activities that are reimbursed or funded. Then, HTA and *coverage with evidence development* models are discussed. Funding and reimbursement – decisions on how, and how much, to pay for a device and the intervention(s) it is used in – are considered next. The focus is on how to best integrate new technology within established financing and reimbursement mechanisms, and on determining the optimal reimbursement rate. This is followed by a short section on using coverage and funding to complement other incentives for appropriate use of health care resources. The focus throughout is mainly on high-risk implantable, diagnostic and therapeutic devices.

2.1. HTA often informs coverage decisions

Once initial market approval is granted, payers must decide on coverage. OECD countries are increasingly using HTA to make coverage decisions for all categories of health care products and services, especially for medicines (Auraaen et al., 2016). HTA is often, though not always, required for a medical device (or its intended use) to be covered by public payers. Depending on the type of medical device, HTA is used to inform coverage decisions relative to either the medical device itself (e.g. implantable devices) or to diagnostic and therapeutic procedures using this device (e.g. imaging or surgery). According to information collected through two surveys, two-thirds of OECD countries use HTA to make decisions on devices or interventions, systematically or "in some circumstances" (Table 4.2).

Table 4.2. **Countries using HTA to make coverage decisions or to set reimbursement level or price for new medical devices**

Type of technology	Use of HTA to make coverage decisions	Countries
Procedures	**Systematically**	Australia, Chile,[1] France, Hungary, Israel, Korea, Netherlands, Poland, Slovenia
	In some circumstances	Austria, Belgium, Canada, Denmark, Finland, Ireland, Italy, Japan, Luxembourg, Mexico, New Zealand, Norway, Spain, Sweden, Switzerland, United Kingdom
	Determine reimbursement level or price	Israel
Devices	**Systematically**	Australia, Belgium, Chile,[1] France, Hungary, Israel, Korea, Poland
	In some circumstances	Austria, Canada, Denmark, Estonia, Finland, Ireland, Italy, Japan, Luxembourg, Mexico, Netherlands, New Zealand, Norway, Spain, Sweden, Switzerland, United Kingdom, United States
	Determine reimbursement level or price	France, Israel

1. Only for products and services to be included in GES ("Garantías Explícitas en Salud"), i.e. covered by all health plans (public and private)).

Source: *2014 OECD Health Benefit Basket Questionnaire* and *2012 OECD Health Systems Characteristics Survey*.

Almost all OECD countries define, at a central level, the range of devices, products, services and interventions covered by government schemes or compulsory health insurance. While this definition can be explicit or implicit and based on positive or negative lists, some trends can be observed: countries with residence-based health coverage tend to define the range of medical services covered in very broad terms, while countries with contributory health insurance systems most often use positive lists to define the range of services covered at the central level, with some exceptions (Auraaen et al., 2016).

In principle, an implicit definition gives more choice to health care providers and patients and does not impose any "regulatory delay" in the adoption of new technologies.

An explicit definition of the benefit package, by contrast, implies the need for "listing decisions". This approach potentially allows a better allocation of resources towards more effective or more cost-effective health care interventions. But listing decisions can take time, potentially delaying adoption of a useful technology.

European jurisdictions, ideally though not always, assess the therapeutic benefit of new medical devices to inform coverage decisions. In some, such as England and the Netherlands, cost-effectiveness against a pre-determined value for money threshold is also assessed, at least in some circumstances (Sorenson et al., 2013). In the United Kingdom, NICE assesses the cost-effectiveness of medical devices with high budget impact to guide their use in the NHS, and evaluations are often conducted after market entry, using information on observed costs. In the United States, coverage determinations by the principal public payer (the Centers for Medicare & Medicaid Services, CMS) are based on therapeutic benefit but do not explicitly require or consider evidence of cost-effectiveness (Chambers et al., 2010). Generally, private insurers in the United States use the same approach, but some are beginning to consider cost-effectiveness in their coverage and pricing decisions (Sorenson et al., 2013).

Medical devices for individual use follow various assessment, coverage and funding pathways depending on country and clinical setting. In Germany, for instance, rules differ for outpatient and inpatient settings. In outpatient care, new medical (or dental) procedures are not included in the catalogue of covered services unless the G-BA (joint association of physicians, dentists, hospitals, patients and statutory health insurance funds) assessed that there is evidence of a clinical benefit for patients. In inpatient settings, by contrast, new procedures are funded unless they have been explicitly banned by the G-BA. The G-BA began considering evidence for controversial services in 2000 and by 2013 only 15 services had been excluded from reimbursement (Olberg et al., 2014). Several stakeholders can initiate a G-BA assessment: federal and regional associations of physicians, the federal association of social health insurance funds, and patients.

In France, manufacturers of new devices must file an application to a specific committee of the national HTA agency if they want their device to be included in the positive list of reimbursed devices. This committee assesses the clinical benefit of the product to issue a recommendation on coverage, as well as the added clinical benefit (five levels, from I, major improvement, to V, no improvement) to inform price negotiations between the manufacturer and the Economic Committee of Medical Products (HAS, 2009).

HTA and coverage decisions often take time and delay patient access to new technologies. Some countries and non-government organisations are exploring ways to shorten this review time. In the United States, for instance, the FDA and CMS implemented a pilot programme in 2011 for "parallel review" of medical devices – where regulatory reviews and coverage determination are conducted simultaneously – to expedite the regulatory and coverage and funding processes (FDA, 2011). To date, only one product has completed the process and shortening the overall review resulted in a preliminary coverage determination that coincided with FDA approval (Ridge and Statz, 2015). In 2015, the FDA and CMS extended their Memorandum of Understanding for information-sharing indefinitely (FDA, 2015a). In 2016, the FDA took the further step of creating a Payer Communication Task Force to invite private payer and HTA entity input on ways to shorten time from FDA clearance to payer coverage (FDA, 2016a). Similarly, Canada is actively exploring the alignment of regulatory and HTA pathways (Box 4.2).

Box 4.2. **MaRS EXCITE Program**

The Medical and Related Sciences (MaRS) Excellence in Clinical Innovation Technology Evaluation (EXCITE) program is a Canadian initiative aimed at helping health technology innovators test their products and generate the required evidence to bring these to market, and to demonstrate the value of the technology. The goal is to generate an "EXCITE Evidentiary Bundle" comprising: 1) a clinical trial or field evaluation, 2) a systematic review of relevant research, and 3) an economic analysis. In addition, the programme offers an analysis of barriers to uptake, patient preferences, usability and human factors, training programmes and longitudinal registry studies.

MaRS EXCITE is part of the MaRS Health portfolio, which supports manufacturers and companies that develop products spanning the full spectrum of health technologies, from health monitoring and disease treatment to information storage and sharing. The programme is based on connecting innovators with experienced and successful researchers to obtain the right evidence and facilitate discussions with relevant stakeholders in the health care system.

Source: www.marsdd.com (consulted on 10 October 2016).

Some health care systems use coverage with evidence development

Regulatory requirements for medical devices and the peculiarities of this type of medical technology sometimes result in limited evidence of clinical performance and utility being available to decision makers at market entry. As with regulation, a lack of sound evidence at market entry presents a challenge for coverage and funding decisions. This can mean coverage of products or procedures that do not represent an improvement on existing practice, at additional cost to payers and to society. Equally, it may result in access to potentially beneficial technologies being denied or delayed.

To respond to the evidence gap, several countries implemented measures to cover promising new technologies that have not yet proven their clinical benefits, under the condition of generating further evidence. Such systems exist in Australia, France (since 2010), Germany (since 2012), the Netherlands (2012), Switzerland (since 1996), the United Kingdom and the United States. In the Netherlands and the United Kingdom, coverage with evidence development (CED) can also be motivated by uncertainty in cost-effectiveness. In most cases only a minority of devices are processed under CED schemes. Except in Germany, where clinical trials are preferred, countries adapt study designs to the context with the aim to obtain the highest level of evidence, through clinical trials or real-life data. CED is primarily applied in publicly funded systems (Olberg et al., 2014), and fits well into the cyclical approach of periodic review illustrated in Figure 4.1. Four examples of CED schemes are provided in Box 4.3.

Countries starting to apply CED schemes are using the approach incrementally and cautiously. Overall, according to the available literature only a small number of devices have been processed using the CED approach so far. The products assessed have a limited amount of pre-market evidence, but show promising characteristics and potential to generate benefit and/or address unmet need. This could be said of most truly innovative new technologies with few or no antecedents. During the CED process, use of the product is generally funded by the payer, while the costs of evidence collection are usually borne by the manufacturer. With the exception of Switzerland, not much information is available yet on the outcomes of

Box 4.3. Examples of Coverage with Evidence Development schemes in OECD countries

The Medicare programme in the **United States** implemented several national coverage determinations (NCDs) with CED conditions in 1995, specifically for certain items in FDA-approved clinical trials. Coverage was restricted to beneficiaries participating in trials for certain devices in 2005, such as cochlear implantation and diagnostic positron emission tomography (PET) scans. The first instance of using evidence from CED to inform a revised coverage determination for a medical device came in 2008, with the reconsideration of PET for diagnosis, staging and restaging of cancer patients. Data from the National Oncologic PET Registry were used. CMS also took on the subject of precision medicine and IVDs in its ongoing CED for pharmacogenomic testing for warfarin response (CMS, 2009). At the time of writing, CMS had 22 active NCDs requiring some form of evidence development, 16 of which pertain to medical devices while the remainder consider medicines and procedures.

In **Switzerland**, CED has been used for medical devices and other non-pharmaceutical technologies since 1996. All coverage decisions were classified as "yes", "no", "yes, in evaluation" (denoting CED status) or "no, in evaluation". The latter meant that the intervention could be provided but not reimbursed by health insurance. The intention behind this rule was that providers would engage in producing and delivering better evidence. In 2004, the "no, in evaluation" category was abandoned, since this label had no practical meaning. A total of 152 "contested medical services" were evaluated by Swiss authorities between 1996 and 2012. A contested designation is applied to devices, procedures and medical services for which reasonable doubt of effectiveness or cost-effectiveness exists, and can be brought forward by "anyone with a legitimate interest, for example, a health insurance provider" (Brugger et al., 2015, p. 2). Of the 152, 46 were assigned CED status. By 2013, a decision was made for 37 of the 46 CED products, of which 22 (60%) were granted reimbursement. A "no, in evaluation" status was assigned to 36 products before 2004, of which 35 had been decided upon by 2013. Reimbursement was granted for 15 (42.9%) of these products. While the introduction of CED in Switzerland enabled access to promising technologies early in their lifecycle, and might have triggered the establishment of registries and research, the impact on patients' outcome and costs is unknown (Brugger et al., 2015).

In **France**, the CED scheme for medical devices was first introduced in 2010 and amended in 2015. It provides coverage of innovative medical devices likely to provide significant benefits to patients pending final assessment. Four criteria must be met for a new device to be considered innovative: 1) the medical device must be novel and not simply an updated version of an existing product used for the same indications; 2) the medical device must only recently have become available on the market and not have been previously reimbursed by the French national health insurance scheme for the indications concerned; 3) the available clinical data for the product must have clearly established the potential risks for patients and users; and 4) the available clinical and/or economic data must have shown that the product is likely to a) provide significant clinical benefit for an unmet or insufficiently covered medical need, or b) decrease health care expenditure due to its cost-effectiveness, although only if the device is at least as effective as the standard treatment without being "similar" (Martelli et al., 2016). Manufacturers apply simultaneously to the Ministry of Health and to the committee in charge of assessing medical devices with a study plan to assess clinical benefit or spending reductions. The final decision must be issued within 120 days. If the CED scheme is accepted, the Ministry of Health determines the amount allocated per patient to cover the use of the medical device ("*forfait innovation*") and related hospitalisation costs where relevant, the duration of CED, the list of health care settings involved and the number of patients to include for the collection of evidence. The company only pays for the costs of generating evidence.

Box 4.3. **Examples of Coverage with Evidence Development schemes in OECD countries** *(cont.)*

In **Germany**, a 2012 reform allowed prospectively testing innovative diagnostic and therapeutic methods (with or without use of a medical device) pending a final decision on coverage. This CED scheme applies to new methods that have the potential to be a viable alternative to the current standard. This "potential" is assessed against the mechanism of action of the new technology and the evidence available. The new method should be potentially more effective, less complicated, less invasive, or less harmful. It could optimise the current treatment or improve it. Companies can apply for such an assessment, as can other stakeholders. If the G-BA considers that the technology has potential to replace the current standard, it issues recommendations for development of further evidence and commissions an independent evaluator. The timeframe is not predefined and may vary across technologies. At the end of the evaluation period, the G-BA assesses the evidence generated and makes a decision about social health insurance coverage. The G-BA final assessment has three potential outcomes: 1) confirmation of patient-relevant benefit; 2) exclusion because of lack of evidence of benefit (i.e. the new technology provides less benefit than standard treatment) or evidence of harm; and 3) suspension of assessment because of lack of evidence, which can lead again to CED. This new CED scheme encourages quicker adoption of innovative technologies since health insurance funds pay for the treatment during the evidence development phase. In outpatient settings, this allows quicker access to innovation while in inpatient settings (where immediate access was the general rule), it improves the level of evidence required to remain funded. In addition, if CED shows that the new technology must be delisted, this is valid for both the outpatient and inpatient sectors (Olberg et al., 2014). Since 2014, several CED assessments have been initiated.

the CED processes – in terms of favourable versus negative decisions – as applied to devices. Solid evidence of the utility of this approach is still emerging.

CED provides a suitable compromise for payers, especially for high-cost and high-risk products, and enables coverage and funding to be approached as a cycle and not an "all-or-nothing" decision (Figure 4.1). This represents a more rational and evidence-based approach. It could also benefit manufacturers of the most innovative products, who often bear the highest levels of risk and the highest costs to produce clinical evidence, at the cost of a reduced market exclusivity period. CED signals to manufacturers that an initial coverage decision is only the beginning of an ongoing process. A product's effectiveness and performance will also be evaluated after it enters routine use and generates revenue for the manufacturer. This would particularly benefit less capitalised SMEs. However, restrictions and careful monitoring must be applied diligently, and patients must be informed of the conditional nature of the product's use.

With the ongoing development of information infrastructure enabled by modern ICT, the type of post-market evidence that can be collected can be expanded and its quality improved. Future CED schemes will be able to draw on Patient-Reported Outcome Measures (PROMs) and other types of patient-generated evidence to assess the real-world effectiveness and utility of interventions. EHRs that enable patients to contribute their own information in a more routine and longitudinal fashion, and that link to other sources such as registries, claims and administrative data, are being implemented. The information generated by these systems will benefit the regulation, coverage and funding of health technology, and make CED based on cyclical review much more reliable and practicable.

Revising coverage decisions downwards is always politically difficult

Many countries face difficulties revising coverage decisions, either to place restrictions on the use of a device or to remove it from reimbursement schedules – a process called delisting or disinvestment (Auraaen et al., 2016). Amendment or reversal of decisions may be necessary due to: 1) new evidence exposing safety problems, a lack of clinical utility or cost-effectiveness of the device or procedure; 2) a new innovation that renders existing technology obsolete or comparatively less cost-effective, no longer justifying its coverage; or (3) a combination of the two. In any case, cyclical review of decisions based on transparent and explicit criteria and informed by CED can enable payers to amend or reverse coverage decisions, and lead to more productive use of resources (recall Figure 4.1). However, payers must consider the resource implications and opportunity costs to effectively design and/or approve evidence collection requirements that will meet future policy needs, as well as the resources to actually review and amend coverage.

2.2. Funding mechanisms are crucial to encourage appropriate use of medical devices

Following the coverage decision payers have to decide how, and how much, to pay for the application and use of medical devices in clinical practice. Funding and reimbursement is challenging and depends on a range of variables: the nature of the device and its intended use (e.g. devices with specific versus broad indication, single- versus re-usable products); the range of diagnoses and conditions it is used for; necessary inputs such as labour; health care setting and operational context; and the overarching health care financing mechanism within which the intervention(s) using the device needs to be incorporated (prospective payment, FFS, global budgets and bundled payment tariffs for cycles of care). Approaches differ, manifesting in considerable variation between countries in prices paid for clinical activity – especially for technology-laden interventions.

Devices are subject to varying financing mechanisms and funding

Medical devices are embedded in virtually all clinical activity and not always reimbursed in isolation, except for medical devices acquired by patients. Rather, the "price" is often incorporated within the reimbursement, payment or tariff of the clinical activity for which the device is used. Reimbursement also includes a range of other inputs: labour, supplies, facility expenses and so on. The funding and reimbursement of devices is therefore inextricably linked to financing mechanisms for the clinical services and activities (diagnostic or therapeutic interventions) enabled by the product.

Funding and reimbursement approaches for devices used in diagnostic or therapeutic interventions differ across the OECD. Funding of devices also varies depending on setting and sector. For example, providers of ambulatory care or clinical laboratories can be paid through capitation, FFS or global budget, while hospitals are most often paid through DRG-type payments or global budget. Table 4.3 summarises the various potential situations based on the three types of devices.

Different funding models exist for devices acquired directly by patients. The United States Medicare programme was mandated by the Medicare Prescription Drug, Improvement, and Modernization Act of 2003 (MMA) to replace the previous fee schedule payment methodology for selected Durable Medical Equipment, Prosthetics, Orthotics and Supplies (DMEPOS) items with a competitive bid process to select vendors and set pricing. The intent was to improve the effectiveness of the Medicare methodology for setting

Table 4.3. **Paying for medical devices covered in health care systems**

	Implantable devices used in medical procedures	Devices used to perform diagnostic or therapeutic procedures	Devices for individual use acquired directly by patients
Funding and reimbursement	The cost of the device can be included in providers' fee, DRG tariff or global budget. The cost may also be paid on top of the fee or tariff (e.g. privately insured in Australia and the United States) as an additional payment (see below).	The cost of the device is generally included in providers' fee, DRG tariff or global budget. Costs of using the device are reflected differently in fees or tariffs depending on the nature of the device (single use vs. multi-use devices).	Reimbursement mechanism and rate set by regulators or payers.
Purchasing	The purchase price of the device for the individual provider results from the procurement process (call for tender or negotiation between the provider and the manufacturer of the device), with some exceptions (see below).	The purchase price of the device for the individual provider results from the procurement process (call for tender or negotiation between the provider and the manufacturer of the device), with some exceptions.	In some countries, the actual price may be higher than the reimbursement ceiling (e.g. France), resulting in a co-payment by the user.

DMEPOS payment amounts, thereby reducing beneficiary out-of-pocket expenses and saving the Medicare programme money while ensuring beneficiary access. However, some have criticised the rate-setting methodology, which sets prices based on the median of all winning bids for an item, as potentially not achieving this objective.

Each financing mechanism bears incentives likely to play a role in the adoption of the technology, and therefore its diffusion.[10] While global budget and capitation provide incentives to reduce costs, FFS and DRG payments provide incentives to reduce the costs per procedure or per admission but also incentives to increase volumes of care. Most financing mechanisms where technology is embedded in a payment to cover an episode or a cycle of care, to a greater or lesser extent, encourage adoption of cost-reducing new technologies but can potentially hinder adoption of new technologies that increase costs.

The hospital sector serves as a useful example. Here, financial incentives for adoption of new technologies depend on: the number of DRG groups (more granularity is likely to better take into account the costs of new technologies where appropriate) as well as the number of complexity levels within DRGs; the frequency of DRG tariff updates (more frequent updates are likely to encourage appropriate use of technologies); and the time lag to cost data[11] (a greater time lag fails to incorporate the use of very new technologies in tariffs). The number of DRG groups varies from about 500 to 2 500 in OECD countries using DRG payments. Although most OECD countries update DRG tariffs annually, the time lag to reference cost data is often two years or more (Table 4.4).

In the longer term, adjustments of DRG classification and/or tariffs are used to incorporate the costs of new technologies in hospital payments. This can be done by splitting existing DRG groups (into separate cases where the new technologies are used), creating new DRG groups and/or adjusting tariffs to include the costs of using a new technology (Quentin et al., 2011).

Additional payments may be needed to encourage adoption of beneficial but costly technology

To allow diffusion of costly but beneficial new technologies, many countries introduced short-term measures (Quentin et al., 2011; Hernandez et al., 2015). These provide financial incentives to adopt these technologies through separate payments for use of the product on top of existing tariffs (or global budgets) before the relevant reimbursement item is adjusted appropriately or created. These mechanisms can take two forms: 1) reimbursement based on the cost of using a specific technology; or 2) earmarked funding to allow providers to acquire or use the new technology. Such systems exist for instance in France, Germany, Japan, the

Table 4.4. **Frequency of updates, time lags and number of groupings for hospital care payment systems in selected countries**

	Classification	Number of groups	Frequency of update of payment rates	Time-lag to cost data
Australia	AR-DRG Classification (Version 8.0)	807	Every 1-2 years	2-4 years
Austria	Katalog medizinischer Einzelleistungen/ MEL for procedures	1 004	Smaller updates every year, complete revision every 7 years	
Belgium	APR-DRG			
Chile	Valued benefit programme	not applicable	Annually	
Czech Republic	Adjusted IR DRG	1 046	Annually	
Denmark	DKDRG 2012	717	Annually	
Finland	NordDRG	500 inpatient, ~900 including out-patients	Annually	0-1 year
France	GHM	~2 500	Annually	2 years
Germany	DRG 2016	~1 220	Annually	2-3 years
Greece	ICD-10	26 main groups with subcategories	Since October 2011: one price revision	
Hungary	HBCs (HCFA-DRG)	728	Continually	
Italy	DRG 24 v	538	3 years	
Japan	ICD-10	2 012 (as of 07/2012)	2 years	
Netherlands	DBC	~700	Irregularly, but often	2 years or based on negotiations
Norway	NordDRG	870	Annually	
Poland	ICD-10 and ICD 9CM.	526	Annually	1 year
Portugal	AP-DRG v21	669	Irregular	2-3 years
Slovenia	ICD-10-AM (AR-DRG V 4.2)	653	Minor modifications can be introduced through the annual contract between payer and provider	
Sweden	NordDRG	983 (in and outpatient, day cases)	Annually	2 years
Switzerland	SwissDRG 1.0	1 052	Annually	3 years
United Kingdom (England)	HRG v4	~1 200	Annually	3 years (but adjusted for inflation)
United States	MSDRGs	~2 400	Annually	2 years

Source: *OECD Health Characteristics Survey 2012*, and Quentin, W., D. Scheller-Kreinsen and R. Busse (2011), "Technological Innovation in DRG-based Hospital Payment Systems Across Europe", in R. Busse, A. Geissler, W. Quentin and M. Wiley (eds.), *Diagnosis-Related Groups in Europe – Moving Towards Transparency, Efficiency and Quality in Hospitals*, European Observatory on Health Systems and Policies.

Netherlands, the United Kingdom and the United States (Table 4.5). Their objectives and scopes differ, as reflected by the number of technologies approved for supplementary funding: the US Medicare programme seems to be more restrictive, while the French system seems the most open.

Additional payments need to consider the potential for incentives to overuse costly technology paid on top of DRG tariffs, where an older, cheaper and equally effective technology could be used. They should be applied prudently and limited to products and interventions for which sufficient evidence exists of superior cost-effectiveness (and value) compared to alternatives.

Funding and reimbursement considerations are critical to appropriate use of medical devices

A particularly challenging aspect of funding of medical devices is setting the right price or tariff for its use within reimbursement for the relevant clinical interventions. This is difficult given the vast array of devices, many of which can be applied in a range of interventions with varying degrees of therapeutic benefit. Devices are often, with time,

Table 4.5. **Examples of additional payments for new technologies**

Country/mechanism	Add-on payments for new technologies
France "Liste en sus"	Aims: Paying for high-cost implantable medical devices, and since December 2015, for high-cost devices used in invasive procedures, which are new or used to treat rare diseases on top of DRG tariffs, pending their inclusion in DRG tariffs. Conditions: These payments are only available for implantable devices included in the national List of Reimbursable Products and Services Payment. Applications for funding are submitted by companies. Payment: A reimbursement price is set by the Economic Committee of Health Products. It involves direct negotiations with the manufacturer that may define payment levels and use. Health insurance covers 100% of the reimbursement price. The hospital signs a contract of "appropriate use" and the reimbursement rate can be reduced up to 30% if the hospital does not comply with this contract. Duration: Up to five years, with possible renewal. Since 2005, more than 3 000 devices have been included in the "Liste en sus".
Germany Supplementary funding for new diagnostic and therapeutic methods (NUB) – inpatient setting only	Aims: Bridge the time lag between adoption of technology and update of DRG payment, and generate data during this interim period to identify the appropriate payment for the technologies in the regular system. Applications are submitted by hospitals. Conditions: The technology must be truly new, which implicitly takes into account the clinical improvements associated with the technology, and involves costs that are inadequately paid under the existing DRG system. The institute in charge of application has discretion to decide whether these criteria are met. Payments are negotiated between hospitals and regional authorities. Duration: One year, renewable until integration in the DRG tariff. The technology might remain paid on top of DRG-tariff, based on national fees or payments negotiated between hospitals and insurers. Since 2005, 234 technologies have been approved for supplementary funding.
Japan Supplemental payment	Conditions: Used for new device technologies used as part of an existing procedure but shown to be a significant improvement (C1 category) or new device technologies resulting in a completely new procedure or therapy (C2 category). Payment: Additional payments can cover the whole procedure or the procedure and the medical device separately. Their amount is set by the Social Health Insurance Medical Council. Since 2002, 265 new technologies have been approved for supplementary funding.
United States (Medicare) New technology add-on payment programme (inpatient hospital)	Aim: Bridge the time lag between adoption of technology and update of DRG payment. Applications for funding are submitted by companies. Condition: Technology is truly novel and represents a "substantial clinical improvement"; the incremental cost of a new technology exceeds the lesser of 75% of the standard MS-DRG payment amount and 75% of one standard deviation above the charge for the MS-DRG or DRGs to which the technology is assigned. Payment: Set at the lesser of 50% of the estimated difference between the hospital's estimated costs and the DRG payment amount and 50% of the new technology cost. Duration: Three years after technology approval and commercialisation. Since 2001, 19 technologies have been approved for add-on payments.
United States (Medicare) Pass-through payment programme (outpatient hospital)	Same aim, conditions and qualitative criteria as add-on payments but for the outpatient setting; thresholds for newness and substantial clinical improvement vary. Payment: Set at 100% of reported cost of the device minus the cost already built into the base reimbursement rate. Duration: Until data reflecting costs can be used to recalibrate appropriate Ambulatory Payment Classification weights (usually 2-3 years following approval).

Source: Hernandez, J., S.F. Machacz and J.C. Robinson (2015), "US Hospital Payment Adjustments for Innovative Technology Lag Behind Those in Germany, France, and Japan", *Health Affairs*, Vol. 34, No. 2, pp. 261-270; Sorenson, C., M. Drummond and L. Burns (2013), "Evolving Reimbursement and Pricing Policies for Devices in Europe and the United States Should Encourage Greater Value", *Health Affairs (Millwood)*, Vol. 32, No. 4, pp. 788-796; ministère de la Santé et des Sports (2009), "Règles de facturation des soins dispensés dans les établissements de santé – Dispositifs médicaux", MSS, *http://social-sante.gouv.fr/IMG/pdf/dispositifs_medicaux-2.pdf* (accessed 13 February 2016); and *www.atih.sante.fr/*.

used in a growing range of indications and diagnoses. Some devices are for single use, while others can be used repeatedly. These factors need to be considered in determining reimbursement levels and prices, which should be based on evidence of clinical utility sourced from clinical trials and subsequently based on RWE.

Prices paid for medical devices and associated procedure should vary over time to reflect changes in productivity or relative utility

Pricing of devices and associated interventions and procedures differs internationally and is partly a function of contextual factors, most importantly financing mechanisms.

Nevertheless, noteworthy variation arises in the prices and reimbursement levels for technology-laden services and interventions, even within the same country (BHI, 2015; OECD, 2010). For example, using US claims data, Cooper et al. (2016) found that prices paid for knee replacement varied four-fold within the same city, while MRI (magnetic resonance imaging) prices varied by a factor of 12 across the country. Prices may reflect quality, case mix and overheads (e.g. remoteness) but it is difficult to conceive that the outcomes of a cataract procedure, hip replacement or MRI scan are several orders of magnitude better in some jurisdictions compared to others. As mentioned previously, prices include other inputs. For example, diagnostic devices (e.g. endoscopes) can be applied by technicians and nurse specialists, whose input labour costs are lower than those of physicians, and can be reflected in lower tariffs or prices for usage of the device. This may affect quality, but without better data on outcomes it is impossible to quantify to what extent.

Prices do not necessarily reflect quality, value for patients or a rational approach to resource allocation. In a normal market, a price is a function of supply, demand, willingness/ability to pay and information. In the regulated health care market, a price – particularly in a high-cost and risk category – reflects what payers are prepared to pay, and what manufacturers of the product, and providers applying it in the clinical setting, are prepared to accept. The figure arrived at is informed by the available evidence but is also highly dependent on institutional and legislative settings, and how these distribute power and leverage in the reimbursement rate-setting process. As all health expenditure is somebody's income, this can be a dissonant mix of public health objectives and powerful interests. This manifests in several ways. As mentioned previously, one of these is the difficulty payers face in delisting outdated interventions with poor cost-utility (Auraaen et al., 2016).

Attempts to refine outdated billing or reimbursement methods can be met with similar resistance. In the United States, IVDs were traditionally reimbursed via a "code stacking" process that detailed each step in the test process (e.g. DNA extraction, amplification and detection). This process provided limited information regarding which test was being performed. In 2011 the American Medical Association introduced new molecular pathology ("MolPath") billing codes, allowing billing – and therefore improved capability for adjudication and data collection – for the entire process of testing for a specific biomarker. The implementation process for payment of these new codes under Medicare caused some confusion, as coverage and payment decisions were made at the regional level based on submitted charges, the cost of resources required to run the test, and payment rates established by other payers. While arguably resulting in more accurate billing, in the short term it often resulted in lower reimbursement rates for particular tests, in addition to short-term confusion regarding coverage and payment status for individual laboratories. Some stakeholders raised the concern that reimbursement may continue to be a challenge for laboratories implementing new technologies such as Next Generation Sequencing (NGS) (discussed in Chapter 5 on precision medicine).

Paying the right price also means that prices should be flexible over time. In ordinary markets, prices adjust in response to more information, users' accumulated experience and the appearance of superior products. A similar flexibility should be exercised by payers through cyclical review of reimbursement based on accumulated evidence of utility and costs gathered through CED schemes or other data collection. The critical importance of collecting evidence of clinical outcomes as experienced by consumers (patients) – the closest approximation to market information – should be quite obvious here. But data are not enough; other enabling institutional requirements are important. Payers also need to be empowered to base decisions on the evidence through appropriate legislation, sound information infrastructure, adequate resourcing, independence and public communications, as discussed in the next section.

In many health care systems, considerable discretion is given to clinicians over what product to choose. Because prices vary considerably between similar items (e.g. hip prostheses), these clinical decisions can strongly influence costs and expenditure. In a system like the United States, which spends over USD 150 billion on medical devices annually (Donahoe and King, 2012), this can amount to a lot of money and resources. In situations where there is little difference in the effectiveness or utility of the product, an expensive choice will undermine value. Yet evidence from the United States suggests that orthopaedic surgeons rarely know the cost of the devices they implant, despite the majority believing that cost should be an important part of the device selection process (Okike et al., 2014). Better information must be provided to clinicians to improve value in systems where clinicians can choose among a range of products.

Developers often respond to pricing adjustments in a positive way, and examples exist where pricing and reimbursement can drive, and determine the direction of, future innovation. Medicare's downward adjustment of reimbursement for dialysis in the 1970s, for instance, prompted innovation by device manufacturers to make dialysis machines more efficient and less reliant on human operation. This resulted in the dialysis machines used today. Had it not been for the change in price, dialysis might still be cumbersome, time-consuming and expensive (Gelijins and Rosenberg, 1994). Systematic empirical evidence of reimbursement driving innovation type and direction for health technologies (including drugs) is more difficult to pin down, however (Bruen et al., 2016).

Different therapeutic indications may require different levels of funding

While some devices are designed for specific and well-defined uses (e.g. a prosthetic hip), many are designed for use across a range of activities. The clinical utility of these "broad-spectrum" devices is determined for each specific indication by the diagnosis, patient characteristics and therapeutic context as much as by the device itself. Diagnostic equipment such as MRI scanners or endoscopes contributes vital information, which is of considerably higher clinical value in certain conditions and (suspected) diagnoses. In other clinical circumstances their use is of little value and may even be clinically inappropriate. Currently, reimbursement is predominantly based on inputs and resources used as opposed to the benefits derived from that particular use of the device. For example, abdominal or brain imaging is reimbursed at different levels than spinal imaging, reflecting the different inputs such as expertise and time. However, little differentiation exists below these categories. For instance, the price paid for imaging of the lower spine does not factor the degree of appropriateness – for example, how long symptoms have persisted, or the likelihood of serious pathology versus a self-limiting, acute complaint.[12]

With time, innovative providers may apply technology with well-defined criteria for use to alternative indications and to an expanding patient population. This can either be through progressively expanded use or through reinvention. The latter concerns alternative uses for a technology that may (or may not) generate new, previously undiscovered benefits in new patient types. For instance, the endoscope has steadily expanded into new disciplines and indications since the device was introduced, with variable therapeutic benefit (Gelijins and Rosenberg, 1994). Expanded use refers to using a technology on a growing patient population with the same illness (usually of progressively less severity). It was discussed in Chapter 2 as a principal factor in diminishing incremental value generated by health technology (Chandra and Skinner, 2012; Shih and Berliner, 2008). For instance, the use of cardiac stents expanded to patients with a less clearly defined presentation as cardiac specialists became more accustomed to inserting them (Shih and Berliner, 2008). But less therapeutic benefit is derived by coronary stenting of patients with stable cardiac disease compared to conservative management (Sedlis et al., 2015). Due to the high cost of the procedure, its value in "new" patients is considerably lower than the alternative low-tech intervention and its use in the narrower patient cohort. Thus depending on the device and its application (and often the practitioner), the clinical benefit in the expanded patient cohort can be enhanced or diminished, as can its cost-utility.

Accurately determining the utility of all applications of a technology, including new ones, is further reason for ongoing collection of post-market RWE – ideally including outcomes as reported by patients – and periodic review of coverage and funding. This is illustrated in Figure 4.2. Not all applications of a multipurpose product should be reimbursed at the same level for all clinical presentations. Reimbursement should reflect the value that the use of the device adds to the episode of care. This can involve creation of several reimbursement categories, and exclusions for products under certain clinical circumstances. It needs to be periodically reviewed in light of new evidence.

Figure 4.2. **Technology diffusion and reinvention in the US context**

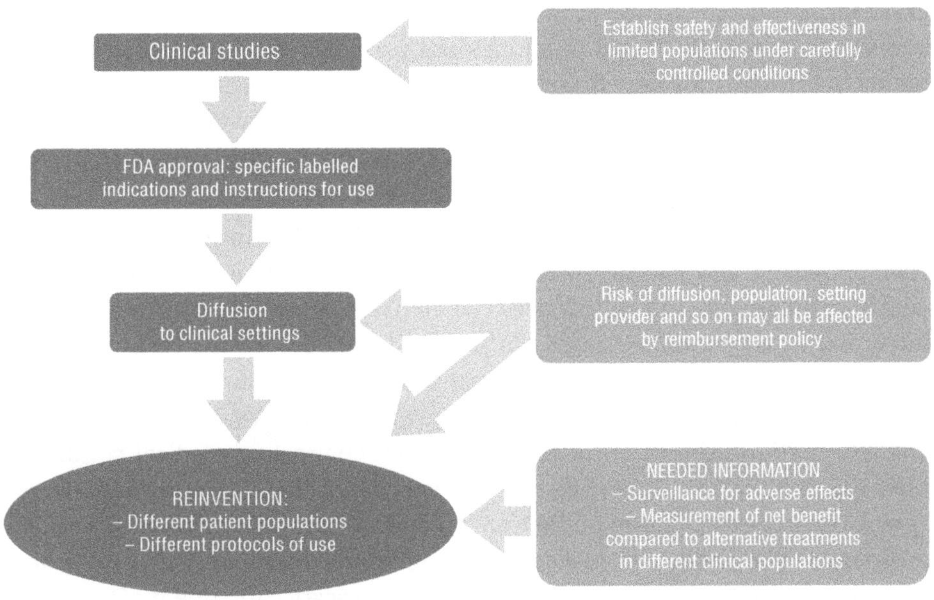

Source: Adapted from Shih, C. and E. Berliner (2008), "Diffusion of New Technology and Payment Policies: Coronary Stents", *Health Affairs (Millwood)*, Vol. 27, No. 6, pp. 1566-1576.

Health care systems are moving towards value- and outcomes-based reimbursement

Value- or outcomes-based reimbursement is becoming an increasingly attractive option for health care payers and is being experimented under various forms. One approach sets different reimbursement rates based on levels of clinical utility. It can also entail differential co-payments by patients and users to nudge behaviour – higher for low-value care and vice versa (Sorenson et al., 2013).

A related approach is to link reimbursement to clinical and patient outcomes, or to base it on appropriate use of a technology. This approach shifts the focus towards value and away from volume. A reimbursement level still needs to be set, and complementary mechanisms such as additional or pass-through payments may still be required to incentivise use of high-value but costly technology.

Health care systems are already implementing innovative payment approaches. As part of its best practice tariffs programme to financially incentivise quality care, England's NHS recently introduced a bonus payment for joint replacement procedures that is based on the results of PROMs as well as submission of data to the relevant registry (NHS England, 2015).

Value-based purchasing (VBP), a component of the Affordable Care Act, is being implemented by CMS in the United States for acute care reimbursement. The initiative rewards acute-care hospitals with incentive payments for the quality of care they provide to Medicare beneficiaries compared to other providers. Financial rewards are based on a composite score comprising: 1) the safety of care provided to Medicare patients (based on a set of measures and indicators including outcomes such as re-admission or nosocomial infection); 2) how closely best clinical practices are followed (e.g. fibrinolytic therapy initiated within 30 minutes of arrival following a heart attack); and 3) how well hospitals enhance patients' experiences of care during hospital stays (results of patient experience surveys). Currently and for the foreseeable future, 2% of hospital revenue is redistributed based on the performance scores (CMS, 2015a). A companion outcomes-based scheme, the Hospital Readmissions Reduction Program, places 3% of a hospital's revenue at risk based on actual versus expected 30-day re-admissions for heart failure, myocardial infarction and pneumonia in Medicare beneficiaries. Current evidence suggests that this programme is starting to have the desired effect (Zuckerman et al., 2016). However, payments for acute care remain principally based on volumes of care and inputs. The proportion of payments linked to outcomes in these schemes is comparatively small.

Value-based reimbursement is complex and challenging to implement. It is highly dependent on reliable and routine outcome data, which are still in their relative infancy for the majority of illnesses and procedures. To envision a model where remuneration is completely based on outcomes seems far-fetched, at least at this stage. However, the feasibility of combining it with current, inputs-based remuneration models will no doubt grow with improved instruments and techniques to collect and analyse these data, a maturing information infrastructure, and concurrent changes in medical culture towards alternative payment models. Collecting post-market evidence and approaching coverage and funding as an ongoing cycle based on RWE are critical as these will enhance payers' ability to make progressively superior and more nuanced reimbursement decisions. New analytical and research techniques to use these data are also a necessary component of these schemes.

Value-based funding engenders a more nuanced approach to reimbursement and price-setting than is currently practised in most jurisdictions. Approaches should be more rational and outcomes-based, and complement other levers to incentivise appropriate care and reduce the unnecessary use of products in clinical circumstances of low utility.

Promoting the appropriate use of devices is critical

The diffusion and use of new technology depends on a complex mix of factors. As discussed in Chapter 2, while supply-side levers such as coverage and funding are important drivers in their own right, they interact with various others including clinical culture, organisational factors and uptake by thought leaders, as well as the type of technology itself and its specific application (Burke et al., 2007; Capellaro et al., 2011; Shih and Berliner, 2008). Nevertheless, coverage and funding can provide useful leverage to complement clinical guidelines, standards and protocols of care to incentivise appropriate, high-value care and to discourage inappropriate application of expensive technology. As described above, this may entail payments triggered only in the presence of a certain diagnosis or procedure, an intervention remunerated only after an alternative has been tried, or a prohibition to use a technology associated with a diagnosis for which little evidence of benefit exists. In addition, payment may be stratified and conditional on the seniority or experience of the clinician applying it.

The National Institute for Health and Care Excellence's (NICE) 2003 and 2008 guidance on coverage and funding of bare metal stents (BMS) versus drug-eluting stents (DES) is a good example of evidence-based, rational decision making that can promote appropriate use. These products are used in percutaneous coronary interventions to treat coronary artery occlusions. Analysis of clinical evidence suggested that the more expensive DES was more effective and cost-effective only in patients presenting with small-calibre arteries and with lesions longer than 15 mm. For these patients, the cost per quality-adjusted life year (QALY) of using DES was under GBP 20 000, whereas for the general patient population with coronary occlusions it was GBP 94 000. NICE made its recommendation to payers accordingly: that DES be covered in the patient subgroup with the specific presentation described above, *but* only up to a price differential of GBP 300 when compared to BMS (NICE, 2008). That said, DES have largely displaced BMS in percutaneous coronary interventions using stents. The UK national audit of PCI shows that 70-90% (depending on the UK constituent country) of PCIs with stenting used DES, and that use of DES has increased over time (Ludman et al., 2014).

2.3. Coverage and funding of mHealth is an emerging challenge

The regulatory challenges of mHealth were discussed above. Coverage and funding is, at this stage, perhaps more relevant for portable devices than apps, given the higher cost of the former. This may change, however, as apps become more complex and more integrated with other technologies and services. Decision-making processes should align with those of regular medical devices. Once the threshold question of safety is addressed, HTA needs to consider the evidence of a product's effectiveness and potential utility. As noted in the regulation section, emerging evidence of the effectiveness of apps and portable devices is mixed. Collection of evidence should continue after the initial approval and reimbursement decision, especially as mHealth products (particularly apps) may be frequently updated. As with conventional devices, payers must also consider how the product integrates with existing clinical activity, and whether it adds value in terms of impact on health outcomes and use of resources.

The utility of mHealth products – particularly those aiming to change behaviours and habits – relies not just on design and functionality but on user-dependent factors: among others, motivation, digital literacy, extrinsic support and if they are used in combination with other interventions or programmes. The science on this is still in its infancy (Quelly et al., 2016). The Commonwealth Fund evaluated apps designed to engage people in their care, and found that 27% of iOS (iPhone and iPad) apps and 27% of Android apps were "likely to be useful" (Commonwealth Fund, 2016). The behavioural factors behind the success or failure of these products – the *how* and the *why* – should therefore be a focus of ongoing evaluation and research.

Individuals' access to and engagement with mHealth requires policy consideration. Using this technology requires a certain level of proficiency and skill. Those lacking in digital literacy – likely older people and/or those with lower levels of education and general literacy – already experience poorer health and access to health care than their digitally literate peers. They may be marginalised in terms of benefiting from mHealth, or could be at risk for not using them properly. Policy makers and providers must therefore be aware of this "digital divide" and ensure that people using mHealth technologies have the skills, or have access to opportunities to improve their skills, to use them effectively. Concerns regarding cost to users of the applications as well as of Internet access must also be considered. If not addressed properly, mHealth could create additional disadvantages for people of lower socio-economic status and/or those who live in regions with limited Internet access.

Policy makers and payers must also ensure that health care reimbursement and financing systems as well as scope of practice and providers' indemnity insurance parameters keep pace with innovation in this field. At a minimum, reimbursement schedules need to be constantly updated to ensure these new technologies are incorporated and their use incentivised properly. As mHealth and the networks and processes within which it is embedded become more complex, new financing models will be needed to incentivise the development, use and equitable adoption of value-adding mHealth technology. Telemedicine provides a useful illustration in this regard (Box 4.4).

Box 4.4. **Telehealth**

Telehealth describes the provision of health care remotely by means of various telecommunication tools including telephones, smartphones and mobile devices. Telehealth has been available for some time. In fact, predictions of long-distance medical consultations began in the 19th century, not long after the invention of the telephone (Blake, 1880, p. 486).

Yet routine use of this technology has been slow to develop in most countries. Its cost-effectiveness has been questioned. Studies show mixed results and the incremental cost-effectiveness ratio (ICER) varies according to the exact approach and clinical specialty area (Mistry, 2012; Pasquel et al., 2015). However, this area is undergoing rapid technological change and improving economies of scale – a telemedicine consultation used to require complex videoconferencing equipment but can now be done via smartphone; and the cost of reliable Internet access is reducing while access grows. The cost-effectiveness assessment of telehealth needs constant updating. Low-cost virtual visits are now offered by an increasing number of health care organisations.

One barrier to adoption is financial. Billing or reimbursement is often absent or set at a level that does not incentivise telehealth consultation by practitioners. Another barrier is the lack of inter-jurisdictional regulatory co-ordination for practitioner licensing. This may reflect poor co-ordination between regulators of health professionals as well as a threat to vested interests (RAND, 2014). The situation is changing, however, as payers institute more attractive reimbursement parameters and jurisdictions enact enabling legislation (Kern, 2015) and remuneration schedules. In 2014 the US Department of Veterans' Affairs provided over 2 million telehealth visits (Dorsey and Topol, 2016). Since 2014, France has piloted telemedicine and remote consultation to improve equity of access to health services. An evaluation of these pilots is being conducted by the Haute Autorité de Santé (HAS).

Box 4.4. **Telehealth** *(cont.)*

Clinical and social barriers also impede telehealth. Questions persist over quality, and it is clear that this modality is not suitable for all types of consultation (e.g. where palpation is required). In this way telehealth should be seen as complementary to, rather than as a replacement for, traditional assessment and treatment. In some ways telehealth represents a reflection of the past – the house call, in which providers visit patients in their home. Seen in this fashion, telehealth has the potential to address some of the social and geographic inequities of access to care. In addition to removing legal barriers and financial disincentives for providers, access to the technology that enables telehealth (e.g. reliable Internet; telecommunication devices) must be an important policy consideration. Too often, those who would benefit most from telehealth are on the wrong side of the "digital divide" (Dorsey and Topol, 2016).

Equally important for policy makers as mHealth begins to disseminate more broadly are considerations of the workflow, remuneration and ethical and legal responsibilities of providers whose practice is subject to change with the proliferation of mHealth. For example, practitioners are starting to receive real-time data feeds of vital signs from an increasing number of their patients. Payers are beginning to embrace coverage and reimbursement of mHealth products and the activities they enable (Dolan, 2013; Kern, 2015).

Finally, the very real possibility that constant monitoring of health status may drive more health care utilisation – with little incremental benefit – must be considered. Although early research suggests that this is not the case, continued investigation and monitoring is advised (Bloss et al., 2016).

3. Institutional requirements for effective regulation, coverage and funding of medical devices

This chapter has so far illustrated the challenges and complexities of regulating and funding medical devices as a category of health technology. As with any public policy, a sound regulatory and funding framework requires a set of institutional requirements, settings and characteristics. The specific focus of this section is two key areas in this regard: information infrastructure and governance.

3.1. *Information infrastructure provides a necessary platform*

This chapter emphasises the importance of approaching regulation and funding of medical devices as a cycle based on RWE of a product's performance. As discussed earlier, the WHO urged member states to engage in regional regulatory networks and to "promote international co-operation, as appropriate, for collaboration and information sharing, including through electronic platforms" (WHO, 2014, p. 3). This approach relies heavily on timely and high-quality information, derived from capturing and analysing data from a range of sources. Sound information systems and infrastructure are a necessary platform to create a harmonised regulatory and funding framework.

Challenges arise in implementing health information systems

Basing regulation on RWE and sharing information with other authorities are not possible without a comprehensive and integrated data infrastructure. Regulatory systems recognise this and are moving towards improving the quality and timeliness of data collection and analysis, but many shortcomings still need to be addressed. A major problem is the failure to gather and use longitudinal evidence of a product's performance to inform cyclical review, principally because data systems and information infrastructure do not enable this. In a sense, the failure to approach regulation and funding as a cycle can be attributed to poor data infrastructure.

In the European Union, since 2011, the European databank on medical devices (Eudamed) has collected information on adverse events linked to medical devices. Reporting of and action on these incidents is said to be variable and of limited utility (Kramer et al., 2012). Eudamed is improving the quality, standardisation, accessibility and interoperability of its data. This has the potential to permit establishment of a more comprehensive and dynamic picture of safety and utility across a device's lifecycle.

In the United States, reporting of adverse events is mandatory for providers and manufacturers, and formal post-market studies are requested for some products. A series of networks was designed to facilitate capture of information on adverse events associated with devices. However, these rules are neither well-enforced nor complied with. This contrasts with the FDA Sentinel Initiative for pharmaceuticals, a comprehensive and integrated surveillance system that links and monitors a range of clinical and administrative data sources. Using "Big Data" analytics, it proactively detects any safety concerns, improving response time and obviating the reliance on spontaneous reporting by actors in the system and the problems this entails (Sorenson and Drummond, 2014).[13] A related initiative is under way for medical devices, named the Medical Device Epidemiology Network Initiative (MDEpiNet).

The problems and shortcomings of information systems in the context of regulating and funding medical devices more effectively and efficiently mirror the broader information issues that health care systems grapple with. These manifest in the inability to track devices by reliably and meaningfully linking various datasets. Longitudinal evaluation of a product's utility from the perspective of users or patients is also lacking. Underlying these are a number of shortcomings and challenges of health data infrastructure, particularly for using health data for secondary purposes such as system performance monitoring, surveillance, research and, of course, regulation and funding of medical technology. These challenges are detailed in Chapter 6, and are explored and discussed in other recent OECD publications (OECD, 2013a, 2015a, 2015b).

Unique device identifiers and data linkage are potential tools

No single data source can capture all information required about the utility and cost-utility of a product. Data linkage is therefore a key requirement of successful surveillance, monitoring and review. The types of datasets that should be linked for this purpose include registries (see below), EHR data, imaging and laboratory results, mortality statistics, financial/claims data, and administrative and clinical activity data. Aided by the requisite analytical techniques, linkage enables aggregation of sufficient information to identify safety concerns quickly, and permits statistically valid observational studies of products' real-world performance, utility and cost. The importance of a unique patient identifier to enable this was mentioned above.

Another key enabler of linkage for the purpose of medical devices is a UDI, a serial number that enables a device to be easily coded and recognised in various datasets. Absence of UDIs prevents a scheme similar to the US Sentinel Initiative from being implemented for medical devices, which would improve the responsiveness and accuracy of safety reporting and the clinical utility of devices. Both the US and European regulatory regimes are at various stages of implementing a UDI (Engelberg Center for Health Care Reform, 2015; Sorenson and Drummond, 2014; Evans et al., 2015). Ideally, UDIs should be internationally consistent.

Patient-reported measures can help improve device value

To truly evaluate whether a device or procedure is worth paying for, and at what price, information about its impact on the user is required. Health information systems are good at collecting data on health care activity but lacking when it comes to collecting information on the results or outcomes of this activity. Some have begun to capture PROMs as well as clinical safety incidents (Patient-Reported Incident Measures, or PRIMs). This information is potentially very valuable to policy and decision makers in all aspects of the health care system, including device regulation, coverage and funding. This work is, however, in its infancy and requires investment of resources for meaningful integration into health information systems.

All of these patient-reported measures are useful in the context of medical devices. PRIMs inform safety concerns, providing extra granularity of information regarding safety failures of a device, which may be due to a range of factors: design, manufacture, application or inappropriate use. PROMs, used to complement conventional clinical outcomes such as mortality or re-admission, may enable payers to more accurately ascertain clinical utility, as outlined previously, and are of importance to patients, carers and citizens. Policy makers must therefore recognise the value of these instruments.

Registries are frequently cited as an important tool for quality, but are difficult to implement

Registries can be used to monitor the safety, clinical utility and impact of a product or intervention over time as it is used in routine clinical practice. A registry is an organised system that uses observational study methods to collect uniform data (clinical and other) to evaluate specified outcomes for a population defined by a particular disease or exposure (Gliklich and Dreyer, 2007). An exposure can be a procedure, drug or medical device. Registries can greatly enhance regulators' ability to track the safety and clinical utility of medical devices and have been instrumental in tracking performance and detecting device failure (Kandala et al., 2015) but their application varies between jurisdictions.

Scandinavian countries are cited as the most advanced in this regard (James et al., 2011). Data from the Swedish Coronary Angiography and Angioplasty Registry (SCAAR) enabled monitoring of the safety and clinical utility of new-generation cardiac stents. This led to several reviews of regulatory decisions, and the insightful finding that differences are explained not by the products themselves but by improved proficiency of clinicians after using the new stents over a prolonged period of time (Lagerqvist et al., 2009; Sarno et al., 2012). In another example, analysis of French and US registries alerted regulators that the number of patients treated transapically for aortic valve implantation far exceeded clinical guidelines and FDA recommendations (Van Brabandt et al., 2012). Similarly, findings from the Australian and UK orthopaedic registries showed that cemented hip prostheses were more performant than non-cemented ones. It is interesting to note, however, that information derived from one country's national registry is not necessarily used in another's. While Sweden quickly adopted cemented prostheses in 98% of hip replacements, France used them in only 51% of cases in 2012 (CNAMTS, 2012).

To optimise the utility of registries, criteria for what devices should be captured in a registry are required. Clear guidelines on methods, data quality and transparency are also needed and should be determined in consultation with stakeholders. To permit evaluation of clinical utility based on outcomes, it is important that, when possible, registries incorporate information generated by patients, such as PROMs and PRIMs. At the international level, the IMDRF's ongoing project defines common principles and methods for registries.

3.2. Governance provides context for approval and funding decisions

Differences in the governance of regulation and funding of medical technology have been highlighted. The result is variation in approval and funding decisions between countries, which has downstream effects on clinical practice, health outcomes and expenditure. This section highlights key aspects of governance that need to be considered and applied according to local context and requirements.

Health care systems increasingly use consultation and stakeholder engagement

Legitimacy of any public policy depends on consultation and stakeholder engagement (Wallner, 2008). Regulating and funding medical devices is not different. Most systems deploy clinical experts and health care providers, biomedical engineers, and experts in health economics, statistics and financing. The growing number of web-enabled products that transmit information on patients' health status, such as smartphone applications and wearable devices, requires data management and privacy experts to be more involved in regulatory decisions.

However, health care has a particularly broad stakeholder catchment, and two groups in particular are increasingly recognised as having essential expertise and potential to contribute:

- patients and sufferers from the illness or disease that the specific product in question aims to ameliorate or manage (and their carers); and
- citizens, who are the principal funders and custodians of health services and who are all potential patients.

The citizen- and patient-centred approach in health care delivery gained traction over the past decade. Including these stakeholders can equally pay dividends in health technology regulation and funding. For example, there is a strong argument that valuing the non-medical effects of care is an important consideration in many interventions, and can only be approached in consultation with these stakeholders (Birch and Donaldson, 2003; Lee et al., 2010).

Health technology regulation is beginning to incorporate this consultative approach. Indeed, countries are increasingly involving citizens and patients to some extent in the assessment and appraisal of medical technologies in health care systems (Auraaen et al., 2016). NICE has a Patient and Public Involvement Program (PPIP) to assist in decisions about specific technology, and a Citizens Council to assist in value judgments required for many regulatory decisions (NICE, 2011). The FDA is increasingly engaging patients and carers in the development and approval of health technologies (Hunter et al., 2015). Proposals to review European regulation in this regard are being considered (Sorenson and Drummond, 2014).

The framework for regulating and funding devices must be founded on a clear and explicit set of principles. This will provide a way to manage tensions between stakeholders appropriately and a foundation for processes to flow more efficiently. It will also promote better outcomes by: 1) providing clear parameters and guidance to stakeholders; 2) increasing the legitimacy of decisions; and 3) offering recourse to fundamentals in the event of decisions generating political controversy. For decisions to be accepted by stakeholders, the principles must align with other objectives of the health care system and broader public policy. Objectives of regulatory and funding aspects of the framework will differ. In each case, they need to be determined in consultation with all stakeholders and the public.

Patient and citizen perspectives differ

The distinction between patients and citizens is important. Both groups can provide invaluable insight and expertise, but they do so from different perspectives. Their preferences can contrast sharply. Patients who may benefit from new technology will have expertise on a product's impact on their treatment, and on the quality of their lives. However, they will generally have a strong personal interest to see products approved regardless of cost. They have a disincentive to consider the indirect impact and opportunity costs to the health care system.

Citizens, on the other hand, have a more detached viewpoint that is more representative of society as a whole. While not providing the granular detail of a product's potential clinical effect, as custodians of the health care system, citizens' contribution can be invaluable when making difficult judgements, weighting various dimensions and setting priorities, and in the inevitable trade-offs that regulation entails. A panel of citizens is better placed than other experts to judge if, for example, a technology to extend the life of the old versus the young should be valued differently. For example, a citizens' jury in Australia deliberated over weighting the health outcomes of indigenous versus non-indigenous people for the purpose of resource allocation (Mooney and Blackwell, 2004).

Involving citizens and patients is a value judgement in itself. Societies may strongly prefer to defer public policy decisions to technical and academic experts only. In such cases, the decision to do so should still be made in consultation with the public. Involving the public serves to legitimise decisions, and is the general direction of regulatory systems worldwide.

Transparency is a requirement of good governance

The worldwide trend in public policy is moving in the direction of transparency (The White House, n.d.). The WHO urged member states to base regulatory systems for medical products on strong legal foundations, with emphasis on transparency in decision making (WHO, 2014). The FDA took steps to improve the transparency of medical device market authorisation in recent years, making information about its activities publicly available, and requiring the disclosure of financial interests of individual investigators (Sorenson and Drummond, 2014). The European regulatory system has been criticised for its lack of transparency. Europe's Notified Bodies, agencies responsible for product approval, have no obligation to make information about certification decisions public (Freemantle, 2011). This effectively makes it impossible for researchers or even policy makers and national authorities themselves to do any kind of systematic research into which devices were approved when and how because the information resides with a fragmented group of notified bodies and there is no centralised database, similar to that of the FDA in the US, information can be retrieved from. Eudamed, the pan-European database for collecting information on device failure and adverse events, is not publicly accessible (Kramer et al., 2012), although some countries' local authorities make this information public (Sorenson and Drummond, 2014). Current developments in Eudamed will improve the transparency and accessibility of information regarding safety and performance of devices in Europe.

Transparency is, of course, an important democratic principle in its own right but its instrumental value becomes most evident following controversial regulatory funding decisions. Combined with recourse to fundamental principles and objectives, transparency is a strong signal about an institution's integrity of process and provides leverage to legitimise actions. It can build public trust and make the politics of regulation and funding easier to manage.

In practice, transparency may involve: publishing outcomes and processes of deliberations and decision making; establishing formal relationships with the media; making information visible and easily accessible; and collaborating with other countries' regulatory systems.[14] The exact nature depends on the culture and values of the country in question, but the underlying principle is that all stakeholders should have access to information regarding health technology regulation.

Resourcing is crucial for effective regulation and reimbursement of medical devices

A comprehensive regulatory and funding system needs to be adequately funded and resourced. The WHO urges member states to consider competencies associated with medical product regulation an integral part of the health workforce, and to develop the regulatory field as a profession (WHO, 2014). It is important that the right expertise is engaged in assessment of device categories; the evolving needs in this regard were discussed earlier. For example, data management and privacy expertise is required to assess mobile applications and wearable diagnostic devices.

To cover expenses, some regimes require manufacturers to pay a fee for the assessment of a product. The European Notified Bodies for device regulation are for-profit organisations. Fees are certainly acceptable practice. However, this report warns against regulatory authorities being for-profit organisations as this is likely to introduce perverse incentives into the system. Regardless of the approach, costs should be seen in the context of minimising risks of harm and in the opportunity to increase a product's value for money through rational and evidence-based funding decisions.

Conclusion

Medical devices encompass a very broad range of products that inhabit a wide spectrum of complexity, risk and costs. Devices are often integrated into clinical activities, and their utility often depends on multiple factors, including providers' skill and experience. The diffusion of uptake of medical technology, including devices, is cited as a principal driver of health expenditure growth. Device regulation, coverage and funding contribute to a safe, high-quality and sustainable health care system. Medical devices present unique challenges for policy makers. A sound framework must balance several objectives: clinical safety and utility with value for money, expediency and encouraging ongoing innovation to help achieve health policy goals – all in an environment comprising multiple interest groups and (sometimes) public and political pressure.

This chapter presented an analysis of medical device regulation and funding, based on a review of the literature and an examination of a number of regulatory systems in OECD countries. While many positive aspects are contained in these, some aspects merit further examination and improvement. Key findings can be summarised as follows.

Regulation followed by coverage and funding decisions are all complementary and mutually reinforcing, and face similar conceptual and evidentiary challenges. Importantly, considerable overlap exists in the evidence, expertise and deliberations required to make regulatory, coverage and funding decisions, particularly if established as a cycle of periodic review. A sound approach incorporates all three within a dynamic framework, and it makes sense to adopt a more integrated approach.

Regulation is concerned with a device's safety and performance or effectiveness. Sound evidence of this is not always complete until the product enters routine clinical use. Market authorisation should be granted with explicit conditions and restrictions for use based on what is known at the time, with periodic review based on accumulated evidence of safety and performance or effectiveness. Regulation and reimbursement are therefore best approached as a cycle comprising collection of RWE, analysis and review (Figure 4.3). To optimise efficiency and expedite outcomes, regulatory processes should be stratified along criteria that include level of clinical risk and potential impact. International co-operation is strongly encouraged to avoid duplication and to promote harmonisation of requirements and standards.

Figure 4.3. **A regulatory and funding framework for medical devices and their use**

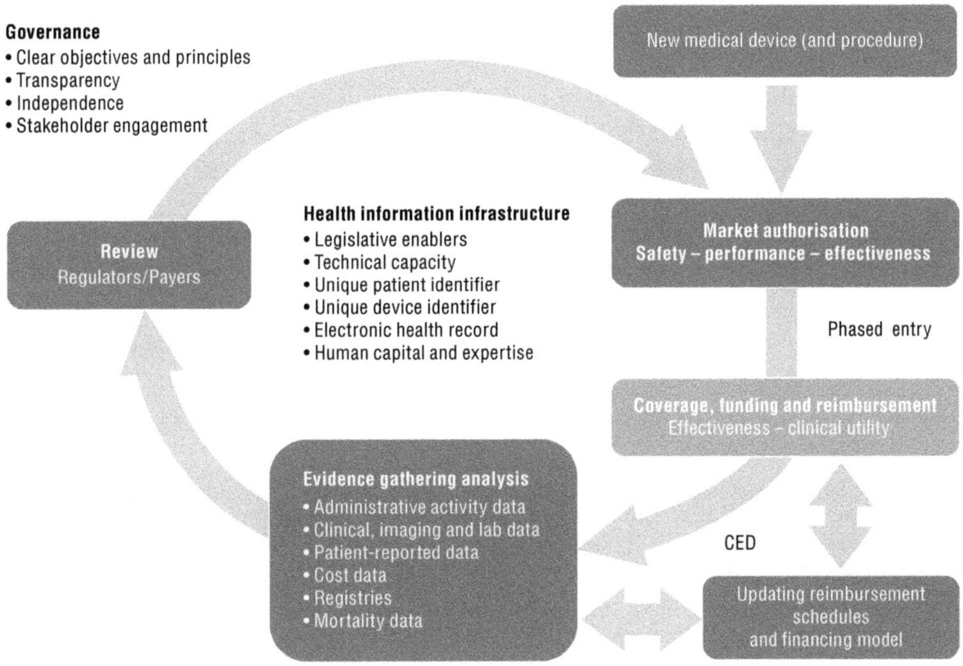

Coverage and funding decisions must consider the cost-utility of a device, its inherent attributes, how it is embedded within clinical activity and the most appropriate financing instrument at payers' disposal. When setting prices for the use of a device, payers must consider the following and set reimbursement levels accordingly:

- the incentives contained within the reimbursement in terms of use and diffusion, and their alignment with broader health care system objectives
- whether the device has a range of applications and, if so, the respective clinical utility of each

- whether some devices can, with time, be used in clinical situations alternative to the one(s) intended at initial approval or market authorisation.

Adjusting funding based on value or outcomes is an option for devices and procedures, particularly for products with multiple uses, some of which may be discretionary and add little clinical benefit. This can be a useful lever to promote appropriate care and minimise unnecessary use.

Coverage and funding decisions rely on good information. Evidence on effectiveness and utility should be accumulated once in routine use and combined with cost data to provide information on cost-utility. This should be used to periodically update coverage and funding decisions. Coverage and funding should, like regulation, be approached as a cyclical process based on the collection and analysis of RWE. A sound regulation and funding framework requires an integrated information system and data infrastructure. This includes a UDI that enables linkage of datasets, and establishment of a series of registries to collect evidence of a product's performance over time.

The regulatory framework relies on strong engagement with all relevant stakeholder groups, including experts in relevant clinical areas, economics, finance and bioethics. Particularly important groups are 1) patients, who bring unique perspectives on the impact of a specific technology, and 2) citizens, who as custodians of the health care system can assist with trade-offs and value judgements required, particularly for coverage and funding decisions.

Processes should be explicit and transparent, and information made publicly available without contravening intellectual property laws or releasing commercially sensitive information. The regulatory framework should be based on a clear and explicit set of principles. These should align with the broader health care system objectives, social preferences, and economic and social policy. Finally, regulatory systems must be adequately resourced.

Notes

1. In some jurisdictions this is referred to as pre-market approval and, in Europe, Conformité Europpéene (CE) certification.
2. Medical device regulation in Europe is in practice defined by three different directives: the Medical Devices Directive (MDD), the Active Implantable Medical Devices Directive (AIMDD) and the In Vitro Diagnostics Directive (IVDD). Each country has a competent authority in charge of ensuring that EU Directives are implemented in national law and to designate Notified Bodies.
3. Perhaps unsurprising given that "the initial primary goal of the EU regulatory system was to harmonise national regulations to reduce barriers to trade, rather than to protect public health" (Campillo-Arrero, 2013, p. 41).
4. In France, medical devices covered by health insurance are re-evaluated every five years by the HTA agency to confirm or discontinue coverage, but there is no direct link with market approval.
5. This is not dissimilar to pharmaceuticals, for which secondary uses are often discovered following widespread clinical use.
6. The most often quoted figure about the length of market exclusivity of medical devices is "18-24 months" (see *www.wto.org/english/tratop_e/trips_e/trilatweb_e/ch3d_trilat_web_13_e.htm*, consulted on 16 October 2016) but no sound estimate was found. In addition, the length of exclusivity period likely depends on the nature of the medical device (small and simple device versus big-ticket item) and levels of patent protection sought by the inventor.
7. *www.imdrf.org/*.

8. In the European Union, for instance, the number of medical devices that received CE Marking in 2014 was estimated to be more than 4 500, around 500 of which were Class III devices (MedTech Europe, 2015).
9. These devices can be purchased or rented.
10. The mix of factors that determine uptake and diffusion are discussed in more detail in Chapter 2.
11. Tariffs are always set by reference to costs observed one or two years before the update of tariffs.
12. To account for this, some payers set different reimbursement rates and co-payments based on the source of the referral. For example, a specialist referral may attract a higher rate or lower co-payment than a general practitioner. This is based on the assumption that the former is able to better identify the severity and clinical need, and that by the time the patient reaches the specialist, persistent symptoms are more likely to warrant further investigation (and perhaps that the specialist will be less inclined to acquiesce to the patient's demand for imaging).
13. Information from the Sentinel Initiative is also publicly available at *www.mini-sentinel.org/Reports/*.
14. Being mindful of commercially sensitive information.

References

ACSQHC – Australian Commission in Safety and Quality in Health Care (2015), *Australian Atlas of Healthcare Variation*, Sydney.

AHRQ – Agency for Healthcare Research and Quality (2010), "Quality, Regulation and Clinical Utility of Laboratory-developed Molecular Tests", Technology Assessment: original 19 May 2010, correction 6 October 2010, United States.

Ardaugh, B., S. Graves and R. Redberg (2013), "The 510(k) Ancestry of a Metal-on-Metal Hip Implant", *New England Journal of Medicine*, Vol. 368, pp. 97-100.

Auraaen, A. et al. (2016), "How OECD Health Systems Define the Range of Goods and Services to Be Financed Collectively", *OECD Working Paper*, OECD Publishing, Paris, *http://dx.doi.org/10.1787/5jlnb59ll80x-en*.

Bach, P. and S. Pearson (2015), "Payer and Policy Maker Steps to Support Value-based Pricing for Drugs", *Journal of the American Medical Association*, Vol. 34, No. 23, pp. 2503-2504.

Baeyens, H. et al. (2015), "Towards a Guided and Phased Introduction of High-risk Medical Devices in Belgium", *KCE Reports No. 249*, Health Services Research (HSR), Belgian Health Care Knowledge Centre (KCE), Brussels.

BHI – Blue Health Intelligence (2015), "A Study of Cost Variations for Knee and Hip Replacement Surgeries in the US" [online], *www.bcbs.com/healthofamerica/BCBS_BHI_Report-Jan-_21_Final.pdf* (accessed 8 March 2016).

Birch, S. and C. Donaldson (2003), "Valuing the Benefits and Costs of Health Care Programmes: Where's the 'Extra' in Extra-welfarism?", *Social Science and Medicine*, Vol. 56, pp. 1121-1133.

Blake, C.J. (1880), "The Telephone and Microphone in Auscultation", *Boston Medicine and Surgery Journal*, Vol. 103, pp. 486-487.

Bloss, C.S. et al. (2016), "A Prospective Randomized Trial Examining Health Care Utilization in Individuals Using Multiple Smartphone-enabled Biosensors", *PeerJournal*, Vol. 4, e1554.

Brennan, Z. (2016), "EU Looks to Improve Data Quality of mHealth Apps" [online], available at: *www.raps.org/Regulatory-Focus/News/2016/01/25/23965/EU-Looks-to-Improve-Data-Quality-of-mHealth-Apps/* (accessed 4 March 2016).

Bruen, B. et al. (2016), *The Impact of Reimbursement Policies and Practices on Healthcare Technology Innovation*, HHS, Washington, DC.

Brügger, U. et al. (2015), "Health Technology Assessment in Switzerland: A Descriptive Analysis of 'Coverage with Evidence Development' Decisions from 1996 to 2013", *British Medical Journal Open*, Vol. 5, No. 3, e007021.

Burke, M., G. Fournier and K. Prasad (2007), "The Diffusion of a Medical Innovation: Is Success in the Stars", *Southern Economic Journal*, Vol. 73, No. 3, pp. 588-603.

Campillo-Artero, C. (2013), "A Full-fledged Overhaul Is Needed for a Risk and Value-based Regulation of Medical Devices in Europe", *Health Policy*, Vol. 113, pp. 38-44.

Capellaro, G., S. Ghislandi and E. Agnessi-Pessina (2011), "Diffusion of Medical Technology: The Role of Financing", *Health Policy*, Vol. 100, pp. 51-59.

Chambers, J., P. Neumann and M. Buxton (2010), "Does Medicare Have an Implicit Cost-effectiveness Threshold?", *Medical Decision Making*, Vol. 30, No. 4, pp. E14-E27.

Chandra, A. and J. Skinner (2012), "Technology Growth and Expenditure Growth in Health Care", *Journal of Economic Literature*, Vol. 50, No. 3, pp. 645-680.

Chen, C., S. Dhruva and R. Redberg (2012), "Inclusion of Comparative Effectiveness Data in High-risk Cardiovascular Device Studies at the Time of Premarket Approval", *Journal of the American Medical Association*, Vol. 308, No. 17, pp. 1740-1742.

Chernew, M. and J. Newhouse (2012), "Health Care Spending and Growth", in M. Pauly, T. McGuire and P. Barros (eds.), *Handbook of Health Economics*, Vol. 2, Elsevier.

Claxton, K. et al. (2015), "Causes for Concern: Is NICE Failing to Uphold Its Responsibilitites to All NHS Patients", *Health Economics*, Vol. 24, pp. 1-7.

CMS – Centers for Medicare & Medicaid Services (2015a), "Hospital Value-based Purchasing" [online], *www.cms.gov/Medicare/Quality-Initiatives-Patient-Assessment-Instruments/hospital-value-based-purchasing/index.html?redirect=/Hospital-Value-Based-Purchasing/* (accessed 7 March 2016).

CMS (2009), "National Coverage Determination (NCD) for Pharmacogenomic Testing for Warfarin Response", NCD No. 90.1, effective date 3 August 2009.

CNAMTS – Caisse Nationale de l'Assurance Maladie des Travailleurs Salariés (2012), "Propositions de l'Assurance Maladie sur les charges et produits pour l'année 2013", Caisse Nationale d'Assurance Maladie des Travailleurs Salariés, Paris.

Cohen, D. (2012), "EU Approval System Leaves Door Open for Dangerous Devices", *British Medical Journal*, Vol. 345, e7173, *http://dx.doi.org/10.1136/bmj.e7173*.

Cohen, D. (2011), "Out of Joint: The Story of the ASR", *British Medical Journal*, Vol. 342, d2905, *http://dx.doi.org/10.1136/bmj.d2905*.

Cohen, D. and M. Billingsley (2011), "Europeans Are Left to their Own Devices", *British Medical Journal*, Vol. 342, d2748.

Commonwealth Fund (2016), *Developing a Framework for Evaluating the Patient Engagement, Quality, and Safety of Mobile Health Applications*, Commonwealth Fund, Washington, DC.

Cooper, Z. et al. (2016), "The Price Ain't Right? Hospital Prices and Health Spending on the Privately Insured", *www.nber.org/papers/w21815* (accessed 19 August 2016).

Cortez, N., G. Cohen and A. Kesselheim, (2014), "FDA Regulation of Mobile Health Technologies", *New England Journal of Medicine*, Vol. 371, No. 4, pp. 372-379.

Council of the European Union (2016), "Proposal for a Regulation of the European Parliament and of the Council on Medical Devices, and Amending Directive 2001/83/EC, Regulation (EC) No. 178/2002 and Regulation (EC) No. 1223/2009", *http://data.consilium.europa.eu/doc/document/ST-9364-2016-REV-3/en/pdf* (accessed 18 July 2016).

Dolan, B. (2013), "WellDoc's BlueStar Secures First Mobile Health Reimbursement" [online], available at: *http://mobihealthnews.com/23026/welldocs-bluestar-secures-first-mobile-health-reimbursement* (accessed 3 February 2016).

Donahoe, G. and G. King (2012), "Estimates of Medical Device Spending in the United States", *http://advamed.org/res.download/291* (accessed 19 July 2016).

Dorsey, E.R. and E.J. Topol (2016), "State of Telehealth", *New England Journal of Medicine*, Vol. 375, No. 2, pp. 154-161.

Engelberg Center for Health Care Reform (2015), "Strengthening Patient Care: Building an Effective National Medical Device Surveillance System", Brookings Institution, Washington, DC.

European Commission (2016a), "Code of Conduct on Privacy for mHealth Apps Has Been Finalised", *https://ec.europa.eu/digital-single-market/en/news/code-conduct-privacy-mhealth-apps-has-been-finalised* (accessed 19 July 2016).

European Commission (2016b), "EU Guidelines on Assessment of the Reliability of Mobile Health Applications (First Draft Guidelines)", *http://ec.europa.eu/newsroom/dae/document.cfm?action=display&doc_id=15353* (accessed 19 July 2016).

European Commission (2016c), "Guidelines on the Qualification and Classification of Standalone Software Used in Healthcare within the Regulatory Framework of Medical Devices", *http://ec.europa.eu/DocsRoom/documents/17921/attachments/1/translations/* (accessed 29 September 2016).

European Commission (2012), "Revisions of Medical Device Directives", *https://ec.europa.eu/growth/sectors/medical-devices/regulatory-framework/revision_en* (accessed 29 September 2016).

Evans, B.J., W. Burke and G. Jarvik (2015), "The FDA and Genomic Tests – Getting the Regulation Right", *New England Journal of Medicine*, Vol. 372, No. 23, pp. 2258-2264.

FDA – Food and Drug Administration (2016a), "Request for Expressions of Interest from Coverage Organizations; Coverage Organizations Interested in Providing Input Regarding Private Payer Coverage to Medical Device Sponsors who Request their Participation in a Pre-Submission Meeting with the Food and Drug Administration", Federal Register 81 FR 9203, Docket No. FDA-2012-D-0530, Document 2016-03909, 24 February 2016.

FDA (2015a), "Memorandum of Understanding between United States Food and Drug Administration and Centers for Medicare & Medicaid Services", MOU 225-10-0010, retrieved from *www.fda.gov/AboutFDA/PartnershipsCollaborations/MemorandaofUnderstandingMOUs/DomesticMOUs/ucm217585.htm*.

FDA (2015b), "What Is a Medical Device?", *www.fda.gov/AboutFDA/Transparency/Basics/ucm211822.htm* (accessed 21 December 2015).

FDA (2012), "Unsafe and Ineffective Devices Approved in the EU That Were Not Approved in the US", HHS, Washington, DC.

FDA (2011), "FDA, CMS Launch Pilot Program for Voluntary Parallel Review of Innovative Devices", available at: *www.fda.gov/NewsEvents/Newsroom/PressAnnouncements/ucm274833.htm* (accessed 8 February 2016).

Free, C. et al. (2013a), "The Effectiveness of Mobile-Health Technology-Based Health Behaviour Change or Disease Management Interventions for Health Care Consumers: A Systematic Review", *PLoS Medicine*, Vol. 10, No. 1, e1001362.

Free, C. et al. (2013b), "The Effectiveness of Mobile-Health Technologies to Improve Health Care Service Delivery Processes: A Systematic Review and Meta-Analysis", *PLoS Medicine*, Vol. 10, No. 1, e1001363.

Freemantle, N. (2011), "Evaluating and Regulating the Device Industry", *British Medical Journal*, Vol. 342, d2839.

GAO – United States Government Accountability Office (2009), "Medical Devices: FDA Should Take Steps to Ensure That High-Risk Device Types Are Approved through the Most Stringent Premarket Review Process", Report to Congressional Addressees, Washington, DC, *www.gao.gov/assets/290/284882.pdf*.

Gelijins, A. and N. Rosenberg (1994), "The Dynamics of Technological Change in Medicine", *Health Affairs*, Vol. 13, No. 3, pp. 28-46.

GHTF – Global Harmonization Task Force (2012), "Clinical Evidence for IVD Medical Devices", GHTF/SG5/N6:2012, 2 November.

Gliklich, R.E. and N.A. Dreyer (2007), "Registries for Evaluating Patient Registries: A User's Guide", AHRQ publication No. 07-EHC001, Rockville, United States.

Gravelle, J.G. and J. Lowry (2015), "The Medical Device Excise Tax: Economic Analysis", Congressional Research Services, Washington, DC.

Grennan, M. (2013), "Price Discrimination and Bargaining: Empirical Evidence from Medical Devices", *American Economic Review*, Vol. 103, No. 1, pp. 145-177.

Hamine, S. et al. (2015), "Impact of mHealth Chronic Disease Management on Treatment Adherence and Patient Outcomes: A Systematic Review", *Journal of Medical Internet Research*, Vol. 17, No. 2, e52.

Hansson, E. (2016), "Update on EU Regulatory Developments", IMDRF 13-15 September, Florianoplos, Brazil.

HAS – Haute Autorité de Santé (2009), "Medical Device Assessment in France – Guidebook", Haute Autorité de Santé, *www.has-sante.fr/portail/upload/docs/application/pdf/2010-03/guide_dm_gb_050310.pdf*.

Hernandez, J., S.F. Machacz and J.C. Robinson (2015), "US Hospital Payment Adjustments for Innovative Technology Lag Behind Those in Germany, France, and Japan", *Health Affairs*, Vol. 34, No. 2, pp. 261-270.

HHS – US Department of Health and Human Services (2016), "ONC Launches New Challenges to Spur Innovation for Market-Ready, User-Friendly Health Technology Apps for Consumers and Providers",

US Department of Health and Human Services, Washington, DC, *www.hhs.gov/about/news/2016/03/01/onc-launches-new-challenges-spur-innovation-market-ready-user-friendly-health-technology-apps.html* (accessed 15 May 2016).

Huckvale, K. et al. (2015), "Unaddressed Privacy Risks in Accredited Health and Wellness Apps: A Cross-sectional Systematic Assessment", *BMC Medicine*, Vol. 13, No. 1, p. 1.

Hunter, N., K. O'Callaghan and R. Califf (2015), "Engaging Patients Across the Spectrum of Medical Product Development", *Journal of the American Medical Association*, Vol. 314, No. 23, pp. 2499-2500.

Husereau, D., D. Marshall and A. Levy (2014), "Health Technology Assessment and Personalized Medicine: Are Economic Evaluation Guidelines Sufficient to Support Decision Making", *International Journal of Technology Assessment in Health Care*, Vol. 30, No. 2, pp. 179-187.

IOM – Institute of Medicine (2011), "Medical Devices and the Public's Health. The FDA 10(k) Clearance Process at 35 Years", National Academics Press, Washington, DC.

James, S., J. Daubert and F. Van der Werf (2011), "Use of Registries to Investigate the Past and Develop the Future", *British Medical Journal*, Vol. 7, No. 7, e1000280.

Kandala, N. et al. (2015), "Setting Benchmark Revision Rates for Total Hip Replacement: Analysis of Registry Evidence", *British Medical Journal*, Vol. 350, h756.

Karhula, T. et al. (2015), "Telemonitoring and Mobile Phone-based Health Coaching among Finnish Diabetic and Heart Disease Patients: Randomized Controlled Trial", *Journal of Medical Internet Research*, Vol. 17, No. 6, e153.

Kern, C. (2015), "CMS Pays Out Nearly $14 Million In Telemedicine Reimbursement" [online], available at: *www.healthitoutcomes.com/doc/cms-pays-out-nearly-million-in-telemedicine-reimbursement-0001* (accessed 3 March 2016).

Kirisits, A. and K. Redekop (2013), "The Economic Evaluation of Medical Devices", *Applied Health Economics and Health Policy*, Vol. 11, pp. 15-26.

Kramer, D., S. Xu and A. Kesselheim (2012), "Regulation of Medical Devices in the US and European Union", *New England Journal of Medicine*, Vol. 366, No. 9, pp. 848-855.

Lagerqvist, B., S. James and U. Stenestrand (2009), "Long-term Outcomes with Drug Eluting Stents versus Bare Metal Stents in Sweden", *New England Journal of Medicine*, Vol. 356, pp. 1009-1019.

Lee, D., J. Neumann and P. Rizzo (2010), "Understanding the Medical and Non-medical Value of Diagnostic Testing", *Value in Health*, Vol. 13, pp. 310-314.

Ludman, P.F. et al. (2014), "National Audit of Percutaneous Coronary Interventions. Annual Public Report January 2013-December 2013", UCL (University College London), London.

Martelli, N., H. van den Brink and I. Borget (2016), "New French Coverage with Evidence Development for Innovative Medical Devices: Improvements and Unresolved Issues", *Value in Health*, Vol. 19, pp. 17-19.

MedTech Europe (2015), "The European Medical Technology Industry in Figures", *www.medtecheurope.org/sites/default/files/resource_items/files/MEDTECH_FactFigures_ONLINE3.pdf* (accessed 15 July 2016).

MHRA – Medicines and Healthcare Products Regulatory Agency, (2014), "Medical Devices: Software Applications (apps)" [online], available at: *www.gov.uk/government/publications/medical-devices-software-applications-apps* (accessed 4 March 2016).

Ministère de la Santé et des Sports (2009), "Règles de facturation des soins dispensés dans les établissements de santé – Dispositifs médicaux", MSS, *http://social-sante.gouv.fr/IMG/pdf/dispositifs_medicaux-2.pdf* (accessed 13 February 2016).

Mistry, H. (2012), "Systematic Review of Studies of the Cost-effectiveness of Telemedicine and Telecare. Changes in the Economic Evidence Over Twenty Years", *Journal of Telemedicine and Telecare*, Vol. 18, No. 1, pp. 1-6.

Mooney, G. and S. Blackwell (2004), "Whose Health Service Is It Anyway? Community Values in Health Care", *Medical Journal of Australia*, Vol. 180, No. 2, pp. 76-78.

NHS England (2015), "2015/16 National Tariff Payment System: Engagement on National Prices", *Monitor*, London.

NICE – National Institute for Health and Care Excellence (2011), "Medical Technologoes Evaluation Programme Methods Guide", National Health Service, London.

NICE (2008), "Guidance TA152: Drug-eluting Stents for the Treatment of Coronary Artery Disease" [online], *www.nice.org.uk/guidance/ta152* (accessed 7 March 2016).

OECD (2016), *Better Ways to Pay for Health Care*, OECD Publishing, Paris, *http://dx.doi.org/10.1787/9789264258211-en*.

OECD (2015a), *Data-driven Innovation: Big Data for Growth and Well-being*, OECD Publishing, Paris, http://dx.doi.org/10.1787/9789264229358-en.

OECD (2015b), *Health Data Governance: Privacy, Monitoring and Research*, OECD Publishing, Paris, *http://dx.doi.org/10.1787/9789264244566-en*.

OECD (2013a), *Strengthening Health Information Infrastructure for Health Care Quality Governance: Good Practices, New Opportunities and Data Privacy Protection Challenges*, OECD Publishing, Paris, *http://dx.doi.org/10.1787/9789264193505-en*.

OECD (2013b), "Toward New Models of Innovative Governance of Biomedicine and Health Technologies", *OECD Science, Technology and Industry Policy Papers*, No. 11, OECD Publishing, Paris, *http://dx.doi.org/10.1787/5k3v0hljnnlr-en*.

OECD (2010), "Comparing Price Levels of Hospital Services Across Countries: Results of a Pilot Study", OECD Publishing, Paris, *http://dx.doi.org/10.1787/5km91p4f3rzw-en*.

Okike, K. et al. (2014), "Survey Finds Few Orthopedic Surgeons Know the Costs of the Devices they Implant", *Health Affairs*, Vol. 33, No. 1, pp. 103-109.

Olberg, B., M. Perleth and R. Busse (2014), "The New Regulation to Investigate Potentially Beneficial Diagnostic and Therapeutic Methods in Germany: Up to International Standard?", *Health Policy*, Vol. 117, No. 2, pp. 135-145.

Pasquel, F.J. et al. (2015), "Cost-effectiveness of Different Diabetic Retinopathy Screening Modalities", *Journal of Diabetes Science and Technology*, Vol. 10, No. 2, pp. 301-307.

Quelly, S., A. Norris and J. DiPietro (2016), "Impact of Mobile Apps to Combat Obesity in Children and Adolescents: A Systematic Literature Review", *Pediatric Nursing*, Vol. 21, pp. 5-17.

Quentin, W., D. Scheller-Kreinsen and R. Busse (2011), "Technological Innovation in DRG-based Hospital Payment Systems Across Europe", in R. Busse, A. Geissler, W. Quentin and M. Wiley (eds.), *Diagnosis-Related Groups in Europe – Moving Towards Transparency, Efficiency and Quality in Hospitals*, European Observatory on Health Systems and Policies.

RAND (2014), *Redirecting Innovation in US Health Care*, RAND Corporation, Washington, DC.

Ridge, J.R. and S. Statz (2015), "Exact Sciences' Experience with the FDA and CMS Parallel Review Program", *Expert Review of Molecular Diagnostics*, Vol. 15, No. 9, pp. 1117-1124.

Sansom, L., W. Delaat and J.H. Horvath (2015), "Recommendations to the Minister for Health on the Regulatory Frameworks for Medicines, Medical Devices, Complementary Medicines and Advertising of Therapeutic Goods", Expert Panel Review of Medicines and Medical Devices Regulation, Australia.

Sarno, G., B. Lagerqvist and O. Frober (2012), "Lower Risk of Stent Thrombosis and Restenosis with Unrestricted Use of New Generation Drug Eluting Stents. A Report from the Nationwide SCAAR", *European Heart Journal*, Vol. 33, No. 5, pp. 606-613.

Sedlis, S. et al. (2015), "Effect of PCI on Long-Term Survival in Patients with Stable Ischemic Heart Disease", *New England Journal of Medicine*, Vol. 373, No. 20, pp. 1937-1946.

Shih, C. and E. Berliner (2008), "Diffusion of New Technology and Payment Policies: Coronary Stents", *Health Affairs (Millwood)*, Vol. 27, No. 6, pp. 1566-1576.

Sorenson, C. and M. Drummond (2014), "Improving Medical Device Regulation: The United States and Europe in Perspective", *Millbank Quarterly*, Vol. 92, No. 1, pp. 114-150.

Sorenson, C., M. Drummond and L. Burns (2013), "Evolving Reimbursement and Pricing Policies for Devices in Europe and the United States Should Encourage Greater Value", *Health Affairs (Millwood)*, Vol. 32, No. 4, pp. 788-796.

Srivastava, D. et al. (forthcoming), "Organisation of Health Care Delivery and Paying for Health Care Provision for Primary Care, Specialist Care and Inpatient Care in OECD Countries – Result from the 2012 Health Characteristics Survey", *OECD Health Working Paper*, OECD Publishing, Paris.

Steinhubl, S., E. Muse and E. Topol (2015), "The Emerging Field of Mobile Health", *Science Translational Medicine*, *http://dx.doi.org/10.1126/scitranslmed.aaa3487*.

Sweet, B., A. Schwemm and D. Parsons (2011), "Review of the Processes for FDA Oversight of Drugs, Medical Devices and Combination Products", *Journal of Managed Care Pharmacology*, Vol. 17, pp. 40-50.

The Age (2015), "Gluten-free Movement May Be Driving Unnecessary Colonoscopies, Doctor Says", 26 Nov. 2015, *www.theage.com.au/victoria/glutenfree-movement-may-be-driving-unnecessary-colonoscopies-doctor-says-20151126-gl8nga.html*.

The White House. Transparency and Open Government (n.d.), *www.whitehouse.gov/the_press_office/TransparencyandOpenGovernment* (accessed 4 January 2015).

Van Brabandt, H., M. Neyt and F. Hulstaert (2012), "Transcatheter Aortic Valve Implantation (TAVI): Risky and Costly", *British Medical Journal*, Vol. 345, e4710.

Wallner, J. (2008), "Legitimacy and Public Policy: Seeing Beyond Effectiveness, Efficiency, and Performance", *Policy Studies Journal*, Vol. 36, No. 3, pp. 421-443.

WHO (2016), "WHO Global Model Regulatory Framework for Medical Devices Including IVDs (21 July 2016) – Revised draft for Comment", *www.who.int/medicines/areas/quality_safety/quality_assurance/2016-07-27ModelregulatoryFramework_MedDev_QAS16-664Rev1.pdf?ua=1* (accessed 10 October 2016).

WHO (2015), *Republic of Korea: Health System Review*, WHO, Geneva.

WHO (2014), "Outcomes of the Sixty-seventh World Health Assembly", WHA67.20, 15.6, WHO, Geneva.

WHO, WIPO and WTO – World Health Organization, World Intellectual Property Organization and World Trade Organization (2012), "III. Medical Technologies: The Innovation Dimension", *Promoting Access to Medical Technologies and Innovation*, WHO, WIPO, WTO (eds.), Geneva.

Zuckerman, D.M, P. Brown and S.E. Nissen (2011), "Medical Device Recalls and the FDA Approval Process", *Archives of Internal Medicine*, Vol. 171, No. 11, pp. 1006-1011.

Zuckerman, R. et al. (2016), "Readmissions, Observation and the Hospital Readmission Reduction Program", *New England Journal of Medicine*, *http://dx.doi.org/10.1056/NEJMsa1513024*.

New Health Technologies: Managing Access, Value
and Sustainability

Chapter 5

Achieving the promise of precision medicine

by
Valérie Paris, Allison Colbert *and* Nicolas Delaunay

Precision medicine (PM) refines our understanding of disease prediction and risk, onset and progression in patients, informing better selection and development of evidence-based targeted therapies and associated diagnostics, by taking into account the patient's genomic and other biological characteristics, as well as health status, medications patients are already prescribed and environmental and lifestyle factors.

This chapter first describes the topic of PM, discussing its current application and challenges. These include establishment of economic incentives to develop biomarker testing and regulatory challenges such as market approval of companion diagnostics and treatments, Health Technology Assessment and coverage and funding decisions. Emerging trends in PM are then discussed, including next-generation sequencing (NGS) testing, patient-centric clinical trials, and sharing of data and knowledge.

We thank country delegates and experts, as well as BIAC members, for their comments on earlier versions of this chapter and during the expert meeting of 22 March 2016 and the OECD Health Committee meeting of 28-29 June 2016. We acknowledge in particular suggestions and material provided by Adrian Towse (Office of Health Economics). We also thank Mark Pearson (OECD) and Michel Grignon (McMaster University) for detailed comments on earlier versions of this chapter.

Introduction

Precision medicine (PM) is defined by the United Kingdom's Programme Coordination Group as "[refining] our understanding of disease prediction and risk, onset and progression in patients, informing better selection and development of evidence-based targeted therapies and associated diagnostics. Disease treatment and other interventions are better targeted to take into account the patient's genomic and other biological characteristics, as well as health status, medications patients are already prescribed and environmental and lifestyle factors" (Innovate UK, 2016).

PM involves using a large body of knowledge and techniques (lab tests, imaging) to better understand development of diseases and how to treat them. Information available at the individual level, notably genetic information, as well as the ability to process that information are increasing at a high pace. PM holds the potential to radically transform medicine, with a change of paradigm from "a medicine of organs (heart, liver)" to a medicine targeting cells, molecules and genes. This could lead to a change of disease taxonomy, but more importantly to more accurate, reliable and safer detection and treatment methods. As an example, a few decades ago, blood cancers were grouped in five categories: chronic leukaemia, acute leukaemia, preleukaemia, indolent lymphoma and aggressive lymphoma. Today, medical science recognises 94 types of blood cancers (WHO, 2016), a refinement that contributed to the development of treatments that have improved five-year survival rates from virtually zero to 70% collectively and as high as 82% for some subtypes (PhRMA, 2015; American Cancer Society, 2016).

Since the first sequencing of the human genome in 2003, advances in technology have been tremendous, shortening the time and reducing the costs of genome sequencing. Several OECD countries have invested in PM (Box 5.1). These research initiatives are expected to increase society's knowledge and its capacity to predict, prevent and treat diseases.

Box 5.1. **OECD country initiatives in precision medicine**

Since 1998, deCode Genetics (purchased by Amgen in 2012) has been analysing the genetic information of a large share of the Icelandic population, in relation to data collected through the health care system. This database allowed identification of disease-related genetic variants, initially for rare and complex diseases, but recent studies based on whole genome and whole exome sequencing are beginning to yield rare variants associated with common diseases. Today, deCode Genetics holds genetic information on 100 000 Icelanders (one-third of the population) and whole genome sequencing for more than 2 200.[1]

Estonia made significant advances in implementing PM at a national level with its government-maintained biobank, established in 1999 with a sample representing 5 per cent of the adult population (Milani et al., 2015). This initiative was codified by the Estonian parliament in the Human Genes Research Act of 2000, which lays out the rights of donors, key biobank processes such as ownership and permissions, data protection, prohibition of

Box 5.1. **OECD country initiatives in precision medicine** *(cont.)*

discrimination, financing and supervision. To date, the Estonian Biobank has focused on epidemiological research and genomics of common diseases, and is moving into patient stratification by disease risk estimates, "omics" data and rare variants. Future directions focus on translating findings into health care, supported by a nationwide electronic health record (EHR) system with full access to individual records for all citizens.

In Canada, several organisations are responsible for funding precision health and personalised medicine initiatives. Genome Canada was created as a not-for-profit organisation in 2000 with a mandate to develop and implement a national strategy in genomics research for the benefit of all Canadians. Genome Canada seeks to deliver on this mandate by investing in large-scale genomics research initiatives in sectors of strategic and economic importance to Canada, including health. Since its creation, the federal government has formally committed CAD 1.2 billion to the organisation for the purpose of supporting genomics research. Genome Canada has also raised over CAD 1.3 billion through co-funding commitments. Half of Genome Canada funding is directed towards health-related genomics research. Co-funding partners include provincial governments and agencies, international non-governmental organisations and research institutes, industry, universities and research hospitals. Since 2012, more than CAD 240 million has funded personalised medicine and precision health research through the Canadian Institutes of Health (CIHR) *Personalized Medicine Signature Initiative* (PMSI). Overall, since 2010, CIHR has directly funded CAD 99 million through priority-driven initiatives (including CAD 85 million through the PMSI alone), and CAD 79 million through investigator-initiated initiatives towards improving clinical health outcomes by working towards a system of predictive, preventive and precision care.

In the United Kingdom, the *100 000 Genomes Project*, launched in 2012 with GBP 300 million, will sequence 100 000 genomes from approximately 70 000 people, all National Health Service (NHS) patients with a rare disease, plus their families, and patients with cancer.[2]

In the United States, the *Precision Medicine Initiative* was launched in 2015 with an initial investment of USD 215 million with the aim to collect genetic and environmental information on a cohort of 1 million people.[3]

France's Cancer Plan for the years 2014-19 has personalised medicine as a key goal, including continued development and clinical trials using next-generation sequencing through its National Cancer Institute (INCa). Discussions are under way at the national level on the costs and ethical issues raised by PM: for example, the National Consultative Ethics Committee recently issued an opinion reflecting on the ethics of high-speed DNA sequencing technology (Basset et al., 2016). The strategic plan *France médecine génomique*, released in 2016 and adopting a wider approach, sets out three broad objectives: consolidate France's leading position in health genomics; implement generic health care pathway with good access to genomic medicines for all patients with cancer, rare diseases or more common diseases by 2025; and ensure 235 000 genome sequencings every year by 2020 for all patients with rare diseases and their families and for 50 000 patients with metastatic/refractory cancer. Strategic objectives are further detailed in operational goals (Aviesan, 2016).

1. *www.wired.com/2015/03/iceland-worlds-greatest-genetic-laboratory/.*
2. *www.genomicsengland.co.uk/the-100000-genomes-project/.*
3. *www.whitehouse.gov/the-press-office/2015/01/30/fact-sheet-president-obama-s-precision-medicine-initiative.*

Section 1 of this chapter analyses the integration of PM in current clinical practice and the specific challenges it raises, focusing on pharmaceutical treatments. Section 2 explores emerging trends and conditions for realising the full potential of PM.

1. Precision medicine in today's practice and associated challenges

Until now, precision medicine has mainly – though not only – found concrete applications in pharmaceutical treatments. In this area, personalised medicine and precision medicine (PM) are often used synonymously (FDA, 2013) and refer to the administration of "the right dose of the right drug to the right person at the right time" (Faulkner et al., 2012). PM involves identification of a biomarker that will be used to guide the therapeutic strategy (Box 5.2). Biomarker tests may be used, for instance: to stratify patients into two categories – those who will get the treatment and those who will not because the evidence shows that they will not benefit from it (stratified medicine); to identify rare diseases for which a treatment is available; or to adapt doses in pharmaceutical treatments.

Box 5.2. **Biomarkers, diagnostic and genomic tests**

A biomarker (biological marker) is a biological molecule found in blood, other body fluids, or tissues that is a sign of a normal or abnormal process, or of a condition or disease. It is also called a molecular marker and a signature molecule.

Different types of biomarkers exist with different purposes: predisposition biomarkers are used to assess the risk of developing a disease; diagnostic biomarkers are used to identify specific diseases; prognostic biomarkers are used to predict the course of a disease; monitoring biomarkers are used to analyse disease progression; and predictive biomarkers are used to predict response or adverse reactions to a pharmaceutical treatment (Bücheler et al., 2014).

Labelling instructions of "personalised" or "stratified" medicines typically include a reference to a biomarker test, as either a recommendation or as a condition of use, essential for the safe and effective use of the product. It can be a test of proteins, metabolites, essential elements, tracers or other categories of in vitro diagnostic (IVD) (Agarwal et al., 2015). In some cases, labelling instructions refer to a specific diagnostic device, most often commercially developed (a "companion diagnostic").

An in vitro companion diagnostic is a specific diagnostic device that provides essential information for the safe and effective use of a corresponding therapeutic product. It is used to identify before or during treatment patients who are most likely to benefit from the corresponding medical product or patients likely to be at increased risk of serious adverse reactions (FDA, 2014). The use of an in vitro companion diagnostic (IVD) device with a therapeutic product is stipulated in the instructions for use in the labelling of both the diagnostic device and the corresponding therapeutic product, including the labelling of any generic equivalents of the therapeutic product. The drug and diagnostic are thus considered co-dependent technologies.

Some analysts also use the term "complementary diagnostic" to refer to "a diagnostic that is utilised by a health care practitioner to assess disease state and assist in diagnosis, patient management and treatment decisions. Unlike companion diagnostics which are tied to one specific drug and are proven to work with and are approved for use only with that drug, complementary diagnostics can be utilised, independent of one specific therapy but useful to guide therapeutic treatment across the classes of therapies" (Garrison et al., 2016).

Box 5.2. **Biomarkers, diagnostic and genomic tests** *(cont.)*

Next-generation sequencing (NGS), also known as high-throughput sequencing, describes a number of different modern sequencing technologies to sequence DNA and RNA much more quickly and cheaply than the previously used Sanger sequencing. As such, NGS has revolutionised the study of genomics and molecular biology.

Whole genome sequencing (WGS) consists of sequencing individuals' entire genetic code, i.e. reading every letter in their DNA. Only some sections of DNA contain genes. Known as "the exome", these make up about 1% of the genome and give instructions to make all proteins in a person's body. Whole exome sequencing (WES) limits investigation to these parts. In contrast with other types of tests, these tests are not designed to capture predefined data points (Evans et al., 2015).

PM is developing rapidly (Ehmann et al., 2015; PMC, 2015a, 2015b, 2016). The PharmGKB[1] lists about 230 medicines with a label that has pharmacogenetic information, approved by the US, European, Japanese and/or Canadian regulatory agency. Labelling instructions specify whether a test is "required" or "recommended" before using a pharmaceutical treatment, or whether the pharmacogenetic information is considered actionable or just informative.[2] For a single product, the role of the biomarker in labelling instructions may vary across countries.[3] The number of new "personalised medicines" approved has increased in recent years, and such treatments accounted for more than 25% of drugs approved by the US Food and Drug Administration (FDA) in 2015 (PMC, 2015a, 2015b, 2016).

Many more personalised medicines are in the pipeline. In 2015, the Tufts Center for the Study of Drug Development surveyed 15 leading companies manufacturing personalised medicines. The share of the pipeline that relies on biomarker data decreases as products move downstream, from 60% in preclinical to 50% in early clinical development and 30% in late development. This may reflect the impact of main challenges reported by companies in the development of personalised medicines; i.e. scientific or regulatory hurdles (such as validating biomarkers for labelling purposes) and reimbursement issues (such as proving clinical utility). The proportion of "personalised treatments" in development is particularly high in oncology, due to a conjunction of scientific and business opportunities, but companies are also increasingly working on treatments for neuropsychiatric disorders, cardiology conditions or immunology and inflammatory conditions (Tufts Center for the Study of Drug Development, 2015; Milne et al., 2016).

1.1. *Companies have incentives to develop personalised medicines*

Economic incentives to develop commercial diagnostic tests and personalised medicines depend on a number of factors, including timing. The development processes of a personalised medicine and its associated biomarker test are not always concomitant. Some predictive biomarker tests exist before the medicine is developed, others are co-developed with the pharmaceutical treatment, and in some cases, the test is developed after the medicine itself. Although an increasing number of products have information on the label that either suggests or requires use of a companion diagnostic,[4] as of 2014 only seven had actually been co-developed (Cohen and Felix, 2014; Agarwal et al., 2015).

The respective timing of development of a treatment and a relevant biomarker affects the associated economic incentives. Identifying a biomarker in the early stages of drug development, thereby allowing stratification of the population into respondents and non-respondents (or people for whom the harm will be higher than the benefits), usually reduces the time and cost of development and increases the chances of success (Jørgensen, 2016). In addition, the manufacturer may be able to claim a high price for the high response rate. By contrast, when a biomarker is discovered after a drug's launch, the manufacturer will not be able to reap these benefits, as prices set at market entry are unlikely to increase in most OECD health care systems – with the notable exception of the United States. This means that companies can only lose market sales (Garrison and Towse, 2014).[5] On the other hand, identifying population targets with a higher response rate may alleviate payers' reluctance to cover a medicine.

Current trends suggest that the development of personalised medicine is attractive for pharmaceutical companies. These companies are increasingly adopting niche strategies, focusing research on medicines developed for relatively small target populations and claiming high prices in an attempt to secure adequate return on investment. In some cases, biomarkers may define a target population so narrowly that the developer qualifies for orphan drug status and the associated development incentives in many OECD member countries.

The incentives for companies to develop commercial biomarker diagnostic tests are less clear. Diagnostic tests typically have a short lifecycle and face competition from "home-brew" laboratory-developed tests (LDT) and they struggle to capture a share of the value of PM (Trusheim and Berndt, 2015). Garrison and Towse (2014) explored several incentive scenarios for developing personalised medicines, varying factors such as pricing policies, timing of development for drug and companion diagnostic, and level of intellectual property rights for diagnostic tests. Assuming that the value created by personalised treatment is equal to or higher than the value of the non-personalised treatment,[6] the authors suggest that payers should pay for tests according to their clinical utility or value instead of paying for production costs, as is the current practice.

1.2. Regulatory challenges must be overcome

PM presents unique challenges for regulatory authorities. Personalised medicines and associated diagnostics all present certain issues and their use in combination raises additional questions for agencies that may have separate divisions to review drugs and diagnostics.

Approval of precision medicines presents challenges for evidence review

The main challenge for approval of PMs is the small size of target populations, which makes recruitment for clinical trials difficult and assessment of results more problematic. Thus traditional development and regulatory paradigms may no longer apply, prompting health care systems to consider new methods for assessing safety and efficacy. In addition, personalised medicines often target severely debilitating or life-threatening conditions for which no treatment is available. As a result, regulators are often urged to provide quick access to medicines even when available evidence might not be sufficient by usual standards.

Although no specific pathway exists for approval of personalised medicines, they often de facto benefit from existing licensing pathways that aim to expedite or facilitate approval (e.g. accelerated approval in the United States and conditional approval in Europe; fast-track approval and scientific advice via free protocol assistance and/or development consultation). For example, in 2015, the FDA noted that among its recent targeted therapy approvals, nearly 60% were approved based on one clinical trial plus supporting evidence, and 90% made use of an expedited pathway (Woodcock, 2015). In certain conditions, personalised medicines may also benefit from an early access scheme, before regulatory approval (Leyens et al., 2015).

Approval of diagnostic tests differs across countries and developers

Regulatory requirements for approval of biomarker diagnostic tests differ across countries but also depend on who develops and performs the test. In Europe and the United States, commercial IVDs need regulatory approval while LDTs or in-house tests are not subject to the same level of requirements (Garrison and Towse, 2014).

In Europe, according to the 1998 EU Directive on in vitro diagnostic medical devices, commercial IVDs need to obtain "CE marking" – which verifies conformity with regulatory requirements – to be placed on the market. For IVDs typically used in PM, a "notified body"[7] is in charge of assessing the performance evaluation data produced by the applicant, which must include clinical evidence that the device achieves its intended purpose without exposing users and patients to further risk. By contrast, "in-house" biomarker tests[8] developed by and used in laboratories do not need CE marking (Bücheler et al., 2014). A new EU Regulation, expected to be adopted in spring 2017,[9] imposes new requirements. Manufacturers seeking CE marking for commercial IVDs typically used in PM[10] will have to provide clinical evidence based on data related to analytical performance, scientific validity and clinical performance, and their mutual relationship, as well as a performance evaluation plan for continuous evaluation of performance. In-house tests need to comply with safety and performance requirements but do not need to obtain CE marking if certain conditions are met, including the health institution justifying in its documentation that the target patient group's specific needs cannot be met at all or cannot be met at the appropriate level of performance by an equivalent device already on the market.

In the United States, the FDA assures both the analytic validity (specificity, sensitivity, accuracy and precision) and clinical validity of commercial diagnostic tests through a premarket clearance and approval process. By contrast, LDTs provided by a laboratory offering testing to the public but not to other providers are not subject to FDA review and approval. The FDA has oversight over analyte-specific reagents (through compliance with Good Manufacturing Practices) and the laboratory needs to have an accreditation according to the Clinical Laboratory Improvement Act (CLIA), which looks at how the lab oversees its operations and ensures the quality of tests results (analytic validity). For now, no formal CLIA-approved proficiency testing programme exists for molecular diagnostics, including NGS. Most NGS are conducted in laboratory, although NGS sequencers are beginning to go through the regulatory approval process. The FDA recently issued two draft guidance documents regarding a regulatory framework for LDTs, including genomic tests. The agency proposes to assure analytic and clinical validity of diagnostic tests through its premarket clearance or approval process, which seems challenging, at least for NGS (Evans et al., 2015).

The reliability of molecular testing is crucial to maximise patient outcomes. One study of 3 244 patients in two French cancer centres analysed the results of genetic testing performed by either the FISH diagnostic device [approved by the FDA as a companion diagnostic for Xalkori® (crizotinib)] or by the laboratory-developed IHC. In this case, genetic testing aims to identify patients with an alteration of the ALK gene. The study found that 150 patients were identified as having this ALK gene alteration by either the commercial test or the laboratory-developed test, but only 80 were identified by both (Cabillic et al., 2014). As false negatives can represent a loss of opportunity or increased risks for patients, this highlights the need for further improvements in test validity and reliability.

1.3. *Clinical and economic assessment of biomarker tests and personalised medicines raises a number of issues*

The clinical and economic assessment of targeted therapies ideally requires a joint assessment of the biomarker test and the medicine. However, in many OECD countries, drugs, medical devices and health care procedures are assessed by separate bodies (Auraaen et al., 2016). To ensure co-ordinated and timely consideration of a medicine and its associated diagnostic (considered co-dependent technologies), two countries developed recommendations to jointly assess a personalised or stratified medicine and the companion test. In 2011, Australia introduced an integrative approach to consider each co-dependent package, in which the claim of co-dependency is assessed in quantitative terms across both their clinical and economic consequences. Similarly, in 2014, the High Health Authority in France published guidelines for the joint assessment of the medicine and the companion test as complementary goods (HAS, 2014). As of summer 2015, HAS had already conducted ten joint assessments under these guidelines. Such assessment allows quantifying the benefits associated with the use of the biomarker test to select patients eligible for the treatment.

Beyond timing and institutional issues and the specific case of pharmaceutical targeted treatments, the economic evaluation of personalised medicine raises a number of methodological issues (Annemans et al., 2013; Buchanan et al., 2013; Hatz et al., 2014; Oosterhoff et al., 2016; Phillips et al., 2014, 2016; Shabaruddin et al., 2015).

- The first issue relates to the research question. While some studies evaluate the incremental cost-effectiveness of a new personalised treatment compared to the standard treatment of reference, other studies evaluate the incremental cost-effectiveness of a test-and-treat strategy, which allows identification of responders (or of patients more likely to experience side effects), compared to a strategy where all patients receive the same treatment. While the first case aims to assess the whole personalised strategy, the second case focuses on evaluation of the test. Box 5.3 illustrates the variety of economic evaluations that can be conducted for a specific biomarker test and a personalised treatment for non-small-cell lung cancer (NSCLC).
- A second issue relates to the biomarker test itself. The performance of the diagnostic test (sensitivity, specificity) must be considered along with its predictive value, which depends on the prevalence of the biomarker in the population. Then, the clinical utility of the test (i.e. the extent to which it is likely to improve patients' outcomes) is a crucial factor to measure cost-effectiveness of personalised medicines. In some cases, the drug label does not refer to a specific diagnostic test, which means that the modelling may need to include several different tests. When the biomarker test produces a continuous measure (rather than a positive/negative result), the need to determine the appropriate cut-off point to stratify the population adds to the complexity. The model can be further complicated if the therapeutic strategy involves several tests, in parallel or in sequence. This complexity increases uncertainty.
- Information gaps exist, as in other types of evaluation but may be even higher when the assessment is conducted in early phases of development, to inform strategic decisions

Box 5.3. The cost-effectiveness of testing for epidermal growth factor receptor mutations in patients with non-small-cell lung cancer

Non-small-cell lung cancer (NSCLC) is an example of how PM has altered the prognosis – and the economics – of a disease. Standard first-line treatment for advanced NSCLC involves platinum-based chemotherapy that prolongs survival without disease progression by 4-6 months. In recent years, researchers discovered retrospectively that a patient subgroup with a mutation to the epidermal growth factor receptor (EGFR) tyrosine kinase (EGFR-TK) gene could benefit more from medicines specifically targeting this pathway, the so-called EGFR-TK inhibitors or TKIs. Notably, this class of therapies is less effective than standard chemotherapy in patients who are negative for EGFR-TK mutations.

Researchers and Health Technology Assessment (HTA) agencies in several OECD countries conducted cost-effectiveness analyses on the diagnostic and care pathways associated with advanced NSCLC. In 2013, NICE in the United Kingdom published diagnostic guidance for EGFR-TK mutation testing in adults with advanced or metastatic NSCLC, which complements the separate guidance documents for individual therapies indicated for patients testing positive for these mutations. The diagnostics guidance recommends EGFR-TK testing in patients with previously untreated, locally advanced or metastatic NSCLC, using one of five CE-marked tests or an LDT designed to detect the same mutations. NICE noted insufficient evidence to make recommendations on five additional testing methods, including NGS, but recommended further research directly comparing different mutation test methods and development of a multivariate prediction model for the response to TKI therapy (NICE, 2013).

In subsequent years, additional cost-effectiveness research was conducted in Japan, Mexico and the United States. The Japanese model estimated the incremental cost-effectiveness ratio (ICER) of the strategy "EGFR mutation testing and gefitinib as first-line therapy for patient testing positive" compared to "no testing and treating all patients with standard first-line standard chemotherapy". The base-case analysis leads to an ICER of USD 32 500 per quality-adjusted life year (QALY) gained and the "test and treat" strategy is cost-effective relative to an (unofficial) ICER threshold set at JPY 5-6 million (USD 48 100-57 700) (Narita et al., 2015).

The Mexican study compared the same strategies and noted the sensitivity of the model to the prevalence of EGFR mutations. Assuming an EGFR positive mutation rate of 34.3%, the ICER of the "test and treat" strategy is USD 3 979 per progression-free month. The ICER is lower (USD 3 630) in a scenario where 50% of patients harbour an EGFR mutation but much higher (USD 4 917) if the prevalence of this mutation is 10% (Arrieta et al., 2016).

The US study compared four strategies: 1) "No Test" and treatment with cisplatin-pemetrexed chemotherapy; 2) "Empiric therapy" strategy where chemotherapy is initiated with concurrent testing and continued for four cycles followed by TKI maintenance treatment in mutation-positive patients; 3) "Empiric switch therapy", with initiation of treatment and concurrent testing, where patients initiated first-line chemotherapy and those with mutation-positive tumours switched to TKI immediately upon return of test results; and 4) "Test-treat" strategy, in which treatment was initiated only after results of testing became available. The model assumed a multiplex biomarker testing for both EGFR mutation and overexpression of the anaplastic lymphoma kinase (ALK) gene. It concluded that "Concurrent EGFR mutation and ALK IHC testing with ALK FISH confirmation for tumors that overexpress the ALK protein prior to initiation of therapy yielded an ICER of USD 136 000 per QALY gained compared to no testing and treatment with chemotherapy alone". Empirical strategies are both dominated (Romanus et al., 2015).

during the process, at a time where many variables are unknown (e.g. the management of adverse events whose occurrence and type are not known).

- All experts call for thorough sensitivity analysis, the use of real-life data, and re-evaluation of cost-effectiveness later in the lifecycle.

1.4. *Personalised medicine is sometimes cost-effective*

Several recently published reviews of cost-effectiveness studies assessed the value of personalised medicines. Phillips et al. (2014) identified 59 English-language studies published between 1998 and 2011 examining the cost-effectiveness of testing to define therapeutic strategies. Cancer was the most examined condition (14 studies), followed by infectious diseases (6 studies). Studies typically report several incremental cost-effectiveness ratios (ICERs) due to sensitivity analyses. Phillips and colleagues analysed the distribution of all ICERs and found that 20% of them were negative (indicating that using the test saves costs) while 8% indicated that the strategy was less effective and more costly. In situations where testing increased both benefits and costs, ICERs were below USD 20 000 per QALY in a majority of cases (31% of all reported ICERs) but were also often higher than USD 50 000 (28% of ICERs). Sixty-four per cent of ICERs would fall under a cost-effectiveness threshold set at USD 50 000, suggesting that the strategy is cost-effective.

Hatz et al. (2014) did a systematic review of evaluations of "individualised medicine", published in English and German. All studies compared strategies including a test to guide treatment with non-guided strategies to answer the question "Is treatment with stratification more cost-effective than treatment without stratification?". They identified 84 studies, half of which were from the United States. A majority of studies (80%) were for drug treatments and almost half (46%) were on cancer. As studies most often report several ICERs due to sensitivity analyses, Hatz and colleagues looked at the distributions of "minimum ICERs", "maximum ICERs" and "median ICERs"[11] computed for the "base-case" strategy (recommended by authors of each analysis). Considering the latter, the test-and-treat strategy was dominant in about 20% of cases and had an ICER ranging between 0 and USD 50 000/QALY in 50% of the cases. Cost-effectiveness was very different depending on the type of test: the median values of individual medicine base-case ICERs for studies that included tests for disease prognosis (USD 10 150/QALY) or screening (USD 8 497/QALY) were lower than the medians for studies including tests to stratify patients experiencing adverse effects (USD 39 196/QALY) and studies including tests to stratify patients for responders and non-responders (USD 37 308/QALY). These differences were not assessed to be statistically significant, however. The authors of the review concluded that "the existing evidence confirms neither the vision that individualised medicine is highly cost-effective nor the fear that it is associated with low benefit at high costs". The median ICER reported for all studies analysed is indeed very close to the median value calculated by Neumann et al. (2009) in their review of cost-utility analyses from 30 years of economic evaluation (around USD 22 000/QALY).

More recently, Garattini et al. (2015) reviewed nine studies in European countries evaluating the cost-effectiveness of trastuzumab (in breast cancer) and cetuximab (in colorectal cancer), which are both targeted therapies linked to a biomarker. They noted that the costs of tests were negligible compared to the costs of therapy, which is generally the case in oncology where medicines are very expensive. Of the nine studies, six concluded in favour of targeted therapy and three against. For the sample of products recently approved and analysed by the OECD, however, HTA agencies struggled to assess benefits and cost-effectiveness (Box 5.4).

Box 5.4. **OECD case studies on precision medicines**

During 2015, the OECD conducted case studies to analyse HTA results and funding decisions for six products in eight countries: Australia, Canada, France, Germany, Italy, Spain, Sweden and the United Kingdom. These countries were initially selected to represent a variety of health care systems and institutional designs for assessment, reimbursement and pricing and according to the availability of information on policies and individual products (HTA reports, prices and reimbursement).

Selected products are either 1) "stratified medicines" where a subgroup of patients to be treated is identified by a biomarker; or 2) highly specialised medicines targeting patients with a rare disease identified by a biomarker. The list of products includes elosulfase alpha (Vimizim®), ibrutinib (Imbruvica®), idelalisib (Zydelig®), obinutuzumab (Gazyvaro®/ Gazyva®), trametinib (Mekinist®) and alipogene tiparvovec (Glybera®). More details are provided in Annex 5.A1. This sample does not cover all treatments associated with a biomarker but illustrates challenges faced by HTA agencies and payers in charge of assessing and making coverage decisions.

For all but one product, biomarker tests were developed and performed by laboratories and no commercial test was available. For Mekinist®, a commercial companion test was available but with no market exclusivity, allowing tests to be performed by laboratory platforms. Two products (Zydelig® and Imbruvica®) have the same biomarker. For some of the medicines of the OECD sample, the biomarker test allows stratifying patients (e.g. chronic lymphocytic leukaemia with a deletion in chromosome 17p or a mutation of the TP53 gene).

HTA agencies struggled to assess benefits and cost-effectiveness

In the sample, three out of the six assessments performed for Vimizim® found no demonstration of clinical benefit. All assessments of Zydelig® concluded that clinical benefit was uncertain or not quantifiable, as was the case for five out of six assessments for Gazyvaro®. Study designs are often inadequate to demonstrate clinical benefit, due to the inexistence of a standard reference treatment (especially when there is a high unmet medical need), to small numbers of patients, and to poorly conceived subgroup analyses.

Incremental cost-effectiveness ratios (ICERs) of selected treatments were estimated with a wide degree of uncertainty. In Canada, for instance, the ICER for Vimizim® ranged from EUR 1.9 to 4.0 million per QALY. The variability in ICERs is explained by several factors: comparators or standard of care are ill-defined (e.g. Imbruvica® in Canada); studies are ill-designed (lack of power or insufficient data (e.g. Zydelig® in England); and outcomes are not well-defined or their link with the disease is not demonstrated (e.g. Vimizim®).

Funding decisions generally followed HTA agencies' recommendations

In Australia, the Pharmaceutical Benefits Advisory Committee (PBAC) considered both Mekinist® and Gazyvaro® twice. After PBAC's initial decision to not recommend listing in each case, both were listed after PBAC subsequently recommended listing; Gazyvaro® with a price arrangement, and Mekinist® with a requirement to provide additional clinical evidence. As observed in other studies, countries using ICERs issued negative recommendations more often than countries not relying on cost-effectiveness analysis to make their decisions.

Managed Entry Agreements (MEAs) were concluded for products selected for case studies. They were generally concluded at the time of reimbursement/pricing decision, as was the case for instance for Vimizim® and Zydelig® in Italy, for Gazyvaro® in England, for Mekinist® in Canada, and for Gazyvaro® and Mekinist® in Australia.

1.5. *Coverage and funding of personalised and precision medicines are often complex*

Coverage decisions and funding streams for personalised medicine are based on a variety of factors, including the necessity to perform (and finance) a diagnostic test, the imperative to provide quick access to patients, sometimes before the end of the evaluation/decision process, and the challenge of high prices claimed by companies.

Coverage and pricing of pharmaceuticals are described elsewhere in this report. Basically, OECD countries have not adopted specific policies for funding or pricing of personalised medicines. These often benefit from pathways used for high-cost treatments (see Chapter 3), including Managed Entry Agreements (MEAs). MEAs are most often used for medicines with variable or uncertain benefits or cost-effectiveness. Some of them consist merely of confidential discounts such as volume-price agreements, but others link the price paid to the performance of the product in real life.

Coverage and funding of the diagnostic test itself are commonly provided through cost-based fees in outpatient care and through regular hospital funding streams when used in inpatient care (see examples in Table 5.1). In some countries, extra-funding is provided on top of diagnosis-related group (DRG) payments to hospitals to encourage adoption of new technologies.

Table 5.1. **Funding/reimbursement of diagnostic tests in selected OECD countries**

	Ambulatory settings	Hospital settings
Canada	N.a.	Hospital laboratories are paid through global budget. Any tests and services offered, including genetic tests, must therefore be subsumed within the available budget. Some provinces provide specific funding for certain designated tests.
France	Code in fee schedule for medical procedures and/or laboratory tests.	Funding through DRG payments or funding through extra-payments on top of diagnosis-related groups (DRGs). Temporary funding by National Institute of Cancer (Ministry of Health and pharma companies) during the diffusion phase and pending regular funding.
Germany	Code in the Uniform Value Scale (fee schedule), reimbursement possible when no code exists by similarity or agreement between the manufacturer and the sickness fund.	Included in DRG payment when a procedure code exists. Temporary funding process pending procedure code through individual applications from hospitals.
Italy	In principle, new codes in the fee schedule, but the fee schedule is not frequently updated. Possible funding from regional budget or from the company selling the medicine.	Included in DRG payments. Extra-funding possible from regional budget or from the company selling the medicine.
Spain	Most tests (including lab tests) are performed in hospital outpatient settings. Hospitals are paid through global budget. The decision to fund the test is made at hospital level. Commercial tests are purchased through calls for tender.	No specific funding. Hospitals are paid through global budgets.
United Kingdom (England)	Laboratories operate with annual budgets. Companies often provide funding for testing in the diffusion phase.	Funding of laboratory tests through global budgets or fee-for-service (FFS).
United States (Medicare)	Code in fee schedule for medical procedures and/or laboratory tests, if covered (transition to MolPath codes in 2014).	Included in DRG payments.

Source: Cohen, J.P. and A.E. Felix (2014), "Personalized Medicine's Bottleneck: Diagnostic Test Evidence and Reimbursement", *Journal of Perzonalized Medicine*, Vol. 4, pp. 163-175. Bücheler, M. et al. (2014), "Personalised Medicine in Europe – Enhancing Patient Access to Pharmaceutical drug-Diagnostic Companion Products", *White Paper*, Luxembourg.

2. Emerging trends in precision medicine

Advances in science and information capacities are pushing for an increased use of next-generation sequencing and a higher integration of research and clinical practices. The sections below describe current trends in these two areas and associated challenges.

2.1. *Next-generation sequencing methods are increasingly used*

Until recently, genetic testing often focused on individual biomarkers or a limited set of biomarkers. Due to massive reductions in the cost of genome sequencing, next-generation sequencing (NGS) technologies are expected to become more effective and potentially more cost-effective than current biomarker tests (Bücheler et al., 2014; Van den Bulcke et al., 2015). The implementation of NGS methods in clinical practice raises a number of challenges. The first challenge for regulatory authorities and payers is to establish the clinical utility of such tests. Whole genome sequencing (WGS) detects more than 3.5 million variants in a typical person, 0.5 million of which are rare or novel. At least 90 to 125 variants would merit further evaluation for clinical significance on the basis of current knowledge, but for most variants, clinical implications, if any, are unknown as yet.[12]

Most often, a diagnostic test is considered clinically relevant when the result can be used by the physician to make a therapeutic decision. Thus, an important consideration for the actionability of a gene-drug relationship is the availability of a therapy. So far, only a small number of the 19 000 human genes are considered to be clinically actionable for germline pharmacogenomics. Beyond "actionability", however, whole exome sequencing (WES) may be a rational diagnostic approach, preferred to conventional genetic testing, for patients with a suspected genetic disease on a "diagnostic odyssey" (Lazaridis et al., 2016). The Canadian College of Medical Geneticists, for instance, made recommendations regarding the use of genome-wide sequencing of germline DNA in the context of diagnosis of monogenic diseases (see Box 5.5.).

Box 5.5. **Recommendations of the Canadian College of Medical Geneticists regarding the use of genome-wide sequencing of germline DNA in the context of diagnosis of monogenic diseases**

The Canadian College of Medical Geneticists recently published a position statement on monogenic diseases to provide recommendations for Canadian medical geneticists, clinical laboratory geneticists, genetic counsellors and other physicians regarding the use of genome-wide sequencing of germline DNA in the context of clinical genetic diagnosis. The statement was developed to facilitate the clinical translation and development of best practices for clinical genome-wide sequencing for genetic diagnosis of monogenic diseases in Canada. It does not address the clinical application of this technology in other fields such as molecular investigation of cancer or for population screening of healthy individuals. The specific recommendations are:

- Clinical genome-wide sequencing is an appropriate approach in the diagnostic assessment of a patient for whom there is suspicion of a significant monogenic disease that is associated with a high degree of genetic heterogeneity, or where specific genetic tests have failed to provide a diagnosis.
- Until the benefits of reporting incidental findings are established, the College does not endorse the intentional clinical analysis of disease-associated genes other than those linked to the primary indication.
- Clinicians should provide genetic counselling and obtain informed consent prior to undertaking clinical genome-wide sequencing. Counselling should include discussion of the limitations of testing, likelihood and implications of diagnosis and incidental findings, and the potential need for further analysis to facilitate clinical interpretation, including studies performed in a research setting. These recommendations will be routinely re-evaluated as knowledge of diagnostic and clinical utility of clinical genome-wide sequencing improves.

Source: http://jmg.bmj.com/content/early/2015/05/07/jmedgenet-2015-103144.full.pdf+html.

Next-generation sequencing is increasingly used in oncology

In oncology, multiplex tests – testing several biomarkers at the same time – are already developing. For instance, three diagnostic tests in breast cancer now allow simultaneous testing for 12, 21 and 70 genes. However, NGS methods are particularly attractive for their ability to compensate for limitations on the quantity of tissue available for testing and to detect most genetic alterations of therapeutically relevant cancer genes in a single assay. NGS may be preferred to individual biomarker tests associated with select treatments. Figure 5.1 represents the expected trends in the use of different types of tests in oncology in France.

Figure 5.1. **Recent and projected number of oncology patients diagnosed using molecular testing in France, 2014-20**

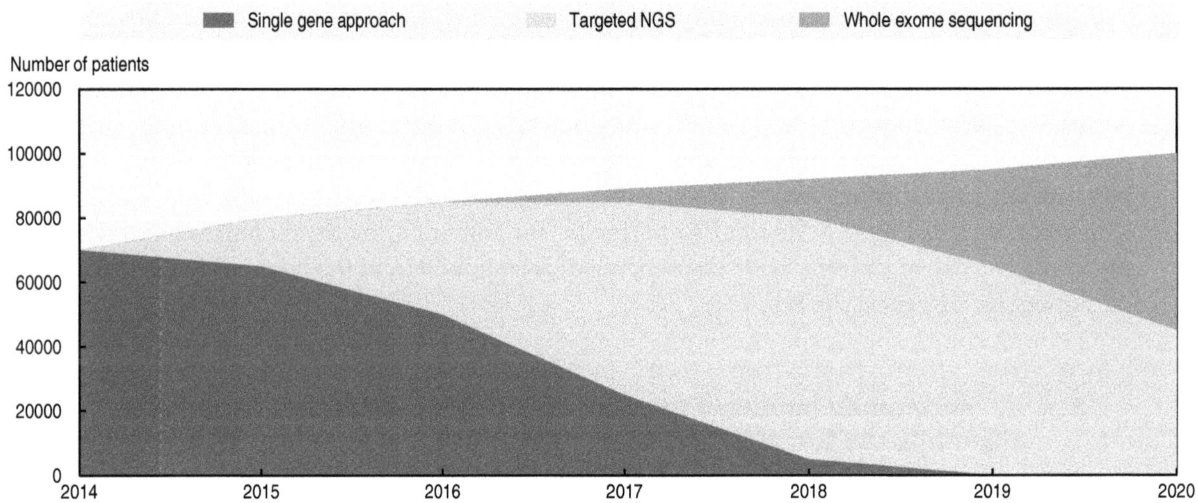

Source: Information provided by the French National Cancer Institute.

StatLink http://dx.doi.org/10.1787/888933442969

In 2015, the Belgian Health Care Knowledge Centre (KCE) conducted research on options to introduce NGS panel tests in oncology and haemato-oncology in the Belgian health care system, including markers for patient selection, targeted therapy, diagnosis confirmation, and prognosis (Van den Bulcke et al., 2015). This research focused on clinical and cost-effectiveness, international policies, and financing options during a period of coverage with evidence development (CED).[13] It reviewed methods for molecular diagnostics and NGS technology and classified biomarkers according to levels of acceptance of their clinical utility. While KCE recognises the opportunities NGS technology provides to realise targeted therapy, it concludes that it is necessary to further standardise the processes for its applications in routine care and in clinical trials. In terms of reimbursement, KCE noted the frequent disconnect between both development and review of a medicine and its companion diagnostic. NGS may replace the recent increase of molecular tests, therefore KCE calculated the projected utilisation and reimbursement rates sustainable at current budget levels in Belgium. The report concluded with a proposed system for the registration and billing of markers for the characterisation of malignancies during the diagnostic workup, including registering the test and its result in KCE's national cancer registry.

Countries need to prepare to further implement next-generation sequencing

Continued implementation of NGS requires a certain number of conditions to be fulfilled. First, providers should provide pre-testing counselling, obtain patient consent, and offer patients the possibility to decline testing or some aspects of reporting. Second, clinicians need to be trained to overcome the current discomfort they experience when using these tools. It is necessary to provide physicians with guidelines on how to interpret and deploy generic variants to improve their prescribing. As an example, the US Centers for Disease Control and Prevention (CDC) publishes guidelines and classifies a number of genomic tests in thirds, according to the level of evidence of their clinical utility.[14] Third, the reporting of incidental findings needs to be regulated, especially for the 56 genes containing mutations considered to be clinically actionable. Finally, reimbursement policies should seek to better understand how technical and professional services should be valued (Deverka and Dreyfus, 2014).

The overall cost of NGS, however, might often be underestimated. Deverka and Dreyfus (2014) noted that the NGS process includes three components: pre-analytics and assay; bioinformatics (database management, data extraction, computational biology and biostatistics); and professional interpretation and services (conveying results to the patient and planning the next course of action). The apparent "value proposition" is based on assumption that NGS represents a cost-effective technology platform substitute for a range of molecular, cytogenetic and histocompatibility testing performed by traditional methods and skilled professionals in the lab today. But if the price of the assay component is declining, a lot uncertainty remains about the cost trends for the two other components and how they should be valued. For each whole genome sequenced, an estimated five hours will be needed to communicate relevant information to the patient. The cost of training practicing clinical scientists or doctors in genetics should also be taken into account, although incorporating these diagnostic tests into medical training will help to reduce costs down the road.

Next-generation sequencing could be used in carrier screening

NGS might be cost-effective in carrier screening. Genetic testing of prospective parents to detect carriers of specific inherited recessive diseases is already part of routine obstetrical practice. Professional organisations recommend testing for a limited number of individual diseases in part based on self-reported racial/ethnic background. A recent study based on simulation models suggests that expanded carrier screening may increase the detection of carrier status for a variety of potentially serious genetic conditions compared with current recommendations from professional societies (Haque et al., 2016). Another simulation, assuming that NGS and conventional genotyping have similar costs, suggests that the former offers greater benefit in clinical outcomes and lower total health care cost for carrier screening of 14 of the recessive disorders for which medical society guidelines recommend screening (Azimi et al., 2016). These studies need to be confirmed with prospective studies.

Consumers are demanding more genetic testing

In addition to development of PM via "traditional" clinical pathways, the digital and genomic eras ushered in an elevated public desire for health information. This has resulted in a number of commercial direct-to-consumer genome sequencing services such as 23andMe, uBiome, DNAfit and VeritasGenetics. Such services offer varying analyses, ranging from genealogy to disease susceptibility, leaving regulators to catch up in terms of validating and enforcing their scientific claims, and in addressing privacy issues. In 2014, the FDA asked the company 23andMe to stop offering these services pending appropriate approval (Annas and Elias, 2014).

The development of next-generation sequencing raises a number of ethical questions

The development of NGS raises a number of ethical issues that will need to be addressed. For instance, who is the owner of the information generated and who has access to it? Can individuals access their own data and share them with specialists over their lifetime? What are the implications for insurance coverage? These questions are not addressed in this chapter but certainly require policy makers' attention.

2.2. The move is towards more efficient research and quicker integration in clinical practice

Precision medicine holds the potential to make research and development (R&D) more efficient and to encourage translational research.

Patient-centric trials are used for therapeutic development

The current model of clinical trials occurs in four phases, with a premium on randomised trials. Biomarkers are now used to drive the selection of patients for trials; however, when a biomarker has a low prevalence, the number of patients to be selected becomes an issue. This limitation has led to new forms of "patient-centric development" (Schork, 2015). Umbrella studies typically investigate a single tumour type selected according to the biomarkers relevant to one or more candidate drugs and patients are directed towards different arms (and different therapeutics) according to the molecular characteristics of their tumour. Basket studies select tumours according to their molecular characteristics and biomarkers but are conducted irrespective of tumour type, focusing instead one or a few specific biomarker(s). Multiplex diagnostic assays are often used to assign participants to different candidate drugs, creating a network of trials (Biankin et al., 2015).

Further integration of research and clinical practice is seen by some experts as an imperative. In cancer for instance, Mahon and Tenenbaum (2015) state that conventional clinical trials are no longer the best solution and that even more innovative approaches, such as adaptive trials, basket trials and umbrella trials, are not enough to reap all the benefits of PM because "with thousands of subtypes of cancer and tens thousands of drug combination to test, there simply are not enough patients to go around".[15] They suggest regarding each patient as an opportunity to learn as much as possible about cancer biology and therapies and switching to "N-of-1" clinical studies.

Mahon and Tenenbaum (2015) propose to implement closed learning loops, based on observational, stratified data, and including the following steps:

- First, patient biopsies should be run through modern, low-cost molecular diagnostic panels to identify potential, clinically actionable mutations (50-100 targets). Clinicians would only report on markers with proven utility and be informed on trial recruitment opportunities. The remaining information should be used for research until clinical utility is established. This step requires patient consent and the funding of the treatment and the test.
- Second, they suggest reporting on treatment and standardised outcome metrics (e.g. tumour progression and survival) in an anonymised central registry. Mining data would allow discovering important signals on responding and non-responding cohorts.

- Third, these cohorts would be referred to in clinical trials and "N-of-1" studies, the results of which would be added to the biomarker panel and database.

The model has many advantages, such as: increased options for patients by facilitating access to stratified trials and special access programmes (e.g. France's molecular diagnostics programme); improvement of health care systems' performance by identifying variations in outcomes, cost and other value metrics; continuous diagnostic improvement; faster and more effective drug development; and a better understanding of the complexity of cancer.

Information sharing would be a crucial element of such an approach (Box 5.6). Mahon and Tenenbaum suggest designing an "open garden", allowing competing interests to collaborate and create novel research and service models (good examples are standardised molecular diagnostics in France through INCa's national laboratory service, and the United Kingdom's taxonomy of cancer treatments). This would require developing a good data infrastructure and solving ethical problems of consent and privacy.[16] Providers and clinicians need electronic decision support tools, while payers need information to support reimbursement policies and optimise the entire care pathway. Such a database could be financed through fees to access data or through a pre-competitive (for-profit) consortium funded by all stakeholders likely to benefit, including pharmaceutical companies and payers. Public-private-partnership (PPP) is seen as a good opportunity to combine results-oriented management and a social mission (Mahon and Tenenbaum, 2015). In any case, co-ordinated efforts are needed, to take stock of ongoing research on personalised medicines, especially in oncology, to avoid duplication of research and concentration of all research efforts depriving other promising avenues of appropriate resources (Tannock and Hickman, 2016).

Box 5.6. **Examples of initiatives to promote data sharing**

The Global Alliance for Genomics and Health was formed to help accelerate the potential of genomic medicine to advance human health. It brings together 427 leading institutions in 41 countries working in health care, research, disease advocacy, life science, and information and communications technology (ICT). The partners in the Global Alliance are working together to create a common framework of harmonised approaches to enable the responsible, voluntary and secure sharing of genomic and clinical data.

The International Cancer Genome Consortium (ICGC) was organised to launch and co-ordinate a large number of research projects that have the common aim of elucidating comprehensively the genomic changes present in many forms of cancers that contribute to the burden of disease in people throughout the world. The primary goals of the ICGC are to 1) generate comprehensive catalogues of genomic abnormalities (somatic mutations, abnormal expression of genes, epigenetic modifications) in tumours from 50 different cancer types and/or subtypes which are of clinical and societal importance across the globe, and 2) make the data available to the entire research community as rapidly as possible, and with minimal restrictions, to accelerate research into the causes and control of cancer. The ICGC facilitates communication among members and provides a forum for co-ordination with the objective of maximising efficiency among scientists working to understand, treat and prevent these diseases.

The Public Population Project in Genomics and Society (P^3G) is an international not-for-profit consortium dedicated to the development and management of multidisciplinary policy infrastructures and research consortia. Through its tools and services, P^3G helps the international research community prepare and propose more effective health care strategies

Box 5.6. **Examples of initiatives to promote data sharing** *(cont.)*

aimed at disease prevention, tailoring of treatments and promotion of the health of individuals, families and communities. P³G's mission is to lead, catalyse and co-ordinate international efforts and expertise to optimise the use of studies, biobanks, research databases and other similar health and social research infrastructures. P³G is committed to: maintaining a global vision of the scientific, technical, ethical, legal, social environmental, economic and behavioural issues that need to be addressed; promoting pre-competitive data sharing while respecting all applicable legal and ethical obligations; and supporting and enabling wide access to research tools and expertise.

Lung-MAP (Lung Cancer Master Protocol) uses comprehensive genetic screening to identify mutations in lung cancer patients to direct them to a specific investigational treatment, all operating under a single clinical trial protocol. Sharing information and resources accelerates drug development and increases trial efficiency, delivering new medicines to patients faster. Lung-MAP is a unique public-private partnership (PPP) between patient and disease advocacy groups, biopharmaceutical companies, the National Cancer Institute in the United States, the Foundation for the National Institutes of Health, and SWOG Cancer Research Consortium. Unlike more traditional study designs, Lung-MAP provides a treatment option for everyone: patients are directed to different treatments so everyone has access to an active therapy.

The Biomarkers Consortium combines expertise and resources to rapidly identify, develop and qualify biomarkers, which will then advance new therapies and guide improvements in regulatory and clinical decision making. Partners include biopharmaceutical companies, the US National Institute of Health, CMS, FDA, and patient and disease organisations.

Source: www.p3g.org/about-p3g, http://icgc.org/, http://genomicsandhealth.org.

Aronson (2015) also insists on the need for HTA to switch from a technology-centred to a patient-centred approach. This would require the development of outcome measurement, comparative effectiveness research, and real-world evidence (RWE). There is a scientific and social interest in maximising the use of data collected.

Additional development is needed to fully realise the potential of pharmacogenomics and precision medicine

According to Relling and Evans (2015), the potential of pharmacogenomics is immense but still needs to be realised. It is now known that the effect of a medicine can be affected by both germline (mainly inherited) and somatic (acquired) genetic variations. In addition, the genetic determinants of tolerance vary across populations. In cancer, both inherited and somatically acquired variants can influence a patient's response to treatment. In infectious diseases, genetic variations can affect a pathogen's sensitivity to antibiotics. Apart from cancer and infectious diseases, genetic variations of interest are primarily in germline DNA. With this in mind, Relling and Evans (2015) analysed the utility of performing early sequencing of the germline genome in patients for use over the lifecycle of new investigations/interpretation. In cancer, they suggest moving from a reactive approach (in which a fresh genetic test is ordered every time it is required) to a pre-emptive approach (in which a single sample is assessed for many likely-to-be-actionable genes at the same time).

In addition to the increasing array of genetic biomarkers affecting diagnosis and treatment of the various conditions discussed above, understanding of the interactions between genes and environment in defining patterns of disease and treatment is also growing. Environmental factors can be internal to the human body (epi-genomics, microbiome) or external exposures (public health factors such as pollution, diet, etc.). As additional data become available to more precisely define these relationships, medicine and health can truly achieve their potential to become more personalised.

Conclusion

PM holds the potential to profoundly transform medicine and health care and enhance population health. While the range of interventions guided by PM is potentially wide, current applications mainly aim to tailor treatments to patients according to their biological characteristics to make them safer and more effective. An increasing number of medicines in development are associated with a biomarker test, used either to select patients to treat or to adapt administration or monitoring of adverse effects. These trends raise a number of challenges that governments and stakeholders must address:

- Clinical trials are taking new, adaptive forms to enable PM. They do so because personalised medicines often target small patient groups, making patient recruitment difficult, but also to be more reactive to new information, which is generated at a high pace. These changes may require adaptations from regulatory science and from regulatory agencies, so that they can fulfil their mission of guaranteeing access to safe and effective treatments.
- The regulation of biomarker tests needs to be improved. Evidentiary requirements differ across settings and across countries and do not guarantee a consistent level of sensitivity/specificity, leading to loss of opportunity or greater risks for patients. International co-operation in the development of evidentiary requirements could benefit both developers and patients.
- Evidentiary requirements for approval of medicines might also benefit from international co-operation. Stratification of patients according to a biomarker is not always based on strong evidence that the medicine would not work in non-selected patients. Differences in labelling instructions of medicines associated with pharmacogenomics biomarkers approved in different regions of the world show that regulatory approval standards are not yet harmonised.
- In many OECD countries, new products or services go through HTA to determine whether they should be covered and at what price. Some countries defined specific pathways to jointly assess stratified medicines and the associated biomarker test (e.g. France, Australia), which is a good step towards ensuring timely assessment of co-dependent products.
- The economic assessment of test-guided therapeutic strategies is more complex than other assessments, notably because of the characteristics of the diagnostic tests (sensibility, specificity, predictive value) and their clinical utility (e.g. ability to improve health outcomes). These higher layers of complexity are usually addressed through sensitivity analyses. Reviews of recent economic evaluation studies suggest that personalised medicine is no more and no less cost-effective than other technologies, however. They are cost-saving in a minority of cases but most often increase both costs and benefits.

- Regulatory and HTA agencies are increasingly co-operating to speed access to new treatments and to send consistent messages to developers about their expectations for evidentiary requirements (methods, outcomes of interest, etc.). International co-operation is developing at the European level (where regulation is regional and HTA national) but could further develop at the international level.
- Health care payers must decide how and how much they pay for diagnostic tests and targeted therapies. While pharmaceutical pricing claims to include some form of value-based pricing, diagnostic tests are often paid through global budgets or fee-for-service (FFS) based on the costs of producing these services. Several experts advocate for value-based pricing for diagnostic tests and propose methods and criteria to account for value beyond cost-effectiveness. But concrete methods to assess such value still need to be defined. Such an approach might be complicated by increased use of multiplex and NGS tests, the clinical utility of which is more difficult to establish.
- Governments and stakeholders need to reflect on new ways to pay for patient pathways to ensure equitable access to personalised treatments and link payments to health outcomes. Effective economic assessment methodologies are key to justifying integration into health care systems.

Realising the full potential of PM requires not only adapting regulation, HTA and coverage, but also efforts to educate doctors and other health care personnel to make them comfortable with using new tools, especially diagnostics and information systems.

Ethical issues need to be addressed, especially those related to genomic testing access and the potential consequences on people's well-being, behaviour and privacy. While populations in individual countries might have differing views on the risks and benefits of personalised medicines, joining forces at an international level to identify these challenges and imagine ways to address them may be fruitful. Access to personal information on people's genomic profiles must be regulated, as discussed in Chapter 6.

Strong information systems that allow linkage of genomic data with environmental and health care information will provide a strong foundation for further development of PM. Such systems would allow more efficient research and quicker integration of R&D results in clinical practice, but would also increase development of knowledge about interactions between personal characteristics, behaviours and environment in the development of diseases and serve public health approaches to enhance population health.

That said, despite the enthusiasm for PM and related investment, policy makers should evaluate and prioritise this among other public health and prevention strategies based on the relative costs and benefits (Bayer and Galea, 2015).

Notes

1. See *www.pharmgkb.org/index.jsp*, consulted on 29 October 2016.
2. Labelling instructions including pharmacogenetic information can be classified in four categories: 1) "Testing is required" when the label states or implies that some sort of gene, protein or chromosomal testing, including genetic testing, functional protein assays, cytogenetic studies, etc., should be conducted before using this drug. This requirement may only be for a particular subset of patients; 2) Genetic testing is recommended when the label states or implies that some sort of gene, protein or chromosomal testing, including genetic testing, functional protein assays, cytogenetic studies, etc., is recommended before using this drug. This recommendation may only be for a particular subset of patients; 3) "Actionable PGx" means that the label does not discuss genetic or other testing for gene/protein/chromosomal variants, but does contain information

about changes in efficacy, dosage or toxicity due to such variants. The label may mention contraindication of the drug in a particular subset of patients but does not require or recommend gene, protein or chromosomal testing; and 4) "Informative PGx" means that the label mentions a gene or protein is involved in the metabolism or pharmacodynamics of the drug, but there is no information to suggest that variation in these genes/proteins leads to different response. See *www.pharmgkb.org/page/drugLabelLegend*, consulted on 29 October 2016.

3. Studies confirm that drug labelling requirements vary across regulatory agencies. Labelling instructions of the FDA and EMA do not exactly match. Looking at 18 medicines approved with a reference to a commercial companion diagnostic by both agencies, Agarwal et al. (2015) observed that the use of the test was required by both agencies in 14 cases but only by one of the two in four cases.

4. As of 10 August 2016, the US FDA lists 26 approved commercial companion diagnostic tests (see *www.fda.gov/medicaldevices/productsandmedicalprocedures/invitrodiagnostics/ucm301431.htm*).

5. In certain cases, the "cut-off points" of the test, which determine both the size of the population to treat and the response rate, are another strategic decision for the firm as these parameters are likely to influence prices (Trusheim and Berndt, 2015) and are bound by ethical constraints (e.g. do not deny treatments to patients who would likely benefit from them).

6. They imagine a situation in which 20% of a population of 100 patients treated are responders. In the absence of a biomarker, the value of the drug is assessed based on the average response when treating 100 patients and the drug company captures 100% of the value created (price x volume). Authors then imagine that a biomarker is identified *ex post*, allowing targeting the 20% of responders. They assume that the total value created is higher, because of the "value of knowing" and also because of reduction of the costs of side effects observed in non-respondents.

7. See Chapter 4 of this publication for further details on "notified bodies" in the European Union.

8. In-house biomarker tests are defined by the IVD Directive as "devices manufactured and used only within the same health institution and on the premises of their manufacture or used on premises in the immediate vicinity without having been transferred to another legal entity". EU rules do not affect the right of member states to subject such activities to appropriate protection requirements.

9. The new regulation will apply five years after the entry into force, i.e. spring of 2022 if the adoption planning works as intended.

10. The new regulation clarifies that "companion diagnostics" and "genetic testing" are within its scope. It also provides a definition of "companion diagnostic" that is very close to that of the FDA. Moreover, a specific conformity assessment procedure is set for these diagnostics, with the involvement of a relevant medicines competent authority.

11. When several studies provided estimates for the same test-treat strategy, results were aggregated in a unique median ICER. Monetary values were all converted in constant 2008 USD, using a health-specific purchasing power parities conversion rate.

12. Increasing server capacity and decreasing procedure costs led to the possibility of so-called "genome-wide association studies" in recent years. That is, a patient's entire genome is tested for common variations in the DNA sequence, and those variations are studied alone and in combination at the population level to analyse their potential impact on the risk of developing common diseases. While this approach has been criticised for not yet explaining more genetic variation in the population, examples at both the country (Milani et al., 2015) and review (Visscher et al., 2012) level demonstrate the ability of this approach to identify reliable disease-associated variants. Opportunities for continued and increased international collaboration should be sought to strengthen the power of such studies.

13. In coverage with evidence development (CED) schemes, a health technology is covered during a predefined period during which further evidence will be accumulated on its effectiveness or cost-effectiveness.

14. See *https://phgkb.cdc.gov/GAPPKB/topicStartPage.do*, consulted on 28 October 2016.

15. "Cancer, it turns out, is a highly complex and adaptive set or rare genetic diseases". Of the hundreds of driver genes discovered, only 13 are mutated in more than 5% of patients across cancer. Most are mutated at frequencies around or lower than 1% of patients.

16. Regulatory and Ethics Working Group of the Global Alliance for Genomics and Health – Framework for Responsible Sharing of Genomic and Health-related Data *https://genomicsandhealth.org/files/public/Framework%20for%20Responsible%20Sharing%20of%20Genomic%20and%20Health-Related%20Data%20-%20Version%2010%20September%202014.pdf*.

References

Agarwal, A. et al. (2015), "The Current and Future State of Companion Diagnostics", *Journal of Pharmacogenomics and Personalized Medicine*, Vol. 8, pp. 99-110.

American Cancer Society (2016), *Cancer Facts and Figures 2016*, American Cancer Society, Atlanta.

Annas, G.J. and S. Elias (2014), "23andMe and the FDA", *New England Journal of Medicine*, Vol. 370, No. 11, pp. 985-988.

Annemans, L., K. Redekop and K.Payne (2013), "Current Methodological Issues in the Economic Assessment of Personalized Medicine", *Value in Health*, Vol. 16, pp. S20-S26.

Aronson, N. (2015), "Making Personalised Medicine More Affordable", *Annals of the New York Academy of Sciences*, No. 1346, pp. 81-89.

Arrieta, O. et al. (2016), "Cost-effectiveness Analysis of EGFR Mutation Testing in Patients with Non-small Cell Lung Cancer (NSCLC) with Gefitinib or Carboplatin-paclitaxel", *European Journal of Health Economics*, Vol. 17, pp. 855-863.

Auraaen, A. et al. (2016), "How OECD Health Systems Define the Range of Goods and Services to Be Financed Collectively", *OECD Working Paper*, OECD Publishing, Paris, *http://dx.doi.org/10.1787/5jlnb59ll80x-en*.

Aviesan (2016), "France Médecine Génomique 2025", Alliance Nationale pour les Sciences de la Vie et de la Santé, Paris, *www.gouvernement.fr/sites/default/files/document/document/2016/06/22.06.2016_remise_du_rapport_dyves_levy_-_france_medecine_genomique_2025.pdf*.

Azimi, M. et al. (2016), "Carrier Screening by Next-generation Sequencing: Health Benefits and Cost Effectiveness", *Molecular Genetics & Genomic Medicine*, Vol. 4, No. 3, pp. 292-302.

Basset, C. et al. (2016), "Réflexion éthique sur l'évolution des tests génétiques liée au séquençage de l'ADN humain à très haut debit", Comité Consultatif National d'Éthique pour les sciences de la vie et de la santé, Avis 124, 21 January 2016.

Bayer, R. and S. Galea (2015), "Public Health in the Precision-Medicine Era", *New England Journal of Medicine*, Vol. 373, No. 6, pp. 499-501.

Biankin, A.W., S. Piantadosi and S. Hollingsworth (2015), "Patient Centric Trials for Therapeutic Development in Precision Medicine", *Nature*, Vol. 526, pp. 361-370.

Buchanan, J., S. Wordsworth and A. Schuh (2013), "Issues Surrounding the Health Economic Evaluation of Genomic Technologies", *Pharmacogenomics*, Vol. 14, No. 15, pp. 1833-1847.

Bücheler, M., B. Brüggenjürgen and S. Willich (2014), "Personalised Medicine in Europe – Enhancing Patient Access to Pharmaceutical Drug-diagnostic Companion Products", EPEMED, *White Paper*, Berlin.

Cabillic, F. et al. (2014), "Parallel FISH and Immunohistochemical Studies of ALK Status in 3244 Non-small-cell Lung Cancers Reveal Major Discordances", *Journal of Thoracic Oncology*, Vol. 9, No. 3, pp. 295-306, March.

Cohen, J.P. and A.E. Felix (2014), "Personalized Medicine's Bottleneck: Diagnostic Test Evidence and Reimbursement", *Journal of Perzonalized Medicine, Vol.* 4, pp. 163-175.

De Saunière, A. (2012), "L'accès aux médicaments orphelins en France : entre besoin des patients, soutien à la recherche et politique de prix", Mémoire de l'EHESP, Paris.

Deverka, P. and J. Dreyfus (2014), "Clinical Integration of Next Generation Sequencing: Coverage and Reimbursement Challenges", *Journal of Law, Medicine and Ethics*, Supplement, Fall.

Ehmann, F. et al. (2015), "Pharmacogenomic Information in Drug Labels: European Medicines Agency Perspective", *Pharmacogenomics Journal*, Vol. 15, pp. 201-210.

Evans, B.J., W. Burke and G. Jarvik (2015), "The FDA and Genomic Tests – Getting the Regulation Right", *New England Journal of Medicine*, Vol. 372, No. 23, pp. 2258-2264.

Faulkner, E. et al. (2012), "Challenges in the Development and Reimbursement of Personalized Medicine – Payer and Manufacturer Perspectives and Implications for Health Economics and Outcomes Research: A Report of the ISPOR Personalized Medicine Special Interest Group", *Value in Heath*, Vol. 15, pp. 1162-1171.

FDA – Food and Drug Administration (2014), "In Vitro Companion Diagnostic Devices – Guidance for Industry and Food and Drug Administration Staff", FDA, Washington, DC, *www.fda.gov/downloads/medicaldevices/deviceregulationandguidance/guidancedocuments/ucm262327.pdf*.

FDA (2013), "Paving the Way for Personalized Medicine, FDA's Role in a New Era of Medical Product Development, Washington, DC.

Garattini L., A. Curto and N. Freemantle (2015), "Personalized Medicine and Economic Evaluation in Oncology: All Theory and No Practice?", *Expert Review of Pharmacoeconomics and Outcomes Research*, Vol. 15, No. 5, pp. 733-738.

Garrison, L.P. and A. Towse (2014), "Personalized Medicine: Pricing and Reimbursement Policies as a Potential Barrier to Development and Adoption", in Anthony J. Culyer (ed.), *Encyclopedia of Health Economics*, Vol. 2, Elsevier, pp. 484-490.

Garrison, L., J. Mestre-Ferrandiz and B. Zamora (2016), "The Value of Knowing and Knowing the Value: Improving the Health Technology Assessment of Complementary Diagnostics", *White Paper*, Office of Health Economics and EPEMED.

Haque, I.S. et al. (2016), "Modeled Fetal Risk of Genetic Diseases Identified by Expanded Carrier Screening", *Journal of the American Medical Association*, Vol. 316, No. 7, pp. 734-742.

HAS – Haute Autorité de Santé (2014), "Test compagnon associé à une thérapie ciblée : Définitions et méthode d'évaluation", Guide méthodologique, Haute Autorité de Santé.

Hatz, M.H.M., K. Schremser and W.H. Rogowski (2014), "Is Individualized Medicine More Cost-Effective? A Systematic Review", *PharmacoEconomics*, Vol. 32, pp. 443-455.

Innovate UK (2016), "Mapping the Precision Medicine Landscape", *www.gov.uk/government/uploads/system/uploads/attachment_data/file/483560/Precision_Medicines_Booklet_Final_Web__002_.pdf* (accessed 19 Oct 2016).

Jørgensen, J.T. (2016), "The Importance of Predictive Biomarkers in Oncology Drug Development", *Expert Review of Molecular Diagnostics*, Vol. 16, No. 8, pp. 807-809, *http//dx.doi.org/10.1080/14737159.2016.1199962*.

Lazaridis, K.N. et al. (2016), "Outcome of Whole Exome Sequencing for Diagnostic Odyssey Cases of an Individualized Medicine Clinic: The Mayo Clinic Experience", *Mayo Clinic Proceedings*, Vol. 91, No. 3, pp. 297-307, *http://dx.doi.org/10.1016/j.mayocp.2015.12.018*.

Leyens, L. et al. (2015), "Available Tools to Facilitate Early Patient Access to Medicines in the EU and the USA: Analysis of Conditional Approvals and Implications for Personalised Medicines", *Public Health Genomics*, August.

Mahon, P. and J. Tenenbaum (2015), "Paths to Precision Medicine – A Perspective", *Journal of Precision Medicine*, *www.thejournalofprecisionmedicine.com/wp-content/uploads/2015/01/MAHON-ARTICLE___new.pdf*.

Meckley, L.M. et al. (2010), "Personalized Medicine: Factor Influencing Reimbursement", *Health Policy*, Vol. 94, pp. 91-100.

Milani, L. et al. (2015), "An Epidemiological Perspective of Personalized Medicine: The Estonian Experience", *Journal of Internal Medicine*, Vol. 277, pp. 188-200.

Milne, C.P., J.P. Cohen and R. Chakravarthy (2016), "Where Is Personalized Medicine in Industry Heading?", *Nature Reviews – Drug Discovery*, Vol. 14, pp. 912-813.

Morrison, C. (2015), "$1-million Price Tag Set for Glybera Gene Therapy", *Nature Biotechnology*, Vol. 33, No. 3, pp. 217-218.

Narita, Y. et al. (2015), "Cost-effectiveness Analysis of EGFR Mutation Testing and Gefitinib as First-line Therapy for Non-small Cell Lung Cancer", *Lung Cancer*, Vol. 90, pp. 71-77.

NICE – National Institute for Health and Care Excellence (2013), "EGFR-TK Mutation Testing in Adults with Locally Advanced or Metastatic Non-small-cell-lung Cancer", *Diagnostics Guidance*, 14 August 2013.

Neumann, P.J., C.H. Fang and J.T. Cohen (2009), "30 years of Pharmaceutical Cost-utility Analyses: Growth, Diversity and Methodological Improvement", *Pharmaco Economics*, Vol. 27, No. 10, pp. 861-872.

Oosterhoff, M., M.E. van der Maas and L.M.G. Steuten (2016), "A Systematic Review of Health Economic Evaluations of Diagnostic Biomarkers", *Applied Health Economics and Health Policy*, Vol. 14, pp. 51-65, *http://dx.doi.org/10.1007/s40258-015-0198-x*.

Phillips, K.A., K. Payne and K. Redekop (2016), "Personalized Medicine: Economic Evaluation and Evidence", *World Scientific Handbook of Global Health and Public Policy*, Vol. 3, pp. 123-150.

Phillips, K.A. et al. (2014), "The Economic Value of Personalized Medicine Tests: What We Know and What We Need to Know", *Genetics in Medicine*, Vol. 16, No. 3, pp. 251-257.

PhRMA (2015), "Value of Personalized Medicine", Chartpack, Spring.

PMC – Personalized Medicine Coalition (2016), "2015 Progress Report – Personalized Medicine at FDA, Washington, DC.

PMC (2015a), "FDA 2014 Novel New Drugs Approved", Washington, DC.

PMC (2015b), "Personalised Medicines by the Numbers", Factsheet, Washington, DC.

Relling, M. and W. Evans (2015), "Pharmacogenomics in the Clinic", *Nature*, Vol. 526, pp. 343-350.

Romanus, D. et al. (2015), "Cost-effectiveness of Multiplexed Predictive Biomarker Screening in Non-Small-Cell Lung Cancer", *Journal of Thoracic Oncology*, Vol. 10, No. 4, pp. 586-594, April.

Schork, N.J. (2015), "Time for One-person Trials", *Nature*, Vol. 520, pp. 609-611.

Shabaruddin, F.H. et al. (2015), "Economic Evaluations of Personalized Medicine: Existing Challenges and Current Developments", *Pharmacogenomics and Personalized Medicine*, Vol. 8, pp. 115-126.

Tannock I.F. and J.A. Hickman (2016), "Limits to Personalised Cancer Medicine", *New England Journal of Medicine*, Vol. 375, No. 13, pp. 1289-1294.

Trusheim, M.R. and E.R. Berndt (2015), "An Overview of the Stratified Economics of Stratified Medicine", *NBER Working Paper* No. 21233, Cambridge, United States.

Tufts Center for the Study of Drug Development (2015), "Personalized Medicine Gains Traction but Still Faces Multiple Dhallenges", *Impact Reports*, Vol. 17, No. 3, May/June 2015.

Van den Bulcke, M. et al. (2015), "Next Generation Sequencing Gene Panels for Targeted Therapy in Oncology and Haemato-oncology – Synthesis", *KCE Reports No. 240Cs*, Health Technology Assessment (HTA), Belgian Health Care Knowledge Centre (KCE), Brussels.

Visscher, P.M. et al. (2012), "Five Years of GWAS Discovery", *American Journal of Human Genetics*, Vol. 90, pp. 7-24.

WHO – World Health Organization (2016), *International Classification of Diseases*, 10th Edition (ICD-10), Version 2016, World Health Organization, Geneva, *http://apps.who.int/classifications/icd10/browse/2016/en* (accessed 6 June 2016).

Woodcock, J. (2015), "FDA Continues to Lead in Precision Medicine", *FDA Voice*, 23 March, Washington, DC.

ANNEX 5.A1

Sample of products selected for the 2015 OECD case study

The sample of products selected covers precision medicines. Selected products are either 1) "stratified medicines" where a subgroup of patients to be treated is identified by a biomarker; or 2) highly specialised medicines targeting patients with a rare disease identified by a biomarker.

Six products were selected using the following strategy. First, the list of medicines authorised in 2014 by the US Food and Drug Administration (FDA) was consulted and products were identified as "personalised medicines" by the Personalised Medicine Coalition (PMC, 2015). From this list, only medicines also authorised in Europe were selected. This first step led to selection of two products (Harvoni® and Vimizim®). To extend this list and given that oncology is a major domain for precision medicine, all oncology products approved by the European Medicine Agency associated with a biomarker were selected, and only those also approved in the United States were kept.

Harvoni®, initially part of this selection, was not studied here, to focus on products with small target populations. Glybera®, not yet approved in the United States, was selected as the first gene therapy approved in Europe. It targets a small population (a rare disease) and is now covered in Germany at EUR 1 million per cure (Morrison, 2015).

Selected products are presented in Table 5.A1.1. All of them were approved through special procedures 1) to recognise their innovative character (breakthrough designation, priority review, accelerated approval) or the fact that they treat rare diseases (orphan designation), and/or 2) to take into account the uncertainty about benefits and risks at the time of marketing authorisation (additional monitoring).

Table 5.A1.1. **List of medicines selected for case studies**

Brand name	Active ingredient	Indications approved	Biomarker	Approval pathway Orphan status
Vimizim®	Elosulfase alpha	Treatment of mucopolysaccharidosis type IVA (MPS IVA, also known as Morquio A syndrome)	Genetic biomarker	EU: Orphan designation, Additional monitoring United States: Orphan designation, Paediatric use, Priority review Australia: Orphan status
Imbruvica®	Ibrutinib	Treatment of adult patients with chronic lymphocytic leukaemia (CLL) who have received at least one prior therapy, or in first line in the presence of 17p deletion or TP53 mutation in patients unsuitable for chemo-immunotherapy. Treatment of adult patients with relapsed or refractory mantle cell lymphoma (MCL). Treatment of adult patients with Waldenström's macroglobulinaemia (WM) who have received at least one prior therapy, or in first line treatment for patients unsuitable for chemo immunotherapy.	Burton's Tysosine kinase/ Genetic biomarker	EU: Orphan Designation, Additional monitoring United States: Orphan designation (MCL), Breakthrough, Accelerated approval and priority review
Zydelig®	Idelalisib	In chronic lymphocytic leukaemia (CLL), Zydelig is used in combination with rituximab in patients who have received at least one previous treatment or[1] in patients who have genetic mutations in their cancer cells called 17p deletion or TP53 mutation that make them unsuitable for treatment with a combination of chemotherapy medicines and immunotherapy (treatments that stimulate the immune system to kill cancer cells). In follicular lymphoma (FL), Zydelig is used in patients whose disease has not responded to two previous treatments.	PI3K δ/Genetic biomarker	EU: Additional monitoring United States: Accelerated approval
Gazyvaro®	Obinutuzumab	Used with chlorambucil to treat adult patients with previously untreated chronic lymphocytic leukaemia (CLL).	CD20/Genetic biomarker	EU: Orphan designation, United States: Orphan designation (CCL), Breakthrough, Priority review
Mekinist®	Trametinib	Used as monotherapy or in combination with dabrafenib as indicated for the treatment of adult patients with unresectable or metastatic melanoma with a BRAF V600 mutation[2] (*BRAF V600E or V600K mutations*).[3]	Genetic biomarker	EU: Additional monitoring United States: Orphan designation, Accelerated approval Australia: Orphan status
Glybera®	Alipogene tiparvovec	Indicated for adult patients diagnosed with familial lipoprotein lipase deficiency (LPLD) and suffering from severe or multiple pancreatitis attacks despite dietary fat restrictions. The diagnosis of LPLD has to be confirmed by genetic testing (LPLD).[4]	Genetic biomarker	EU: Orphan designation, Additional monitoring

Note: Indications that are not approved in all countries are in italic.
1. Non-applicable for US and Canadian approval.
2. Indication only available in US and Australian approval.
3. Precision only available in US approval.
4. EMA approval only.
Source: PMC, EMA, FDA, TGA and Santé Canada websites.

New Health Technologies: Managing Access, Value
and Sustainability

Chapter 6

Digital technology: Making better use of health data

by
Luke Slawomirski *and* Jillian Oderkirk

Modern health care systems produce mountains of electronic data, which are now also generated outside health care systems as most aspects of human activity and interaction become digitalised in the modern global economy. The information potentially residing in these data can be very useful to promote health, and to improve health care – a particularly information- and knowledge-intensive industry. This chapter describes various opportunities for harnessing health data, citing examples where the potential is being realised. It discusses the challenges of using health data and sets out a policy framework for managing risks while realising the benefits of health data. The costs of implementing digital technology across societies and health care systems are discussed. This is followed by a more in-depth discussion of the electronic health record (EHR), an important foundation of health information infrastructure. Drawing on the findings from a 2016 study of EHR development and use in 30 OECD countries, health care systems' readiness to use EHR data collected for various purposes – performance monitoring, quality improvement and research – is examined.

The statistical data for Israel are supplied by and under the responsibility of the relevant Israeli authorities. The use of such data by the OECD is without prejudice to the status of the Golan Heights, East Jerusalem and Israeli settlements in the West Bank under the terms of international law.

We thank Ronni Gamzu for his contribution to this work. We thank country delegates and experts, as well as BIAC members, for their comments on earlier versions of this chapter and during the expert meeting of 22 March 2016 and the OECD Health Committee meeting of 28-29 June 2016. We acknowledge in particular suggestions and material provided by Stefano Bonacina (Karolinska Institutet) and Iñaki Gutiérrez Ibarluzea (Osteba).

Introduction

Technological progress has been a defining feature of human history. The last three centuries in particular were punctuated by several advances: combustion engines, mechanisation of industrial processes, and generation of electricity for mass consumption. These leaps in innovation, enabled by new technology, fundamentally changed the way societies and economies are organised – the way people live, work and relate to one another. Humanity is currently experiencing another fundamental technological transformation – the digital age. Just as electrification did in the 20th century, digitalisation is reshaping societies in a profound and far-reaching way in the 21st (OECD, 2016).

The term "digital" describes generating, storing and processing data in a way that is considerably faster and more efficient than any previous means at society's disposal. Data can be described as parcels of raw and unorganised information. Digital technology thus enables meaningful and useful information to be generated and shared, potentially creating much utility and value.

Data are the lifeblood of the modern economy and are increasingly seen as a new factor of production in addition to labour, capital and natural resources (The Economist, 2010; Murdoch and Detsky, 2013). A range of industries across all sectors – police services, commerce, transportation and logistics, finance and politics – recognise the opportunities presented by electronic data, and are using increasingly sophisticated analytical techniques to improve efficiency and value and to tailor services to customers. In a well-known, if slightly disconcerting example, the US retail chain Target is able to ascertain if a woman is pregnant, and accurately estimate the due date based on the purchase data of a small number of products (Duhigg, 2012).

Health care is a particularly information- and knowledge-intensive industry. Some years ago it was foreshadowed that "knowledge is the best enemy of disease [...] the application of what we already know will have a bigger impact on health and disease than any drug or technology likely to be introduced in the next decade" (Pang et al., 2006). Yet health care systems are still said to be "data rich, information poor". The mountains of health-related data generated within health care systems and across societies are not used to their full potential in generating valuable information to help achieve health care system objectives. The health sector seems to be lagging behind other industries in harnessing this potentially transformative technology.

This chapter approaches the use of health data as a potentially transformative and far-reaching process innovation that can improve the way health services function, their outcomes and the value generated across entire systems.[1] The opportunities associated with health data are discussed first. These span all aspects of, and activities within, a health care system. The challenges and risks of using the growing amount of health data are then discussed, including policy implications of managing the risks while maximising the opportunities. These include governance and legislative changes, infrastructure and human capital investment, and socio-technical changes associated with this transformation. The costs and benefits are also discussed, although not much empirical evidence exists about this aspect of digital technology.

The final section includes a more in-depth discussion of the electronic health record (EHR), which refers to the longitudinal electronic record for an individual patient that contains or virtually links together records from multiple electronic medical records (EMRs) that can then be shared (i.e. are interoperable) across health care settings. The EHR aims to contain individual patients' history of contact with the health care system, and is a fundamental component of a health care system's information infrastructure. Countries' readiness to use data collected by EHR systems for various purposes, including performance monitoring, quality improvement and research, is examined. The section presents the findings from a 2016 OECD study into the development and use of EHRs in 30 OECD member and partner countries.

1. Promise and opportunities for health data

Health care systems, both public and private, are generating increasing amounts of electronic data in multiple streams – clinical, diagnostic, administrative, financial, genetic, demographic, behavioural and environmental. For example, more than two billion megabytes are produced annually from mammograms in the United States alone (OECD, 2015d). The proliferation of mobile health (mHealth) innovations – described in Chapter 4 of this report – as well as the digitalisation of just about all facets of human endeavour produce vast amounts of electronic data on health and wellness. Every day, people generate these data in a range of ways: using apps, biosensors, social media and web browsing and simply by tracking their movements and activity with smartphones or portable electronic devices. It is said that individuals now generate their own "digital phenotype" (Jain et al. 2015). This process of datafication – both within and outside of conventional health care system boundaries – will continue (Box 6.1).

Box 6.1. **Big Data**

Big Data is a term used to describe "data whose scale, diversity and complexity require new architecture, techniques, algorithms and analytics to manage them, and to extract value and hidden knowledge from them" (Smith and Suresh-Kumar, 2013). Big Data not only refers to the volume of data in question (although little consensus exists on how "big" the data have to be) but also to their complexity, heterogeneity of format and structure, and the speed at which they are produced. The largest component of Big Data is unstructured (e.g. free text, images, video) and contains considerable amounts of "noise" and uncertainty (e.g. social media data). In short, Big Data is characterised by high volume and velocity and variety of structure and format. Its quality and veracity is questionable (Gandomi and Haider, 2015).

The Big Data phenomenon is slowly encroaching into health care, and some examples cited in this section do entail Big Data analytics and methods. However, the majority of the opportunities and challenges described herein concern conventional health data generated routinely by health services and health care systems. Managing the risks and challenges posed by conventional health data provides a useful platform for dealing with Big Data.

Potentially valuable information is waiting to be uncovered within these mountains of data. The difficulty is that the data are messy and unstructured, continue to flow in multiple streams and are stored separately. For example, a vast amount of information is contained in free text of clinical records, and in diagnostic images. Unstructured data have traditionally been difficult to organise, manage and analyse. This has changed with the confluence of three technological advances:

- Storage: Data can now be stored and managed more efficiently and cheaply.
- Computational capacity: Hardware and software to process data are vastly improved – an example is natural language processing (NLP) and semantic analysis, especially useful for clinical data.
- Machine learning: Algorithms can absorb and learn from raw data without human oversight or instruction.

The opportunities presented by health data concern extracting additional knowledge and information to add value across all aspects and activities of a health care system. These opportunities can be categorised into four overlapping themes: 1) improving patient care; 2) managing the health care system; 3) surveillance and population health; and 4) enabling research (OECD, 2015a). These are discussed below. Their interdependence and complementary nature must be emphasised as the lines between clinical care and disease management, health maintenance, system management and research are increasingly blurring (Aronson and Rehm, 2015).

Realising these opportunities while managing the risks and challenges of using health data, as discussed later in this chapter, can advance the hitherto elusive ideal of a "learning health system" (Olsen et al., 2007). While there is still some way to go, the following sections illustrate how these opportunities are beginning to be realised, and how some health care systems, while (technically speaking) not drawing on the full extent of Big Data yet, are certainly moving in that direction. The examples used below as well as additional examples from a number of sources, including semi-structured interviews with health services, hospitals, payers and insurers, are presented in Box 6.2.

Box 6.2. **Examples of applying health data analytics to improve outcomes**

Kaiser Permanente (KP) United States

- Analysed 15 years of maternal and neonatal data (608 014 live births) to develop a risk-stratification tool enabling detection of sepsis in neonates. This tool significantly reduced antibiotic administration within the 24 hours following birth.
- Used data from 391 000 acute episodes to develop an algorithm predicting the comparative risk of 30-day mortality, enabling more accurate and timely clinical decision making at the bedside and at discharge.
- Used a large acute inpatient dataset to create a bedside alert system for patients at risk of clinical deterioration and transfer to intensive care.
- Studied patterns of screening adherence and glycaemic and blood pressure control among overweight and obese patients using about 165 000 records, with results channelled back to clinical teams to optimise management of diabetic patients.
- Drawing on analysis of outpatient behaviour using ancillary services data, developed a system where patients prescribed cholesterol-lowering drugs are sent automated phone and e-mail reminders. This increased therapeutic adherence and improved cholesterol control across this patient cohort.

Box 6.2. **Examples of applying health data analytics to improve outcomes** *(cont.)*

- Using information derived from the EMR and ancillary datasets, targeted expensive hepatitis C drugs only at patients with the appropriate genetic and clinical indications, aiming to reduce unnecessary spending and maximise clinical outcomes.
- Using a large pathology dataset, found that the national standard of three red blood cells per high power field (HPF) was less predictive of urologic cancer than was four red blood cells, resulting in release of new practice guidelines, and significantly reduced unnecessary exposure to radiation from diagnostic procedures.

Clalit Health Service (CHS) Israel

- Developed an algorithm using integrated patient data to identify multimorbid elderly patients at highest risk of deterioration, enabling a customised and integrated nurse-led intervention currently undergoing clinical trial with very promising results.
- Developed a predictive score for renal failure to identify the most high-risk patients with stage-3 chronic kidney disease. An intervention targeting high-risk patients using customised alerts and quality measures is under way.
- To improve appropriate antibiotic use, linked datasets on episodes of care, antibiotics prescribed/dispensed, pathology results and antibiotic resistance. Information regarding inappropriate use of antibiotics is provided at the clinical level down to individual physicians. Reporting and decision support tools are currently being implemented.
- Analysed data on 400 000 members of lower socio-economic status for disparity in care quality. Implemented a suite of interventions to deliver culturally competent care targeted at this cohort, achieving a 60% improvement in the disparity-associated quality indicators score.
- Used 500 000 records to develop a re-admission risk rating for older patients. This rating is given to patients upon emergency department (ED) admission, alerting caregivers to the risk, enabling effective intervention such as digital discharge plans with direct hospital-clinic communication, and customised alerts. After one year, re-admissions reduced by 5%.

Multiparameter Intelligent Monitoring in Intensive Care (MIMIC)

- Collects raw structured clinical data from over 40 000 ICU admissions including continuous physiologic readings, time-stamped treatments, dosages and clinical conditions. The data are openly shared with researchers from 32 countries.
- Given the data collected, the MIMIC allows analysis and modelling of individual dynamic responses to a physiologic malfunction and to medical interventions. The system is online and freely shared with 600 researchers from 32 countries that have free access to the clinical data under data use agreements (Herland et al., 2014).

Emory University Hospital and Seattle Children's Hospital

- Stream "real-time" data analytics in the intensive care unit (ICU) to enable faster and more reliable detection and clinical decision making, alerting clinicians to trends such as respiratory failure, abnormal heart rhythms and serious infections.
- Use high velocity data analytics to identify medically complex children and to detect clinical deterioration.

Box 6.2. **Examples of applying health data analytics to improve outcomes** *(cont.)*

Data Alliance Collaborative (Carolinas Healthcare System, IBM and Premier Healthcare Alliance)

- Analysed clinical, billing and claims data on over five million patients to create a predictive tool for re-admission risk within 30 days of discharge, and to identify patients at risk for various future complications. The tool has 80% accuracy.
- Geisinger Health System and IBM
- Used language processing code to identify risk of heart failure (HF) using EHR and clinical notes, resulting in a 92.5% positive prediction value with 89.6% sensitivity for HF (Byrd et al., 2014).
- Using 400 000 primary care visits, predicted future HF from asymptomatic presentation, resulting in significantly higher prediction accuracy than ordinary mechanisms (Sun et al., 2012).

FDA Mini-Sentinel Surveillance of Adverse Drug Events

- Uses 380 million person-years of data and over 100 million people to inform post-market surveillance and faster identification of patient safety concerns related to new and existing medical technology. Helps scientists to better understand the potential safety issues associated with medical products.

Boston Children's Hospital

- Uses an algorithm to capture, archive and analyse information to create new critical care best practices and procedures.

Sick Kids Hospital, Toronto

- Analyses streaming data from the ICU to detect medically significant conditions before the clinically detectable onset of medical complications. The platform assists in discovering relationships between physiological data, streamed events and latent medical conditions.

Source: Unless specified, semi-structured stakeholder interviews conducted in 2015.

1.1. *Primary and secondary data use can improve patient care*

High-quality health care is safe, effective and person-centred. Many failures to deliver quality care are caused by problems in providing the right information at the right time to the right person or actor – patients, carers, providers or administrators. Ensuring that the relevant information about a person flows to the right people at the right time enables more accurate, timely and co-ordinated decision making in all care settings. This is known as primary use of health data. It is greatly enabled by access to an integrated EHR. It can improve patient outcomes at, potentially, modest incremental cost if implemented intelligently.

All other uses of health data discussed from here are secondary – i.e. the information derived from them is not deployed in the care of the person to whom they pertain, but for other purposes. Secondary uses can be just as valuable in clinical care. For example, by using a wide range of variables and large datasets that link processes and outcomes of care, predictive statistical modelling can anticipate which patients are likely to deteriorate during acute care, when people may be at risk of re-admission to hospital, or what treatment may be most optimal for a patient in a specific situation (Frankowvich et al.,

2011). Kaiser Permanente, an integrated health service organisation in the United States, combined 15 years of maternal and neonatal data (608 014 live births) to develop an algorithm to predict the probability of neonatal sepsis. Incorporating this with a newborn's clinical data to derive a sepsis risk score enables providers to more accurately determine need for and dosage of antibiotic administration. National implementation of this algorithm would reduce the administration of antibiotics in an estimated 240 000 newborns annually in the United States (Escobar et al., 2014).

IBM and the New York Genome Center recently announced a project to sequence the DNA of individual patients' tumours to better personalise their treatment. While personalised cancer therapies traditionally focus on 30 to 50 genes, this undertaking will involve sequencing the entire 22 000 or so genes in the body and will look at many different aspects of DNA. One aspect of the analysis will involve comparing DNA from tumour cells with DNA from other parts of the body. The amount of data analysed for each patient is in excess of 1 terabyte (1 million million bytes), roughly equivalent to 2 million average-sized photo files. The information could, for instance, enable oncology teams to predict if a certain type of chemotherapy may be extra toxic for a particular individual or if a different drug may be more effective (Cha, 2016).

Sweden uses various data sources to undertake assessment and re-assessment of clinical care guidelines that inform physicians and health care professionals about the most appropriate interventions for patients with different and complex health profiles and problems. The clinical areas covered include cardiac and stroke care, several cancers, and dental, diabetes and mental health care. Every resident of Sweden has a personal identity number (OECD, 2013a), which permits linking a number of different databases. It enables following patients – in a digital sense – through the entire cycle of care, evaluating the extent to which guidelines are followed and measuring the real-world health outcomes of care. This evidence is then used to revise the clinical care guidelines, completing an ongoing cycle of quality improvement (OECD, 2015a).

Combining mHealth with Big Data analytical techniques opens a new frontier in home-based care and health maintenance. Smartphones or portable devices act as a portal to access remote (or cloud-based) processors able to integrate individuals' information with vast amounts of other data from various sources to guide, in real time, treatment and management of disease. This could be especially helpful for the growing number of people with multimorbidity, every one of whom has a unique set of needs based on his disease profile, demographic characteristics, genetic make-up and personal preferences. Only analytical techniques drawing on Big Data are able to access and process the various types of fast-flowing data to enable this type of information to be generated in a timely manner. More examples are provided in Box 6.2.

1.2. Data can be used for better health care system management

Health data can be used to monitor, manage and improve health care system performance and inform decisions regarding resource allocation, planning and policy. Sophisticated data analysis can be used to predict and manage future health care demand, identify missed opportunities, and optimise service alignment and use of resources. Health data from various streams and sources are used to actively monitor quality and system performance (Bates et al., 2014). Analysis using NLP free text in medical records has been shown to have a higher accuracy in identifying post-operative complications compared with patient safety indicators based on discharge coding (Murff et al., 2011).

In Finland, for example, data are collected on the entire population's contact with the health care system across all sectors and settings – from admission to hospital to care by their community doctor to the medications prescribed and deaths. These data are continuously analysed to monitor interventions' quality and cost-effectiveness for a range of conditions[2] (OECD, 2013a). Hospital-level results are publicly available and improvements in performance – based on quality of care indicators – have been observed (OECD, 2015a).

Korea links population-wide health insurance data across people's entire pathway of care and services to periodically report on a range of quality indicators including: mortality and re-admission after hospital procedures; inappropriate prescribing in primary care; and outcomes following discharge from mental health facilities. This approach enables system managers to identify poor performance in terms of inappropriate care, address variations in practice, and take steps to maximise efficiency and value. Authorities report on the quality of services provided by physicians, clinics, hospitals and long-term care providers by particular patient groups, including diabetic, heart and cancer patients (OECD, 2013a).

Health data from a range of sources can provide real-world evidence (RWE) to evaluate the effectiveness and utility of clinical interventions. As discussed in more detail in other chapters of this report, evaluating the utility of a health technology in normal patient populations can be enhanced by collecting and analysing RWE (Eichler et al., 2015). A sufficient volume of data coupled with modern analytical techniques can complement existing evidence regarding the effectiveness of interventions. RWE, particularly if based on large datasets, can complement information derived from clinical trials. This not only improves care quality, but enables payers to conduct more accurate Health Technology Assessments (HTAs) and make informed regulatory and reimbursement decisions for more consistent funding and better value and allocative efficiency. The opportunity for people to contribute their own data enabled by other information and communications technology (ICT) innovations such as the smartphone may enhance the collection of RWE.

1.3. *Health data contribute to surveillance efforts and population health issues*

Analysis of disparate databases and other data streams can be used to better understand and monitor population health and the burden of illness, and to manage and evaluate public health interventions such as health promotion and disease prevention programmes. This can range from surveillance of viral outbreaks, to national and global monitoring of antimicrobial resistance, to timely identification of side effects and safety concerns of pharmaceutical products. Here, integrating conventional health data with those generated in other domains such as social media and web browsing can be said to truly draw on Big Data concepts and analytics. Big Data analysis can be especially useful in the area of health promotion and prevention of chronic disease through targeted management of risk factors such as obesity. Combining health, socio-economic and social care data with data on daily activities (such as shopping) and physical movement and activity levels (tracked by smartphones or wearable devices) can potentially generate valuable information about behaviour, health and a range of other variables. For example, geographic and temporal trends in behavioural risk factors and their interaction with other variables that impact health and health care systems can be valuable to policy makers and researchers.

In mental health, combining clinical data with web and telecommunications data offers great opportunities for monitoring and surveillance. A number of innovative technologies combine the smartphone functionality with sophisticated data analytics, language processing and sentiment analysis to detect patterns and meaning, and to monitor changes in individuals' mental well-being. This enables suitable responses in crisis situations, and generates useful knowledge in the longer term (Darcy et al., 2016; Parikh et al., 2016).

Another example is the United States Food and Drug Administration's (FDA) Mini Sentinel Initiative to monitor the safety of approved medical technology. This project harnesses information from multiple EHR systems, administrative data and insurance claim records – these data include demographics, enrolment history, drug dispensing, encounters, vital signs, lab results, diagnoses, procedures and mortality. The project involves multiple data partners across the United States and encompasses a vast amount of data: 2.9 billion drug dispensing encounters, and 2.4 billion unique medical encounters, including 38 million acute inpatient hospital stays (FDA, 2015). Patient details are not collected centrally. Instead, using a common data model, standardised common input files are generated locally by each data partner, and sent in de-identified and encrypted format to a central database for evaluation and analysis. The combined data are then assessed to identify safety failures (OECD, 2015a).

1.4. *Technological advances in data collection and analysis enable research*

Biomedical research has traditionally been limited by the need for special settings and facilities, which are not only highly expensive, but are also normally limited in terms of the number of cases studied, in their diversity, and in the speed of results and feedback. In the era of digitalisation, modern data analytics and algorithms can reduce these limits. Research drawing on the massive amounts of data now generated can be faster, deeper and of considerably larger scale than previously possible. The situation offers the potential to scale up scientific enquiry, create a sufficient evidence base, and complement existing methods such as randomised controlled trials (RCTs) to solve difficult problems in a relatively inexpensive way.

Sharing information at international level and integrating numerous data platforms, such as molecule libraries, early phase research data and clinical trial databases, can assist with research and innovation effort to, for example, identify new antimicrobial agents (Checchini et al., 2015). Great opportunities also arise in global efforts to progress research in dementia (OECD, 2015c). Biobanks are also opening new opportunities in research, while going some way to circumvent some of the legal challenges regarding privacy and consent. In the United Kingdom, a Biobank was developed comprising biological, behavioural and environmental data of 500 000 adults. This information can be linked to health care records, registered cancers and deaths for research projects to understand the epidemiology of diseases more deeply and to discover which treatments work better for which types of patients.

Shah et al. (2015) examined the association of proton pump inhibitors (PPIs) – used to treat gastroesophageal reflux disease (GERD) – with adverse cardiovascular effects, which were previously recognised among PPI users with pre-existing cardiovascular problems. The investigators sought to examine such a link in the general, uncomplicated population. Using a deep data-mining algorithm, they analysed two independent datasets containing 2.9 million individual patient records spanning 1994-2011. Results suggest a previously unknown association between PPI use and an elevated risk of heart attack in the general population, including the young (Shah and Pathak, 2014). As each year 113 million PPIs are prescribed globally, the implications of this research are profound.

The powerful storage and processing capabilities that have enabled Big Data analytics are shaping the health research landscape. Advances in genetic sequencing and the remarkable decrease in its cost are an example. Analysis of health data can continue to provide a powerful way to advance the understanding of health, disease and the complex interaction between therapies, individuals and the environment (OECD, 2015a). Research drawing on Big Data requires specific skills and expertise and it has limitations that require specific methods and approaches to minimise risks of inaccurate or even false results (Frakt and Pizer, 2016). However, it is a (comparatively) low-cost approach that can complement more targeted studies and trials, enhancing the evidence base and improving clinical and public health practice.

2. Challenges, risks and policy implications of using health data

Fulfilling the potential of health data entails overcoming some key challenges and managing multiple risks. The datafication of health, as well as technological advances, techniques and methods to store and analyse these data, create several tensions that are challenging the existing institutional frameworks of health care systems. As already discussed, the distinction between clinical and secondary use of health data is becoming vague (Aronson and Rehm, 2015). Data ownership is also increasingly unclear, and the boundary between public and private domains is blurring. Data taxonomies and definitions are an increasingly important concern. New actors and experts with different corporate cultures and institutional approaches are entering, and disrupting, this space, requiring a new perspective on collaboration and partnerships (Vayena and Gasser, 2016).

Several policy considerations emerge from these tensions. Health data – particularly in the context of Big Data – are not just sitting there ready for information to be extracted from them. To generate any value, they must be combined, harmonised, managed and analysed. This requires investing in technical infrastructure and human capital, as well as enacting the requisite legislative enablers. Given the sensitivity of these data, the risks and consequences (e.g. breach of privacy, discrimination in employment or insurance coverage) are arguably greater than those faced in other industries and sectors. The challenges cover the entire public policy spectrum – from technical and administrative to cultural and political. The institutions deployed to hold, manage and analyse health data must be trusted by all stakeholders, including (and perhaps especially) the public. All of this can be complex, time-consuming and expensive, but the dividend is better health outcomes, more efficiency and greater value. Health care systems need to develop a comprehensive governance framework that encompasses all the technical, legal and resourcing aspects of data management. Such a framework is presented at the end of this section.

Most importantly, however, getting the most out of data in health requires a transformation in culture and mindset by all actors and stakeholders: governments, policy makers, providers, administrators and the public. Data need to be seen as a core asset of health care systems, societies and the global community, not as a by-product of clinical and other health service activities such as administration and billing (Murdoch and Detsky, 2013). Without this cultural change the challenges outlined below will not be overcome and the potential of health data will remain largely unrealised.

Due in part to these challenges, the health sector has been slower than others to recognise the value of data, but its application is gaining policy traction. WHO Europe recently released its updated eHealth report based on a global survey to which 47 of 53 regional member states responded. Among the report's findings: 70% of respondents have a national eHealth policy or strategy; 59% have a national EHR system, with half of respondents reporting that funding is the most important barrier to implementing such a system; 13% have a national policy or strategy regulating the use of Big Data in the health sector; and 80% have legislation to protect the privacy of an individual's health-related data in electronic format (an increase of nearly 30% since 2009) (WHO Europe, 2016). The European Commission is midway through its eHealth Action Plan 2012-2020 (European Commission, 2012).

2.1. Data interoperability and linkage must be established for maximum value

To grasp the importance of digital interoperability, it is perhaps useful to imagine a world where personal computers and other devices such as smartphones or tablets could only exchange information with those produced by the same manufacturer or software developer. That this scenario seems quite improbable is testament to the fundamental importance of digital interoperability (and how much it is taken for granted). The current situation in most health care systems when it comes to sharing data is quite different. Information is captured in separate silos as it is simply not possible to store all relevant data (clinical, administrative, financial, registry, mortality, demographic and environmental) in the same repository. While health care systems have access to an ever-increasing number of information technology products, many of these systems cannot "talk" to each other and health information exchange remains a problem in the majority of countries. If information systems cannot communicate, data will not meet its potential in the health care system.

Much of this can be attributed to the legacy of traditional medical culture. Health care systems grew considerably in size and complexity over the past century (owing, in large part, to the proliferation of medical technology – see Chapter 2). Concurrently, the needs of the populations served by these systems evolved – both clinically (e.g. chronic diseases and multimorbidity) and culturally (e.g. information and empowerment). This growth and change was not matched by the necessary evolution in health care system structure and governance. Barring some notable exceptions, traditional silos of clinical practice, administrative control and communication are the same now as they were in the 1950s. Beyond the fact that immense amounts of data are still collected and stored in paper form, in the digital era this has manifested in gatekeeping, protection and claims of ownership over data (Schneeweiss, 2014; Groves et al., 2013; Murdoch and Detsky, 2013).[3] This in turn manifests in more systemic barriers such as misaligned incentives of actors within the health care system, legal impediments, and difficulty quantifying the value of – and making a strong business case for – investment in data analysis.

Data interoperability and linkage are therefore key policy issues that must be addressed to get the most from health data and realise the opportunities outlined previously. This may shift the resolution of underlying problems concerning disease- and specialty-based care provision to a more person-centric, inter-professional approach. Equally, changes in this aspect of medical culture can make data linkage, information sharing and, above all, transparency the rule rather than the exception.

Based on a 2013/14 survey of 22 OECD member and partner countries, health care systems still tend to analyse data separately. Key datasets are not routinely linked to generate more valuable information about health care quality and performance than can be extracted from them separately (Figure 6.1). In many cases the technical pre-requisites are in place, meaning that the real reasons are related to governance, legislation and culture (OECD,

Figure 6.1. **Extent of linkage across relevant databases in 22 OECD countries, 2013/14**

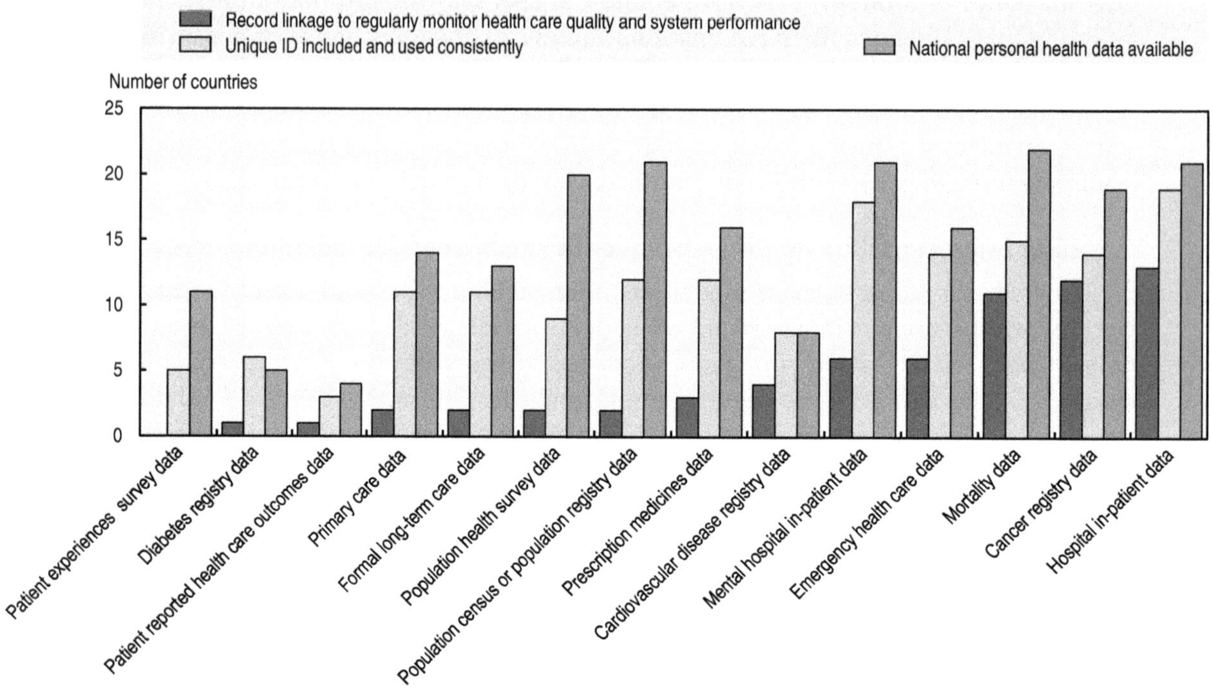

Source: OECD (2015), *Health Data Governance: Privacy, Monitoring and Research*, OECD Health Policy Studies, OECD Publishing, Paris.

StatLink http://dx.doi.org/10.1787/888933442975

2015b). Nevertheless, the quality, consistency and reliability of health data are important challenges in this regard. These are a function of standards and interoperability.

In practice, interoperability means having common protocols and common ontologies that define the basic mechanisms by which users and resources negotiate, establish, manage and exploit data sharing. It means sharing not only data but anything that connects to the data's production and processing, including computing tools, applications, methods, software, metadata and workflows across different platforms. A fundamental requirement is use of a unique patient identifier that enables people's contact with health services to be connected and ultimately linked with other information sources. Other strategies to address interoperability include terminology standards, incentives and/or penalties relating to adoption and use, certification of software vendors and auditing (OECD, 2013a).

A key challenge concerns the EHR, which is likely to become one of the biggest repositories of health information as its implementation advances (see Section 3 for more detail). EHRs need to be designed thoughtfully with the user in mind. Policy makers must create the right regulatory framework, one that encourages innovation to promote good design yet ensures adequate functionality and the capacity to link with other sources of information. Ensuring that electronic records can be transferred or shared among a patient's primary care physician and specialists is an issue that has yet to be addressed. This problem is common to all OECD countries, even those where deployment of EHRs is making good progress (Oderkirk, forthcoming). In systems with multiple EHR platforms – most likely developed by different vendors – it is essential that these are interoperable with other systems and datasets. Actors involved in developing EHRs, inputting the data and using them are primarily motivated by very different incentives. Laws or regulations mandating adoption and use of EHR systems that conform to standards to improve data quality and coverage are required. Technical solutions such as NLP must be engaged.

2.2. *Privacy and security are sensitive issues*

The collection and use of personal health data present a number of important risks to individuals' privacy. Not only can this be damaging for individuals, it can also undermine public confidence in government and social institutions (OECD, 2013b). Yet equally significant risks to individuals and to societies arise when health information assets are not developed, remain unused, or are very difficult to use. Both sets of risks can be conceptualised as a spectrum, and the balance between them is illustrated in Figure 6.2. The risks should be viewed from the individual as well as a societal perspective. A situation where no data is collected and used minimises the risk of individual privacy breaches, and the broader risk of undermining confidence in public institutions. However, this scenario elevates other risks regarding the safety, quality and performance of health care systems, which also manifest at individual and societal levels. Individuals and societies are likely to wish to trade off eliminating all privacy risks for improved quality of healthcare, and other, services. The challenge for policy makers is to manage the different risk dimensions in a manner that optimises outcomes and benefits, while maintaining the confidence and trust of the public. A governance framework to enable better decision making in this regard provided in section 2.7.

Figure 6.2. **Risks associated with the collection and use of personal health data**

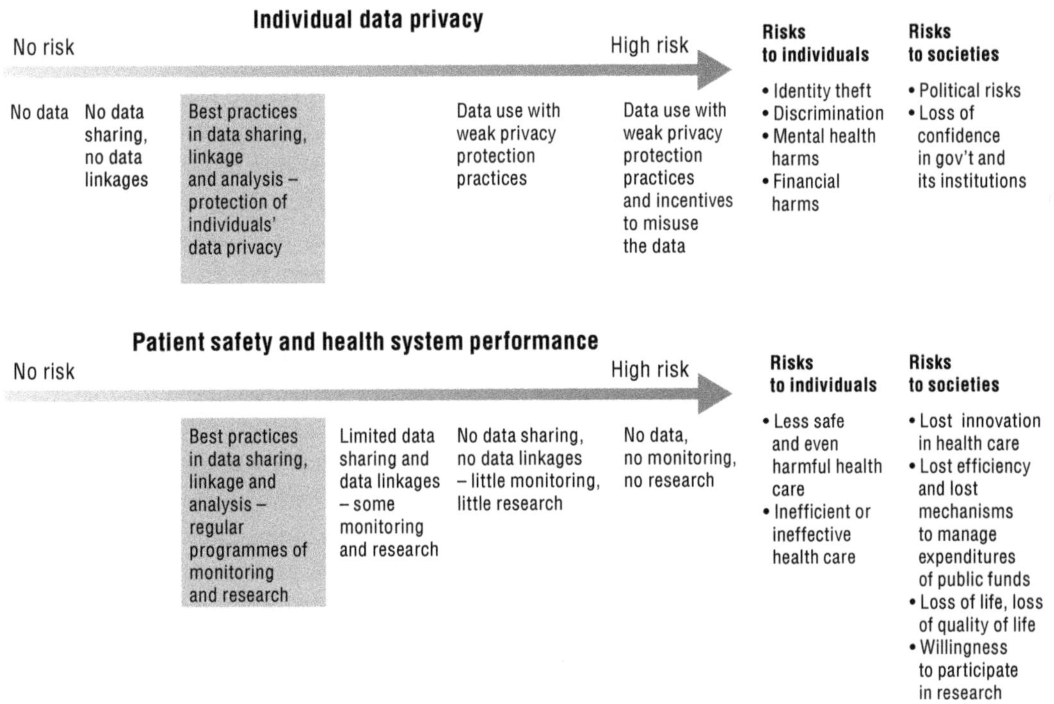

Source: Adapted from OECD (2013), *Strengthening Health Information Infrastructure for Health Care Quality Governance: Good Practices, New Opportunities and Data Privacy Protection Challenges*, OECD Publishing, Paris, *www.oecd.org/publications/strengthening-health-information-infrastructure-for-health-care-quality-governance-9789264193505-en.htm.*

Considerable advances in privacy-enhancing technologies provide additional avenues to meet both health care data use and privacy protection needs (OECD, 2013b). A growing number of approaches to data anonymisation exist, such as data de-identification and data pseudonymisation. De-identification involves removal of key patient-identifying information, such as names, patient numbers, exact addresses and key dates. Pseudonymisation replaces key patient identifiers with a meaningless code that can, for approved purposes, allow re-identification. These practices need to be implemented before data are made available for research and analysis, but in a way that is context-specific and considerate of any unintended consequences. However, data de-identification techniques rarely remove all risk that a dataset could be manipulated or combined with other data to rediscover the identity of data subjects (OECD, 2015b). This is especially relevant in the context of Big Data, where removal of *all* identification risks may become increasingly difficult.[4]

Some countries such as Belgium, Finland and the United Kingdom, implemented data governance mechanisms that provide added security to protect de-identified data. These include: independent review bodies that evaluate data use proposals for public benefits and adequacy of data security; contractual agreements that bind data receivers to required data security and disclosure practices; and security audits and follow-up mechanisms to ensure compliance with contractual obligations (OECD, 2013a). A range of conditions of access to data can enhance the safeguarding of data. For example, on-site "reading rooms" enable data to be extracted and analysed without being exported.

Significant differences in approaches to the protection of data subjects' privacy among OECD countries resulted in some countries (New Zealand, Sweden and the United Kingdom) advancing the generation of health data – particularly for research and statistical purposes. Others restrict data collection, sharing and use (OECD 2015b). These differences are significant and can be attributed to differences in risk-benefit evaluations based on legal, technical and political factors. The OECD developed a risk-benefit evaluation tool to assist institutions with these challenges. This tool is based on 32 questions to assess the societal risks and the societal benefits of processing personal health data. Questions concern key factors such as expected impact and beneficiaries, consistency with acceptable practice, potential to use aggregated data, consent processes, data transfer requirements, and vulnerability to breaches (see Annex 6.A1).

Attention is needed to ensure that individuals are informed about the immediate and potential future use of their data. In some cases individuals may choose to restrict or withdraw their data from their contribution to research and statistics. While this may be reasonable in some cases, in others this may undermine the objectives of the use of the data, and bias results with potentially significant consequences in terms of societal benefit. Care must be taken that the withdrawal or restriction does not compromise data integrity, or that withdrawn data are not used for research purposes. Technical and legal mechanisms to enable consent are evolving and form an important part of an overarching data governance framework (OECD 2015b, 2013a, 2013b).

2.3. *Legal and legislative challenges need to be resolved*

Many OECD countries report legislative barriers to the use of personal health data, including enabling data linkages and developing combined databases from information contained in the EHR. Some of these countries have decentralised administration of health care systems, and have not reached a consensus within the country on how the levels of government could work together. A principal challenge is the lack of clarity on how to translate into practice legislation concerning the protection of data privacy, including informed consent at the national and subnational levels. This includes the legality of data sharing among public authorities and that of providing access to personal health data for research (OECD, 2015b). This complexity extends to multicountry data-sharing initiatives. The result is that such initiatives remain rare, challenged by concerns regarding differences in data privacy protection laws and whether shared data will be adequately protected in the receiving country.

A key problem is that the legislative instruments governing data, privacy and security predate the digital era. The lines between primary and secondary use of health data are blurring. Participation in research can lead to direct benefit in outcomes for the same person. The continuous capture of clinical data has effectively expanded the generalisable stock of knowledge at society's disposal. Legal mechanisms enabling the use of health data therefore need to be updated. An example of a current legal question is specifying the parameters for ownership of health data once they are authorised for secondary uses. European countries have made the most progress among OECD members, having recognised in law that foreign entities can apply and be approved for access to data when the legal protection of information privacy in the foreign country adequately matches that of the home country. However, lack of resources to evaluate the adequacy of foreign laws continues to pose barriers to data sharing between European and other countries (OECD, 2015a).

The OECD Council Recommendation on health data governance can assist countries to maximise the potential and minimise the risks of using personal health data to advance public policy objectives. The Recommendation comprises 12 measures for establishing and implementing a national health data governance framework, including a recommendation on how governments can support interoperable trans-border sharing of personal health data (OECD, 2017).

2.4. *Infrastructure and human capital must be reinforced to keep pace with technological advances*

Realising the potential of data requires investment in technical infrastructure and human capital and expertise. Infrastructure is very important as it can dictate the quantity and quality of the data, and how well they can be shared, extracted and analysed. An important technical issue is analysing unstructured data, most often comprising free-flowing text using the vocabulary of a person's choice. Unstructured data are very difficult to analyse and investment in professional human coders is essential. Sophisticated NLP algorithms are necessary to "read" through the large volumes of unstructured data to try to create structure by searching for words that could refer to the same concept (Liao et al., 2015). Given that reliable and routine NLP may still be some way off, it is important to specify minimum datasets and standards for health data (see Section 3).

Equally important is to have personnel with sound communication skills, and health care providers at ease with the fundamentals of data science and computing. Involving all stakeholders in the development of processes and applications of data is important. Only in this way can providers and managers be better equipped to work with ICT professionals towards developing useful tools. This will avoid situations where a detailed specification is given to a programmer who works alone to try to develop the product, often to the dissatisfaction of the end user.

Another benefit of building expertise among health care providers is to overcome professional reluctance to change and to embrace the opportunities presented by better use of data in health. Uptake of clinical decision-making algorithms may be resisted due to fears about professional autonomy. Knowledge of how analytics works and how it can enhance practice without removing autonomy, and involvement in the development of these tools can all help allay this anxiety.

Data scientists need to be trained and recruited. The training must ensure that data scientists have the collaboration skills to partner with health care professionals. Adapting education and training programmes for other health care professions to guarantee at least a minimum degree of skill development in statistics and programming is another objective, both to build a generation of clinical data scientists and to increase appreciation for data and high-quality recordkeeping within the health care professional community (OECD, 2015a).

Human and financial resource challenges are limiting data use. For example, in a 2016 survey of 30 OECD countries on the implementation and use of EHR systems, 12 countries reported that lack of technical and financial resources limit dataset development and accessibility of data for research and statistical purposes (Oderkirk, forthcoming). This is principally due to financial investments required. Specific resource issues include:

- investments to address a diversity of record formats, terminologies and other interoperability problems [Canada, Denmark, Spain, the United Kingdom (Scotland) and the United States]
- resources for dataset pseudonymisation so that patients' privacy can be protected when data are made accessible for analysis and research purposes (Denmark and Latvia)
- resources and other investments to address the lack of staff skilled in creation, analysis and visualisation of data from EHRs [Canada, Estonia, Mexico, Norway and the United Kingdom (Scotland)]
- investments to set strategic priorities and manage competing demands for statistical and research uses of data [Canada and the United Kingdom (Scotland)]
- solutions to address high financial charges levied by ICT system providers that limit the creation of registries from EHRs (Finland).

2.5. *How well stakeholders are engaged can determine success*

Transitioning health care systems to make the most from data requires establishment of trust among stakeholders. In many countries, considerable community unease surfaces over the use of personal health information, as illustrated by the *care.data* initiative. With over 50 million records, this initiative to integrate England's health and social care data is potentially the largest data repository of this type in the world. The *care.data* strategy focused on legislative and technical planning and preparation. However, public release of the strategy caused a backlash that effectively derailed the initiative, setting it back a number of years.

Denmark has hundreds of clinical registries containing potentially valuable data on diseases, patient groups and interventions. A co-ordinated effort has begun linking these data and combining them with health information from other sources, including primary and acute care, and data from physiological monitoring devices. Approximately 16 million episodes of care spanning 18 years are currently being analysed for association between bed occupancy, time of admission and mortality. Critically, officials are investing considerably in managing stakeholder and public relations, and ensuring the risks and benefits are communicated in a way that will minimise community unease and reduce the likelihood of public backlash. The initiative is being framed as a means to ensure that the government can fulfil its responsibility to provide high-quality care.

In a 2012 OECD survey of 25 countries, 13 reported having involved groups of stakeholders in their efforts to govern development and implementation of their national EHR system, either through the groups' representation within the governing body or through consultation, or both. Groups included, for example, clinicians, pharmacists, professional associations, patients, insurers, ICT professionals, lawyers and policy makers (OECD, 2013a). The follow-up 2016 survey of 30 countries indicates growing recognition that stakeholder engagement is a critical aspect of good governance and implementation (Oderkirk, forthcoming).

It must be recognised that health data initiatives are a political as well as a technical exercise. Commensurate thought and planning need to be devoted to stakeholder management, communication and public relations. Engaging with all interested stakeholders would appear to be the best strategy for ensuring that all voices are heard and a consensus is reached on data use. An open, transparent public communication strategy can go a long way towards demystifying this topic, opening data for secondary purposes and generating positive public discourse about risks and benefits. Ideally, the strategy would enable all stakeholders to know what data are being collected; how they are being used; how and with whom to apply for access to them; the conditions of approval; data security requirements; and details of research projects that are approved. It is also important that policy makers engage with stakeholders across the public and private sectors. Only this way can the necessary innovation, expertise and partnerships be established to successfully begin using health data to maximum effect.

2.6. *Costs and resourcing for digital health technology must be carefully evaluated*

It is often observed that health care is the only sector where new technology and innovation – drugs, devices and the interventions they enable – result in higher expenditure (Chandra and Skinner, 2012; Sorenson et al., 2013; Scannell et al., 2012). Implementation of digital technologies and processes requires up-front and ongoing investment in infrastructure and human capital, but can it have the opposite effect? That is, can it improve the efficiency, performance and sustainability of health care systems' work to improve the health and well-being of people and populations? As the majority of the data described here are routinely generated anyway, greater cost may be incurred by not creating the systems, processes and institutions to extract and use information from them.

In an exploration of the productivity effect of digital technology in business, Brynjolffson (1993) and Brynjolffson and Hitt (1998) describe how digitalisation often failed to generate workplace efficiency until the nature of the work was re-configured as well. They note that "[t]he unmistakable lesson was that purchasing computerised equipment was the smallest part of the overall cost ... The biggest costs were in changing the organization" (Brynjolfsson and Hitt, 1998, p. 54). This may also be the case for digitalisation and datafication in health care because of the profound socio-technical transformation it entails.

Introduction of digital technology into England's National Health Service (NHS) can deliver up to an estimated GBP 13 billion in savings per annum, and ensuring interoperability between electronic data platforms in the United States would result in aggregate savings approaching USD 100 billion (Digital Health, 2015; Walker et al., 2005). While these are just projections that do not factor in the costs of complete digitalisation, evidence is emerging that ICT in health is already generating efficiencies, economies and savings in a number of health services and systems (Parikh et al., 2016). The potential value-enhancing effect of digital technology compared to conventional health care technology may be because, fundamentally, it does not involve introduction of new and costly biomedical interventions, procedures or devices into health care. Rather, it enables the application of existing medical technology in a more efficient way, and flows across most if not all health and health care activities.

However, the clinical and economic benefits of data – and digital health technology more broadly – need to be studied more rigorously. One difficulty is that because ICT flows across all aspects of health care provision and system management, it is very difficult to disentangle its effects into quantifiable parcels. Shoehorning this area into conventional research methods may not reveal much. New investigative approaches need to be devised and tested for the costs and benefits of ICT in health to be adequately analysed. This also requires investment but it is important because this evidence can be used to convince the public and decision makers of the importance of harnessing health data.

2.7. A data governance framework would promote realisation of health data benefits

To maximise the benefits of health data (better care, greater value, more knowledge) while minimising the risks associated with privacy and misuse, a governance framework that encompasses and addresses the challenges described above should be implemented. Such a framework was developed by the OECD (Figure 6.3). The framework should include the following key elements (OECD, 2015b):

1. The health information system supports the clinical use of data, monitoring and improvement of health care quality and system performance, as well as research innovations for better health care and outcomes. Such systems are accessible for secondary purposes, subject to safeguards. They are developed within a framework and parameters that reflect societal values regarding rights to privacy as well as to health. They are developed through open and transparent consultation with stakeholders.
2. The processing and the secondary use of data for public health, research and statistical purposes are permitted, subject to safeguards specified in the legislative framework for data protection. Such legislative frameworks reflect basic privacy principles outlined in the OECD Privacy Framework (OECD, 2013b), and cover all data sources, custodians and processors. Legal frameworks are renewed to reflect evolving societal values and the changing health technology landscape.
3. The public and other stakeholders are consulted upon and informed about the collection and processing of personal health data. This includes regular, clear and transparent communication with the public about the use of personal health data including the benefits as well as the risks, and how the latter are managed. It necessitates periodic review of the roles and responsibilities of various stakeholder groups (including identification of emerging stakeholders), particularly in countries with multiple jurisdictions.
4. A certification/accreditation process for the processing of health data for research and statistics is implemented. This involves setting standards and norms of data governance, and limits processing of personal health data to entities that are certified and accredited against these standards, reducing the risk of malfeasance and unintended security lapses.[5]

Figure 6.3. **Health data governance framework**

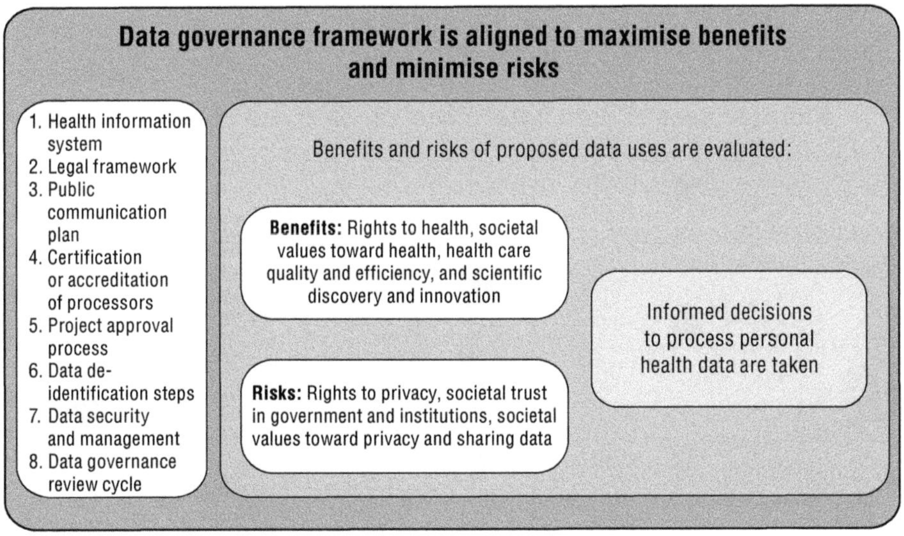

Source: OECD (2015), *Health Data Governance: Privacy, Monitoring and Research*, OECD Health Policy Studies, OECD Publishing, Paris, *www.oecd.org/publications/health-data-governance-9789264244566- en.htm.*

5. The project approval process is fair and transparent and decision making is supported by an independent, multidisciplinary project review body. Processes follow criteria that consider both the societal and personal risks and benefits for proposed uses of health data. A standardised way of assessing these risks and benefits is recommended.
6. Best practices in data de-identification are applied to protect patient data privacy. This includes documenting data de-identification methods, and engaging data privacy expertise in the development or review of methods. Processes and protocols are updated periodically in line with best practice and technological development.
7. Best practices in data security and management are applied to reduce re-identification and breach risks. This includes controlling and monitoring physical and virtual data security, limiting data transfers to secure channels, and using alternative ways of transferring data, such as custom-made data centres or secure portals.
8. Governance mechanisms are periodically reviewed at an international level to maximise societal benefits and minimise societal risks as new data sources and new technologies are introduced. Data governance requires continual assessment and renewal. The volume, velocity and variety of data are growing, and the technologies used to communicate, store and process data are evolving (e.g. cloud services). This creates a dynamic environment where risks as well as benefits continuously evolve.

The OECD Council Recommendation on health data governance should enhance countries' ability to make the most of health data while managing the risks associated with their secondary use (OECD, 2017).

3. EHR systems' readiness to contribute to secondary uses of health data

The EHR can be viewed as the foundation of a sound health information infrastructure. Countries that develop EHR systems that combine or virtually link together data to capture patients' health care histories have the potential to realise an unprecedented advancement in health care quality, efficiency and performance and in the discovery and evaluation of preventive care and treatments, including precision medicine. The depth and breadth of such data far exceed that available from traditional survey, administrative or research sources and support new Big Data research techniques that can search for patterns and anomalies in populations (Figure 6.4).

Figure 6.4. **Multiple uses of data within clinical electronic health record systems**

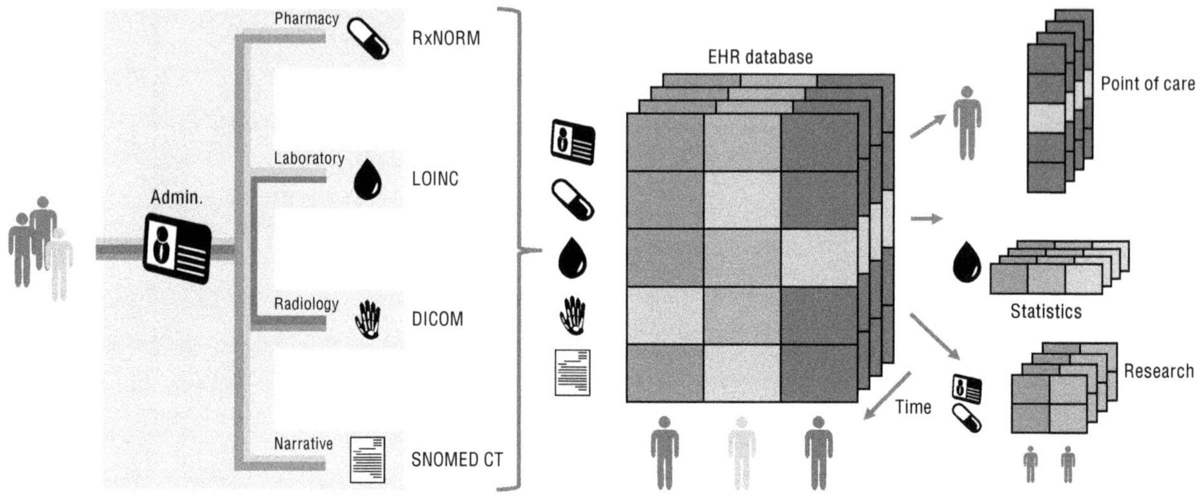

Source: Adapted from Jensen, P.B., L.L. Jensen and S. Brunak (2012), "Mining Electronic Health Records: Towards Better Research Applications and Clinical Care", *Nature Reviews – Genetics*, Vol. 13.

The opportunities of health data outlined in Section 1 encompass the EHR. When longitudinal EHR data can be linked to information about treatment costs and deaths, these data support: detecting unsafe health care practices and treatments; rewarding high-quality and efficient health care practices; and detecting fraud and waste in the health care system. When EHR data can be linked to patients' behavioural, environmental and biological (genetic) characteristics, these data can potentially support: identifying optimal responders to treatment; personalising care for better patient outcomes; and discovering and evaluating new health care treatments and practices. If such data are available for very large and representative patient populations, they can support: selecting cohorts of patients for clinical trials; and conducting long-term follow-up of clinical trials (OECD, 2013a, 2015a, 2015c).

All countries are investing in development of EHRs, but only some countries are actively progressing the possibility of data extraction for research, statistics and other secondary uses. Those progressing towards analytical uses of data are overcoming challenges ranging from ensuring adequate financial and human resources, to managing culture change, to effective engaging the public, to ensuring data usability, quality, security and privacy protection.

In 2016, the OECD Health Care Quality Indicators (HCQI) Expert Group conducted a study of 30 countries[6] to explore the data governance and technical and operational factors that would support them in the development of national health information and research programmes from data held within EHRs (see Annex 6.A2).[7] Results identified nine countries with both high data governance readiness and high technical and operational readiness: Canada, Denmark, Finland, New Zealand, Singapore, Sweden, the United Kingdom (England and Scotland)[8] and the United States.

These nine countries are very well-positioned to capitalise upon the opportunity to develop world-class health information systems that not only support their countries' information needs regarding health care system quality, efficiency and performance reporting, but also create a firm foundation for scientific research and discovery. All of these countries, however, still face important challenges that may limit their future success; and several other countries are moving forward with strategic plans to overcome obstacles and to eventually match or exceed the above-mentioned countries' current capabilities.

3.1. *EHR data governance readiness varies greatly among countries surveyed*

The study explored several key indicators of the readiness of national health data governance frameworks to support the use of EHR data to fulfil national health information and research objectives. These indicators include: 1) having a legal framework that would allow data within EHR systems to be extracted for statistical and research purposes, subject to suitable safeguards; 2) having a national EHR plan or policy that includes the statistical and research uses of these data; 3) engaging in the extraction of data from EHR systems to create national datasets; and 4) analysing data extracted from EHR systems for key national monitoring and research objectives.

While EHR data governance readiness is low in many countries, the top-tier countries provide key examples of how such governance can be successfully developed to advance national health information systems (Figure 6.5 and Table 6.A2.1).

Figure 6.5. **Data governance readiness among OECD member and partner countries surveyed, 2016**

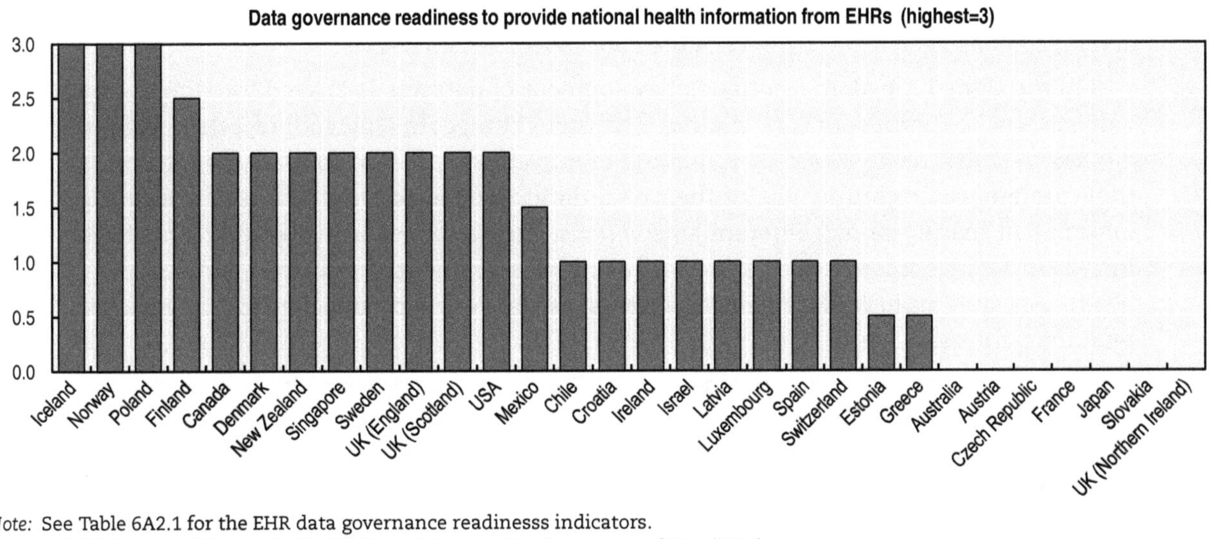

Note: See Table 6A2.1 for the EHR data governance readinesss indicators.
Source: HCQI Survey of Electronic Health Record System Development and Use (2016).

StatLink http://dx.doi.org/10.1787/888933442989

National EHR plans and policies include statistical and research uses of the data

An important health data governance factor is existence of a national policy or plan to develop the EHR system that discusses the importance of secondary data uses (statistical and research) for key national information objectives. Statistical and research uses of data must be given consideration when EHR systems are first developing to avoid decision making that will create obstacles to data uses and that will be costly to address after the fact.

The six key information objectives in national plans and priorities for EHR systems are: 1) public health, 2) health care system performance, and 3) patient safety monitoring; plus 4) research to advance population health and health care, or 5) contribute data to clinical trials; and 6) allowing physicians to query data to inform their decisions about the treatment of individual patients. Ten countries (Canada, Denmark, Estonia, Iceland, Norway, Poland, Singapore, Sweden, the United Kingdom (England and Scotland) and the United States) include at least five of these objectives in their national EHR plans and priorities. Other countries with three or four of these information objectives are: Chile, Croatia, Finland, Iceland, Latvia, Luxembourg, the Slovak Republic and Switzerland.

Legislative framework permits statistical and research uses of data within EHRs

The second key health data governance factor is assuring that the legal framework that protects patients' privacy and data security within EHR systems does so in a manner that still allows data to be extracted for approved statistical and research purposes. Many of the top-tier countries have specific legislation that authorises datasets to be created from data extracted from the EHR system. This is not to suggest, however, that no legislative challenges remain to be addressed in the top-tier countries.

For example, in Finland, data can be extracted from the EHR system to create legally authorised registries; however, the law authorising the EHR system does not allow the data within the national EHR repository to be accessed directly for research purposes. Data within local EHRs, however, may be used for research purposes. Poland reports unresolved issues regarding the legality of access to data within the EHR system for statistical or research purposes. National health registries in Iceland are defined by law and regulations. Hence, if the Directorate of Health needs to add a new database for health monitoring, existing law and regulations need to be changed before data collection can begin.

In the United Kingdom (Scotland), development of datasets is limited by cultural and data governance barriers to data sharing. The United Kingdom (England) reports a need to demonstrate that data processing is fair and to implement a means for patients to express their preferences regarding use of their own data. Sweden reports difficulties securing information sharing among different jurisdictions. Further, as reporting requirements have increased with respect to health and data quality measurement, the costs of administering health care systems have also risen and there is resistance to reporting data for statistical or research purposes.

Among countries that are members of the EU, there is an opportunity to consider and potentially address unnecessary legal limitations to data use as the new 2016 *EU Data Protection Regulation* is implemented.[9]

Legislative prohibitions and other governance obstacles limit the use of data extracted from EHR systems

Several countries reported that their national EHR systems are only legally authorised to share personal data with health care providers for medical treatment purposes [Austria, France, Ireland, Japan, Switzerland and the United Kingdom (Northern Ireland)]. Spain reports a limitation to the extraction of data from the EHR system at the national level.

Australia, Israel and Ireland reported efforts towards legislative reforms that are under way. Ireland is currently drafting a new Health Information and Patient Safety Bill (HIPS) that will facilitate the ability to develop datasets from EHR systems. Australia is developing a secondary use framework that will enable the System Operator (currently the Secretary, Department of Health) to make informed decisions about the benefits, risks and costs of options presented for secondary uses of *My Health Record* system data. Further, Australia recently introduced legislation that adjusts the national EHR from an opt-in to an opt-out patient consent model. This change will improve the population coverage of the EHR system, increasing the viability of data from this source to contribute to statistics and research. Israel is launching a Big Data strategy that will explore the potential secondary use of EHRs through the national health information exchange.

Spain does not have national legislation or regulation to allow extraction of data from the national EHR system for national research or statistical purposes. As a result, databases must be administered by each Healthcare Authority (region). Spain also faces data governance barriers that limit researchers' access to electronic clinical data. These include a strong bureaucracy and a lack of written policies regarding how applicants may apply for access to data within EHR systems. Some ICT providers are reluctant to provide access to data for research and/or apply financial charges for accessing data that may limit data accessibility.

Canada reported that legislation protecting privacy in some jurisdictions may be limiting some secondary uses of data. Other data governance issues in Canada include defining the potential secondary uses of data and securing recognition within the health care system that data uses should be a policy priority. Further work is needed to address concerns of physicians and other stakeholders about the appropriateness of data privacy protections and the benefits of data uses. Canada must also address the legacy of specific programmes "owning" their data and, as a result, creating silos of unshared information; an issue also highlighted by the United Kingdom (Scotland).

In Singapore, health care organisations contributing to or accessing data in the National Electronic Health Records System are bound by a Data Sharing Agreement. In addition to the use of data for patient care, under the Data Sharing Agreement, the Ministry of Health may approve data use for research or statistical purposes, provided relevant ethical and legal requirements are met. Health care quality monitoring in Singapore is currently limited to specific, legally authorised activities, such as clinical quality assessment. Other important aspects of health data governance that require further work in Singapore include assuring patient, provider and public acceptance of data uses.

The development of datasets from data extracted from EHR systems is restricted in Japan and Switzerland. However, both countries recently authorised national cancer registries. In these countries the data will be first collected by regions and then submitted to the national registry. The data submitted to the registry will likely be extracted from local areas' electronic clinical record systems. These national initiatives could potentially advance future national discussions of the benefits and protections necessary to enable dataset creation for other key diseases and patient groups.

Meeting national health information needs with data from EHRs

A third aspect of governance is investing in health information development from data within EHR systems. Sixteen countries indicated that data within EHRs are currently being used to create datasets for health or health care monitoring and analysis and ten countries provided details about datasets and statistical projects under way at the health care system level (see Table 6.A2.3). For example, the Directorate of Health in Iceland builds many national datasets that rely on data extracted from the EHR system, including the Cancer Registry, Birth Registry, Registry of Contacts with Primary Health-Care Centres, Hospital Registry, Pharmaceutical Database, Communicable Disease Registry, Adverse Events Database, Database on Accidents and Cardio-Vascular Disease Database.

In the United Kingdom, for example, data from Scotland's EHR system are routinely extracted to develop many national datasets and registries. For instance, the NSS Discovery project in Scotland is an information system developed from the EHR system that provides approved users with access to a range of comparative information to support health care performance and quality improvement. In England, the National Tariff System captures EHR data from acute care providers to support statistics and reimbursement. The Calculating Quality and Reporting Service (CQRS) in England extracts data from primary care EHR systems to support monitoring, such as indicators for reporting progress against Quality and Outcomes Frameworks.

In Sweden, about 100 clinical research databases and Quality Registries have been developed from electronic clinical records, and several national health databases include patient data from EHRs. Sweden developed an ICT tool to detect health care-associated infections. When antibiotics are prescribed in Sweden, the cause is recorded in EHRs for follow-up and inclusion in databases for monitoring and improvement. Similarly, Norway's Medical Quality Registries and its National Patient Registry depend on data extracted from its EHR system. Norway also has municipal registries created from extraction of data from local EHRs. In Singapore, the *National Registry of Diseases Act* mandates health care institutions to notify the government of cases of reportable diseases and to furnish patient data for stipulated disease registries. The required information can be obtained through direct data extraction from the NEHR. For more detail regarding the results of this survey, see Annex 6.A2 and Oderkirk (forthcoming).

Several countries reported making significant use of data extracted from EHR systems to inform key national information objectives. Denmark, Norway, Sweden and the United Kingdom (Scotland) indicated that data extracted from EHR systems: contribute to monitoring public health, health care system performance and patient safety, and to health and health care research; facilitate and contribute to clinical trials; and support physicians' treatment decision making. Canada, Israel, New Zealand, Poland, Singapore and the United Kingdom (England and Northern Ireland) reported that four or five of these information objectives are currently supported through data extracted from EHRs.

3.2. Technical and operational factors supporting secondary uses of EHR data reveal key differences

The 2016 study examined a set of key technical and operational factors supporting the development of EHR systems that will contain high-quality data suitable for national monitoring and for research. These are among the same factors that would be considered when evaluating the quality of data within any statistical system and include data coverage, completeness, accuracy and usability. Countries with the highest technical and operational capacity are in the best position to develop national health information from data within EHRs (Figure 6.6).[10]

Use of electronic clinical records in physicians' offices and hospitals is high in many countries

OECD countries vary greatly in the degree to which primary care physician offices, medical specialist physician offices and hospitals use electronic clinical records. Eighteen countries reported that at least 70% of both primary health care providers and hospitals are capturing diagnoses and treatment information within EHR systems (Annex Table 6.A2.2). Conversely, Croatia, Mexico and Poland reported that less than one-third of primary care

Figure 6.6. **Technical and operational readiness in OECD member and partner countries surveyed, 2016**

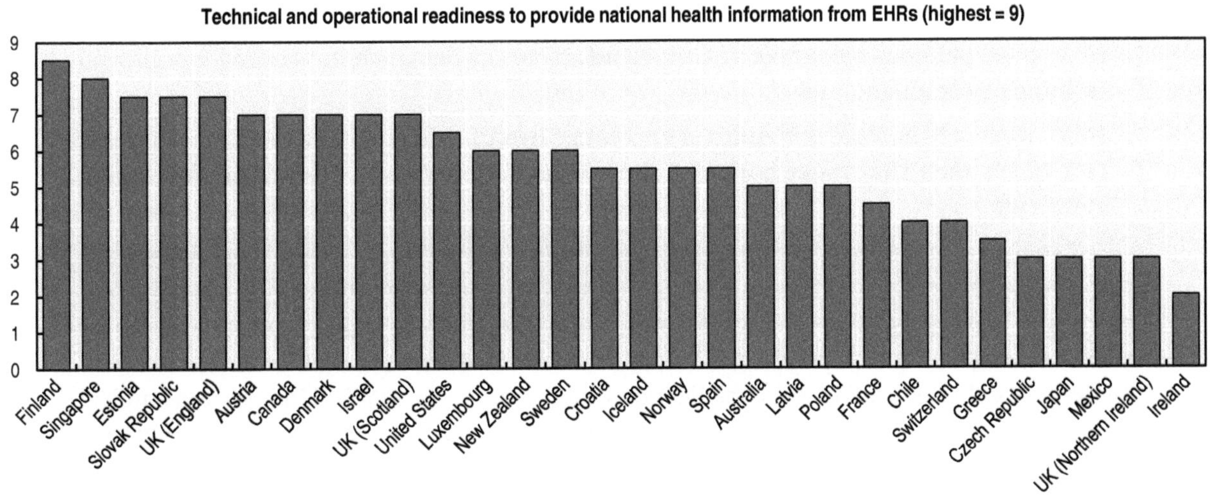

Note: See Table 6.A2.2 for the technical and operational readiness indicators.
Source: HCQI Survey of Electronic Health Record System Development and Use (2016).

StatLink http://dx.doi.org/10.1787/888933442999

physician offices use EMRs and Australia reported that less than one-third of hospitals use electronic patient records for inpatients. Further, several countries lacked the data to estimate the penetration of electronic clinical recordkeeping.

Most countries are implementing a national EHR system

Twenty-three countries reported that they are implementing a national-level EHR system (Table 6.A2.2). Eighteen countries reported comprehensive record sharing within one "countrywide" system designed to support each patient having only one EHR. A few countries have one national EHR system, but within it, some key aspects of record sharing are subnational only, such as within provinces, states, regions or networks of health care organisations (Austria, Canada, Spain, Sweden and Switzerland). Among them, all but Canada have implemented or are implementing a national information exchange that enables key elements to be shared countrywide.

Seven countries indicated that they are not aiming to implement a national-level EHR system at this time (Chile, Croatia, Czech Republic, Denmark, Japan, Mexico and the United States). Croatia and Denmark report aspects of record sharing that are comprehensive at the national level. In the other countries, sharing arrangements differ among health care organisations or regions.

Requirements on data structure and content standards vary

Countries were asked about the degree to which key data elements within EHRs are structured data elements. Data elements are structured by using a controlled vocabulary (a terminology standard) such as SNOMED-CT.[11] Data are entered, for example, using boxes, menus, codes or other aids to ensure they are entered the same way for each patient. Structured data can be easily extracted for monitoring and research uses because the data elements are comparable. Unstructured data predominantly comprise free-flowing text and are difficult to analyse (see Section 2.4).

The key factors supporting structured data are that:

- A national organisation is responsible for setting national clinical terminology and electronic messaging standards;
- All or most patients' electronic health records have key data elements coded to a clinical terminology standard; and
- Policy levers are in place to require or encourage health care providers to adopt electronic record systems that meet national clinical terminology and electronic messaging standards.

Twenty-one countries participating in this study reported that a national organisation is responsible for setting or recommending national standards for clinical terminology and electronic messaging. Electronic messaging standards, such as HL7, permit records to be shared among health care providers. Twenty-one countries reported that for at least three of five key data elements (diagnosis, medications, laboratory tests, medical images and surgical procedures), all or most patient records follow a terminology standard. Eight countries reported that this is true for all five key data elements [Denmark, Estonia, Finland, Iceland, Japan, New Zealand, Singapore and the United Kingdom (England)].

Ten countries reported that they use at least two of three policy levers (legislation, certification and financial incentives) to require or encourage health care providers to adopt EHR systems that conform to national standards for clinical terminology and electronic messaging (Austria, Chile, Estonia, Finland, Luxembourg, Singapore, the Slovak Republic, the United Kingdom [England and Scotland] and the United States).

Seven countries reported having legislation that requires health care providers to adopt EHR systems that conform to clinical terminology and electronic messaging standards (Austria, Denmark, Estonia, Finland, Luxembourg, Poland and the Slovak Republic). Eleven countries reported a certification process for the vendors of EHR systems that requires them to conform to national clinical terminology and electronic messaging standards and to use structured data (Chile, Croatia, Finland, France, Luxembourg, Mexico, Singapore, the Slovak Republic, the United Kingdom [England and Scotland] and the United States). Thirteen countries reported financial incentives to encourage health care providers to adopt EHR systems conforming to national standards for terminology and electronic messaging.

Almost all countries use national unique identifiers for patients and health care providers

Unique patient identification is essential to the development of a longitudinal EHR for patients that is complete and reliable while containing input from multiple health care providers over time. Unique identification of both patients and health care providers supports data quality checks and facilitates the linkage of EHR data to other health-related datasets for approved statistical and research projects.

Virtually all countries reported using a national unique patient identifying number (27 countries) in EHRs. The only exceptions were Chile,[12] Japan and the United States. Most countries (24 countries) also reported using a unique national health care provider number to identify health care providers who are entering data into EHRs.

Minimum dataset is defined but not adhered to in most countries surveyed

Countries were asked if they have defined a minimum set of data that could be shared among physicians treating the same patient. Minimum datasets are developed to promote standardisation of shared information so that clinically relevant and important information may be easily understood by treating professionals. The standardisation required for a minimum dataset also supports extraction of consistent information for monitoring or research.

Twenty-six countries reported defining or implementing a national minimum dataset (Table 6.A2.2). Very few countries, however, reported that EHRs of at least 90% of patients contain this minimum dataset [Australia, Croatia, Denmark, Finland, Iceland, Israel, Singapore and the United Kingdom (England)].

Data quality challenges and their solutions are tackled differently by surveyed countries

Countries that are investing in developing their health information systems with data from EHRs and in making these data available to advance health and health care monitoring and research encounter numerous technical and financial challenges. Ten countries reported that more than one definition of a minimum dataset is in use in their country, such that the content of the data is inconsistent among electronic record systems in different regions, different states or different networks of health care organisations [Australia, Austria, Canada, Chile, Ireland, Norway, Poland, Sweden, the United Kingdom (Northern Ireland) and the United States].

Reasons for this heterogeneity include: decentralised health care systems where different regions, states or health care networks implement their own minimum datasets and conform voluntarily to nationally recommended standards; a lack of national standards, leading to different software vendors offering different minimum dataset specifications; existence of more than one nationally defined minimum dataset (such as general and disease-specific specifications); and inconsistency in completion of required national dataset elements.

Seventeen countries expressed concerns with the quality of data within EHR systems and 14 countries indicated that these concerns limit their ability to develop datasets for monitoring or research. Specific concerns raised by countries include:

- lack of, or inadequate, terminology standards or the use of different terminology standards for the same terms (Canada, Croatia, Norway, Spain, Sweden and the United States)
- incomplete records or records that are not kept up-to-date (Iceland and the United Kingdom [England])
- variable quality of provider-level recordkeeping (Finland, Singapore and the United Kingdom [Scotland])
- lack of provider-level quality checks (Iceland and the United Kingdom [Scotland)]
- low-quality disease or procedure coding by some health care providers (Israel and Mexico)
- incomplete coverage of providers (Spain and Switzerland)
- incomplete coverage of structured patient summaries/minimum dataset (Estonia and Finland)
- inability to assure the data will be fit to fulfil multiple purposes (Australia)
- legacy systems that are difficult or impossible to adjust to required structure or standards (Austria, Canada)
- lack of standard formats and structure for dataset creation (Canada)
- inadequate patient identification for record matching across providers (the United Kingdom [Northern Ireland])

- transitional difficulties resulting in having to maintain duplicate paper and electronic records (Spain).

Solutions adopted in some jurisdictions that have already been described in this report could potentially address some of these data quality concerns. These include setting national terminology and interoperability standards; creating a nationally standardised minimum dataset; and using policy levers (legislation, certification, financial incentives) to encourage or require health care providers to adopt and use EHR systems that adhere to national requirements.

Auditing clinical record content is another key quality-improvement strategy that can help to reduce inconsistencies in record-keeping practices among providers. Nine countries reported instituting quality audits of the clinical content of records (Australia, Estonia, Iceland, Israel, New Zealand, Norway, Singapore, Spain and the United Kingdom [England]).

3.3. *Many countries are investing in EHRs to strengthen national health and health care monitoring and research*

Several countries noted specific recent strategic investments to investigate the potential for the health care system to gain valuable information to improve health and health care from the data within EHRs. Others reported regular processes to continuously evaluate and improve upon the health information already available from EHRs.

The United States *Meaningful Use Electronic Health Records (EHR) Incentive Program*'s Public Health Objective, Measure 3, encourages health care providers to submit data for specialised registry reporting. This programme enables the National Center for Health Statistics to develop national datasets to monitor health care quality and health care system performance. The United States also engages in and sponsors research to make easier the routine capture of health and clinical data in standard formats and terminologies that could eventually reduce the need to require structured data entry while still enabling record interoperability and statistical uses of data.

Israel is launching a new Big Data strategy that will consider how to better govern, integrate and benefit from large volumes of current, de-identified, personal health data from multiple sources. This strategy is intended to address barriers to the systematic use of data in the national health information exchange for research by examining different research scenarios. Australia is developing a secondary data use framework that will examine the benefits, risks and costs of enabling the data within the *My Health Record* system (an EHR) to contribute to national health and health care information and to research.

In Norway, the Directorate of eHealth, commissioned by the Ministry of Health and Care Services, recently evaluated the usability of electronic clinical data for statistics and research purposes. The results support an initiative called *One Patient – One Record* and are described in a report submitted to the ministry in January 2016. In Denmark, a national programme aims to increase accessibility of EHR system data in a secure manner across sectors for relevant statistical and research purposes.

France introduced a law to modernize the health care system that facilitates the use and sharing of health data for projects within the public interest. To facilitate its implementation, a reflection group was launched in 2015 to shed light on the development challenges associated with "Big Data" and on the emerging analytical methods to analyse such data. The group will present its findings in the second half 2016. France also has a committee monitoring studies about the use of medicines in the population using a variety of data sources, such as clinical cohorts, registers, health insurance data and EMRs. The committee periodically reviews obstacles to the realisation of these studies.

New Zealand has a national policy and processes in place to improve the sharing and use of electronic health data among government agencies.

In Iceland, real-time data are currently being collected and stored within the national hospital database. In the summer of 2016, real-time data from primary health care clinics were collected on a national level, creating new opportunities for monitoring and research. In Singapore, data are currently manually extracted from the national EHR system to create legally authorised disease registries and studies are under way to determine the feasibility of automating data extraction. Chile is developing a strategy for a national data warehouse populated with data extracted from EMRs. From the data warehouse, "datamarts" (data subsets) will be created for specific purposes. In the meantime, specific datamarts have been developed. Mexico also reports initiatives to build information products from EHRs for statistical, epidemiological and health care system planning purposes.

Sixteen countries reported having processes in place at the national level to regularly assess the usability of EHR data for dataset creation and analysis. When assessing potential data sources for national information systems, both Canada and the United Kingdom (England) reported conducting pilot studies at the point of care or at a local level. Canada also noted that it is essential to assess the readiness of jurisdictions to contribute data from EHRs and the readiness of the Canadian Institute for Health Information (CIHI) to manage new data. The Slovak Republic is planning a future process to evaluate the usability of electronic health data for statistics and research.

3.4. Countries' outlooks for the future reflect their position in the current continuum of health data use readiness

The results of this study indicate that many countries are poised to make significant advancements in both national health information and research as a result of the considerable investments they are making in EHR systems and in associated policy-relevant data and information products. While most countries were at the beginning of a journey to advance the statistical and research uses of data from EHR systems in 2012 (OECD, 2013a), many countries now report having developed datasets and published health information from EHRs to support better-quality health care and improved health care system performance (Table 6.A2.3). Countries are at very different points on this journey, however. Some demonstrate high data governance and technical and operational readiness to capitalise on this opportunity. Other countries are advanced in only one of these two dimensions, and a small group of countries are not advanced in either dimension (Figure 6.7).

Countries responding to this study were asked to provide their assessment of the likelihood that, over the next five years, any data from EHRs would contribute to regular national monitoring of health care quality. Countries reporting high data governance readiness and high technical and operational readiness also reported that it was likely or very likely that EHR data would contribute to national monitoring of health care quality over the next five years. The exception was the United States, where the outlook was uncertain.

Many other countries also expressed optimism that sufficient political and financial support will exist to overcome any remaining challenges to benefitting from EHR data for national monitoring of health care quality over the next five years. A few countries were uncertain as to whether sufficient progress would be made over the next five years to

Figure 6.7. **Data governance and technical/operational readiness to develop national information from EHRs in countries surveyed, 2016**

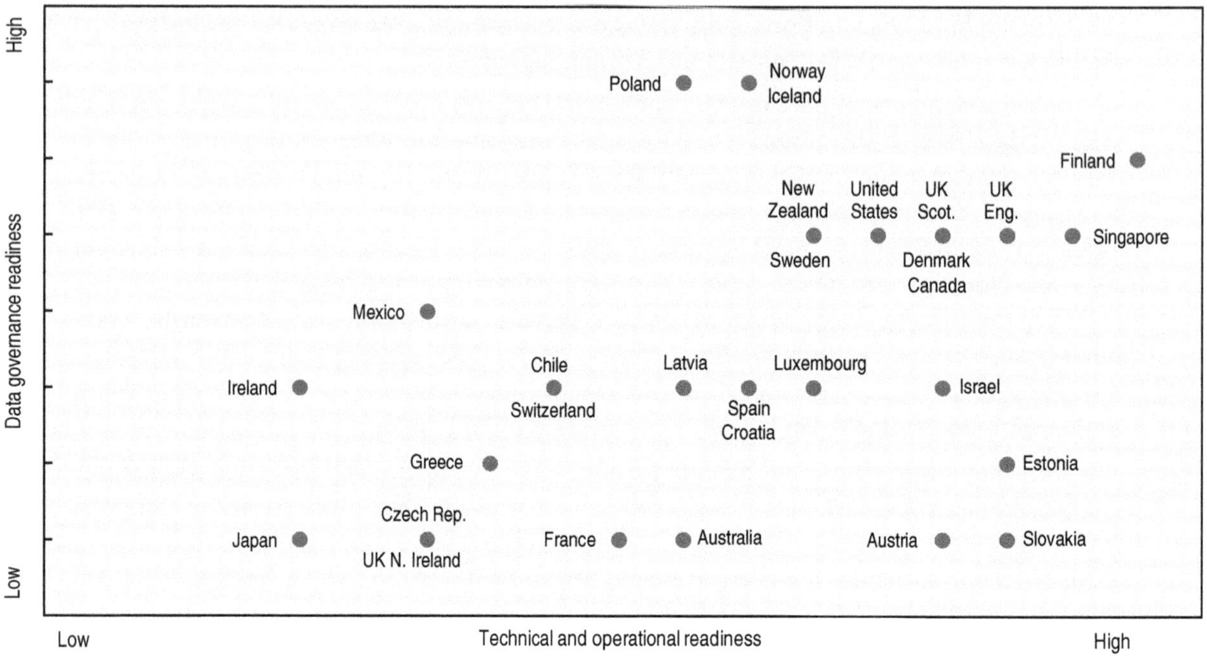

Source: HCQI Survey of Electronic Health Record System Development and Use, 2016.

StatLink http://dx.doi.org/10.1787/888933443009

enable this data use (Czech Republic, Israel, Latvia and the Slovak Republic). Six countries indicated that this data use is unlikely (Austria, France, Greece, Japan, Mexico and Switzerland). Reasons given included that the EHR system is not advanced enough and the use of data from the EHR system is not a policy priority.

Conclusion

The development and proliferation of digital technology represents a seismic, worldwide transformation that is comparable to previous technological revolutions. The lifeblood of this digital transformation is data. Increasingly vast amounts of electronic data related to health and wellness are produced by health care systems, by government and private sector services, and by individuals though daily digital activities. These data – including what is referred to as Big Data – collectively hold much potential information that can foster improvement in all health care system activities, from clinical care to population health, to research and development in the life sciences industry. Taken together, more intelligent use of data can go some way to realising the ideal of the "learning health system".

To realise the potential of health data, several challenges need to be overcome and risks managed. These include facilitation of interoperability and linkage between datasets, security and privacy of personal health data, legal and legislative concerns, human capital and expertise, and management of stakeholders, including providers and the public. At the health care system level, this involves complex socio-technical transformation, cultural change and political engagement. Implementing digital technology and the optimal management of data require considerable investment of resources. The return on this investment will very much depend on how changes are implemented and managed in terms of the challenges and risks described in this chapter. A governance framework comprising eight elements is provided to assist policy makers to maximise the benefits and manage the risks of health data. The OECD Council Recommendation on health data governance will boost countries' ability to get more from health data while protecting the privacy and dignity of individuals and groups (OECD, 2017).

A fundamental part of a health care system's information infrastructure is an EHR. A recent survey of 30 OECD countries suggests that much activity and investment in governance as well as technical and operational aspects of the EHR are currently under way. Countries are at very different stages of implementing and using EHRs to make the most of the health data they generate and contain. Some demonstrate high data governance and technical and operational readiness to capitalise on this opportunity. Other countries are advanced in only one of these two dimensions, and a small group of countries are not advanced in either dimension.

Notes

1. Other aspects of digital technology in health such as mobile health (mHealth) – smartphone apps, biosensors, wearable devices and (modern) TeleHealth – are discussed in Chapters 1 and 4. Chapter 5 is devoted to the data and information aspect of digital technology.
2. Stroke, hip fracture, breast cancer, schizophrenia, heart attack, premature newborns, hip and knee replacement surgery and invasive heart surgery.
3. In fact, many of the broader problems facing Big Data analysis have their epistemological roots in the previous two centuries (Robertson and Travaglia, 2016; Floridi, 2012).
4. Consent becomes an important consideration, and is discussed in the sections on legal and legislative challenges, and on stakeholder engagement.
5. The General Data Protection Regulation (GDPR) of the European Commission (Regulation EU 2016/679) encourages establishment of a certification mechanism for the purpose of demonstrating compliance. See *http://ec.europa.eu/justice/data-protection/reform/files/regulation_oj_en.pdf.*
6. The data governance and operational and technical capacities of members of the United Kingdom have important differences that are of interest to OECD countries and, as a result, they are presented separately.
7. The information in this section is based on countries' responses to the 2016 and 2012 surveys received by the OECD Secretariat. For more detail see Oderkirk (forthcoming).
8. The data governance and operational and technical capacities of members of the United Kingdom have important differences that are of interest to OECD countries and, as a result, they are presented separately in this report.
9. The Data Protection Regulation (EU) 2016/679 ("General Data Protection Regulation") will replace national laws transposing Directive 95/46/EC as of 25 May 2018. This Regulation provides for uniform rules regarding the processing of personal data, including sensitive data, which include health, genetic and biometric data.
10. This is not to indicate that all of these countries intend to advance the statistical or research use of EHR data, nor that they have the financial resources or plans in place to move forward. These aspects are discussed in the next section.
11. SNOMED-CT is one of several unified medical nomenclatures and vocabularies.
12. Chile uses a unique national number to identify citizens/residents. From it, a nationwide Master Patient Index service will be generated and provided to the health sector for use within information systems.

References

Aronson, S. and H. Rehm (2015), "Building the Foundation for Genomics in Precision Medicine", *Nature*, Vol. 526, pp. 336-342.

Bates, D. et al. (2014), "Big Data in Health Care", *Health Affairs (Millwood)*, Vol. 33, No. 7, pp. 1123-1131.

Brynjolfsson, E. (1993), "The Productivity Paradox of Infomration Technology", *Communications of the ACM*, Vol. 36, No. 12, pp. 67-77.

Brynjolfsson, E. and L. Hitt (1998), "Beyond the Productivity Paradox", *Communications of the ACM*, Vol. 41, No. 8, pp. 49-55.

Byrd, R. et al. (2014), "Automatic Identification of Heart Failure Diagnostic Criteria, Using Text Analysis of Clinical Notes from Electronic Health Records", *International Journal of Medical Infomratics*, Vol. 83, No. 12, pp. 983-992.

Cecchini, M., J. Langer and L. Slawomirski (2015), "Antimicrobial Resistance in G7 Countries and Beyond: Economic Issues, Policies and Options for Action", OECD, Paris, *www.oecd.org/els/health-systems/Antimicrobial-Resistance-in-G7-Countries-and-Beyond.pdf.*

Cha, A. (2016), "IBM and New York Genome Center's New Cancer Tumor Repository Aims to Revolutionize Treatment" [online], *www.washingtonpost.com/news/to-your-health/wp/2016/02/25/ibm-and-new-york-genome-centers-new-cancer-tumor-repository-aims-to-revolutionize-treatment/* (accessed 29 February 2016).

Chandra, A. and J. Skinner (2012), "Technology Growth and Expenditure Growth in Health Care", *Journal of Economic Literature*, Vol. 50, No. 3, pp. 645-680.

Darcy, A., A. Louie and L. Weiss-Roberts (2016), "Machine Learning and the Profession of Medicine", *Journal of the American Medical Association*, Vol. 315, No. 6, pp. 551-552.

Digital Health (2015), "IT Could Save NHS £13.7bn a Year: Kelsey" [online], *www.digitalhealth.net/news/29961/it-could-save-nhs-%C2%A313.7bn-a-year:-kelsey* (accessed 29 February 2016).

Duhigg, C. (2012), "How Companies Learn Your Secrets" [online], *www.nytimes.com/2012/02/19/magazine/shopping-habits.html?_r=0* (accessed 29 February 2016).

Eichler, H.G. et al. (2015). "From Adaptive Licensing to Adaptive Pathways: Delivering a Flexible Life-span Approach to Bring New Drugs to Patients", *Clinical Pharmacology & Therapeutics*, Vol. 97, No. 3, pp. 234-246.

Escobar, G. et al. (2014), "Stratification of Risk of Early-Onset Sepsis in Newborns ≥34 Weeks' Gestation", *Pediatrics*, Vol. 133, No. 1, pp. 30-36.

European Commission (2012), *eHealth Action Plan 2012-2020 – Innovative Healthcare for the 21st Century*, Brussels.

FDA – Food and Drug Administration (2015), "Sentinel Initative" [online], *www.fda.gov/Safety/FDAsSentinelInitiative/ucm2007250.htm* (accessed 29 February 2016).

Floridi, L. (2012), "Big Data and their Epistemological Challenge", *Philosophy of Technology*, Vol. 25, No. 4, pp. 435-437.

Frakt, A. and D. Pizer (2016), "The Promise and Perils of Big Data in Healthcare", *American Journal of Managed Care*, Vol. 22, No. 2, pp. 98-99.

Frankowvich, J., C. Longhurst and S. Sutherland (2011), "Evidence-Based Medicine in the EMR Era", *New England Journal of Medicine*, Vol. 365, pp. 1759-1759.

Gandomi, A. and M. Haider (2015), "Beyond the Hype: Big Data Concepts, Methods, and Analytics", *International Journal of Information Management*, Vol. 35, No. 2, pp. 137-144.

Groves, P. et al. (2013), *The "Big Data" Revolution in Healthcare*, McKinsey & Company, Washington.

Herland, M., T. Khoshoghoftaar and R. Wald (2014), "A Review of Data Mining Using Big Data in Health Informatics", *Journal of Big Data*, Vol. 1, No. 2, *http://dx.doi.org/10.1186/2196-1115-1-2*.

Jain, S. et al. (2015), "The Digital Phenotype", *Nature Biotechnology* Vol. 33, pp. 462-463.

Jensen, P.B., L.L. Jensen and S. Brunak (2012), "Mining Electronic Health Records: Towards Better Research Applications and Clinical Care", *Nature Reviews – Genetics*, Vol. 13.

Kaye, J. et al. (2015), "Dynamic Consent: A Patient Interface for Twenty-first Century Research Networks", *European Journal of Human Genetics*, Vol. 23, No. 2, pp. 141-146.

Liao, K.P. et al. (2015), "Development of Phenotype Algorithms Using Electronic Medical Records and Incorporating Natural Language Processing", *British Medical Journal*, Vol. 350, h1885.

Murdoch, T. and A. Detsky (2013), "The Inevitable Application of Big Data to Health Care", *Journal of the American Medical Association*, Vol. 309, No. 13, pp. 1351-1352.

Murff, H. et al. (2011), "Automated Identification of Postoperative Complications within an Electronic Medical Record Using Natural Language Processing", *Journal of the American Medical Association*, Vol. 306, No. 8, pp. 848-855.

Oderkirk, J. (forthcoming), "Readiness of Electronic Health Record Systems to Contribute to National Health Information and Research", *OECD Health Division Working Paper*, OECD Publishing, Paris, forthcoming.

OECD (2017), "Recommendation of the Council on Health Data Governance", OECD Publishing, Paris.

OECD (2016), "Ministerial Declaration on the Digital Economy – Cancún Declaration" [online], *www.oecd.org/sti/ieconomy/Digital-Economy-Ministerial-Declaration-2016.pdf* (accessed 11 July 2016).

OECD (2015a), *Data Driven Innovation for Growth and Well-Being*, Chapter 8: "The Evolution of Health in a Data Rich Environment", OECD Publishing, Paris, *www.oecd.org/sti/data-driven-innovation-9789264229358-en.htm*.

OECD (2015b), *Health Data Governance: Privacy, Monitoring and Research*, OECD Health Policy Studies, OECD Publishing, Paris, *www.oecd.org/publications/health-data-governance-9789264244566-en.htm*.

OECD (2015c), *Dementia Research and Care: Can Big Data Help?*, OECD Publishing, Paris, *www.oecd.org/health/dementia-research-and-care-9789264228429-en.htm*.

OECD (2015d), *The Proliferation of 'Big Data' and Implications for Official Statistics and Statistical Agencies*, OECD Publishing, Paris, *www.oecd-ilibrary.org/science-and-technology/the-proliferation-of-big-data-and-implications-for-official-statistics-and-statistical-agencies_5js7t9wqzvg8-en*.

OECD (2013a), *Strengthening Health Information Infrastructure for Health Care Quality Governance: Good Practices, New Opportunities and Data Privacy Protection Challenges*, OECD Publishing, Paris, *www.oecd.org/publications/strengthening-health-information-infrastructure-for-health-care-quality-governance-9789264193505-en.htm*.

OECD (2013b), "The OECD Privacy Framework", OECD, Paris, *www.oecd.org/sti/ieconomy/oecd_privacy_framework.pdf*.

Olsen, L., D. Aisner and M. McGinnis (2007), *The Learning Healthcare System*, Institute of Medicine (US) Roundtable on Evidence-Based Medicine, National Academies Press, Washington, DC.

Pang, T., M. Gray and T. Evans (2006), "A 15th Grand Challenge for Global Public Health", *The Lancet*, Vol. 367, No. 9507, pp. 284-286.

Parikh, R., M. Kakad and D. Bates (2016), "Integrating Predictive Analytics into High-value Care: The Dawn of Precision Delivery", *Journal of the American Medical Association*, Vol. 315, No. 7, pp. 651-652.

Robertson, H. and J. Travaglia (2015), "Big Data Problems We Face Today Can Be Traced to the Social Ordering Practices of the 19th Century", *London School of Economics and Political Science – The Impact Blog*, *http://blogs.lse.ac.uk/impactofsocialsciences/2015/10/13/ideological-inheritances-in-the-data-revolution/* (accessed 20 July 2016).

Scannell, J.W. et al. (2012), "Diagnosing the Decline in Pharmaceutical R&D Efficiency", *Nature Reviews Drug Discovery*, Vol. 11, No. 3, pp. 191-200.

Schneeweiss, S. (2014), "Learning from Big Health Care Data", *New England Journal of Medicine*, Vol. 370, No. 23, pp. 2161-2136.

Shah, N. and J. Pathak (2014), "Why Health Care May Finally Be Ready for Big Data", *Harvard Business Review*, 3 December.

Shah, N. et al. (2015), "Proton Pump Inhibitor Usage and the Risk of Myocardial Infarction in the General Population", *PLoS One*, Vol. 10, No. 6, e0124653.

Smith, T. and V. Suresh-Kumar (2013), "Applications of Big Data in Data Mining", *International Journal of Technology and Advanced Engineering*, Vol. 7, No. 3.

Sorenson, C., M. Drummond and B. Khan (2013), "Medical Technology As a Key Driver of Rising Health Expenditure: Disentangling the Relationship", *Clinicoeconomics and Outcomes Research*, Vol. 5, pp. 223-234.

Sun, J. et al. (2012), "Combining Knowledge and Data Driven Insights for Identifying Risk Factors using Electronic Health Record", *AMIA Annual Symposium Proceedings*, pp. 901-910.

The Economist (2010), "Data Data Everywhere" [online], *www.economist.com/node/15557443* (accessed 11 July 2016).

Vayena, E. and U. Gasser (2016), "Strictly Biomedical? Sketching the Ethics of the Big Data Ecosystem in Biomedicine", in B. Mittelstadt and L. Floridi (eds.), *The Ethics of Big Biomedical Data*, Springer.

Walker, J. et al. (2005), "The Value of Health Care Information Exchange and Interoperability", *Health Affairs (Millwood)*, Jan-Jun, Suppl. Web Exclusives, pp. W5-10-W5-18.

WHO Europe – World Health Organization (2016), *From Innovation to Implementation: eHealth in the WHO European Region*, WHO, Geneva.

ANNEX 6.A1

Risk-benefit evaluation tool for decision making about the processing of personal health data

Table 6.A1.1. **Risk-benefit evaluation tool for decision making about the processing of personal health data**

	Societal benefits		Societal risks
1)	Is the data use a/an:	7)	What is the Identifiability of the data required to successfully undertake the project?
	a) Ad hoc/one-time only research or statistical project?		a) Aggregated data that could be made public (anonymised data)
	b) Part of an on-going programme of scientific research?		b) Anonymised micro data treated to protect against re-identification that could be made public (public-use micro data)
	c) Part of regular reporting of statistics or indicators for monitoring?		c) De-identified micro data where ID numbers and other direct identifiers are encrypted or suppressed, and potentially identifying variables have been treated (aggregation, masking, swapping, suppression)
	d) To create or enhance an on-going data-set or registry?		d) De-identified micro data where ID numbers and other direct identifiers are encrypted or supressed
2)	Is the data use consistent with acceptable uses of the data?		e) Micro data with identifiers included (fully identifiable data)
3)	What will be the potential benefits of the project? Will results improve:	8)	Could the objectives of the study be realized if at any stage of the project, individual data are aggregated, stored and exchanged in aggregated format only?
	a) Health outcomes?	9)	Could a sample be drawn from the data or is full population data necessary?
	b) Treatments?	10)	Have data subjects consented to the processing?
	c) Patient health care experiences?	11)	Is the collection of informed consent of data subjects practicable to successfully undertake the project?
	d) Quality of health care?	12)	Is an exemption to patient consent requirements legally permissible?
	e) Efficiency, cost or affordability of health care?	13)	Are all elements necessary to grant an exemption to patient consent requirements fulfilled?
	f) Management or governance of the health sector?	14)	Is it necessary to seek the advice of a research ethics board or committee?
	g) Profits or market share for individual health system actors?	15)	Has a research ethics board rendered a positive decision?
	h) Growth of the health care industry or the economy?	16)	Is it necessary to seek the advice or decision of a data protection authority?
	i) Progress of science, research, or innovation?	17)	Has the data protection authority rendered a positive decision?
	j) Quality of health statistics?	18)	Have the custodians of the data involved rendered a positive decision?
	k) Expense or respondent burden of alternative data collection methods?	19)	Has a risk analysis (meeting appropriate standards) been done?
	l) Transparency or accountability of government programmes?	20)	Does the applicant have a track record of privacy protective data use?
4)	Who are the potential beneficiaries of the project results? Are they	21)	Would the data recipient fall under any legal requirements to protect the privacy of data subjects?
	a) Multiple societies/global population?	22)	Are there legal sanctions that could be applied if the data was misused by the requestor?
	b) Society/whole population?	23)	If a foreign applicant, does the legislative framework for the protection of data privacy in the foreign country adequately meet the legal standard of the home country?
	c) Patient groups?	24)	Is it necessary to transfer the data requested to the data recipient?
	d) Government/policy makers?	25)	Could a research data centre or secure remote data access system be used to provide the recipient with access to the data?

Table 6.A1.1. **Risk-benefit evaluation tool for decision making about the processing of personal health data** *(cont.)*

	Societal benefits		Societal risks
	e) Research community?	26)	If it is necessary to transfer the data….
	f) Health care industry?		a) How will the data be protected during the transfer process?
5)	What may be the potential impact of the project results on beneficiaries?		b) Are the data requestor's physical security and security policies and practices sufficient to mitigate risks?
6)	Are the proposed data sources and methods appropriate to realise the potential benefits?	27)	How vulnerable is the data to an outside attack during the transfer process?
		28)	How vulnerable is the data to an outside attack on the data security environment of the data requestor?
		29)	If there was a successful attack from the outside, how difficult or expensive would it be for the hacker to identify or re-identify data subjects?
		30)	What could be the harms incurred if an outside attack were successful?
		31)	How long will identifiable data (or data with a high re-identification risk) be kept before it is either anonymised or destroyed?
		32)	If approved, what will be the process used to follow-up with the data requestor to ensure that all of their legal and contractual obligations have been respected?

Source: OECD (2015), "Health Data Governance: Privacy, Monitoring and Research", OECD Health Policy Studies, OECD Publishing, Paris, *www.oecd.org/publications/health-data-governance-9789264244566- en.htm.*

ANNEX 6.A2

Key results from the 2016 HCQI study of electronic health record system development and data use

With a mandate from the 2010 meeting of OECD Health Ministers, the Health Care Quality Indicators Expert Group (HCQI) began surveying countries in 2011 regarding the development of national health data assets and their use to improve health, health care quality and health care system performance (OECD, 2013a). While all countries are investing in data infrastructure, significant cross-country differences were found in data availability and use, with some countries standing out with significant progress and innovative practices enabling privacy-protective data use, and others falling behind, with insufficient data and restrictions that limit access to and use of data, even by government itself.

This project included a survey of countries' development and secondary use of data from electronic (clinical) health records in 2012. Significant differences were uncovered in the design, implementation and governance of EHR systems between the 13 countries whose national plans or policies called for at least four different data uses and the 12 countries that were planning on fewer or no secondary data uses.

In 2016, this survey was administered again to report on the current status of EHR implementation and data use and to monitor progress since 2012. Twenty-eight countries responded to the survey: Australia, Austria, Canada, Chile, Croatia, the Czech Republic, Estonia, Finland, France, Greece, Iceland, Israel, Japan, Latvia, Luxembourg, Mexico, New Zealand, Norway, Poland, Singapore, the Slovak Republic, Spain, Sweden, Switzerland, the United Kingdom and the United States.

Three members of the United Kingdom are included in this study: England, Northern Ireland and Scotland. The data governance and operational and technical capacities of members of the United Kingdom have important differences that are of interest to OECD countries and, as a result, they are presented separately in this report.

Eighteen countries took part in this survey in both 2012 and 2016: Austria, Canada, Denmark, Estonia, Finland, France, Iceland, Israel, Japan, Mexico, Poland, Singapore, the Slovak Republic, Spain, Sweden, Switzerland, the United Kingdom (England and Scotland) and the United States. For these countries, results from 2016 are compared with those of 2012, where appropriate, in a forthcoming OECD Health Division working paper (Oderkirk, forthcoming).

The following tables summarise the key findings from the 2016 study. The detailed findings upon which these summary tables are based are published in the working paper (Oderkirk, forthcoming).

Table 6.A2.1. **Data governance readiness to generate health information from EHRs**

	Legal issues impeding creation of datasets and/or analysis of data from EHRs[1]	Three or more key secondary data uses included in national plans or priorities[2]	Creating datasets from EHR records[3]	EHR data contributes to three or more key monitoring or research domains[4]	Total (max = 3)
Australia	n.r.	0	0	0	0
Austria	n.r.	0	0	0	0
Canada	-1	1	1	1	2
Chile	n.r.	1	0	0	1
Croatia	n.a.	1	0	0	1
Czech Republic	0	n.r.	0	0	0
Denmark	-1	1	1	1	2
Estonia	-1	1	0	0.5	0.5
Finland	0	1	1	0.5	2.5
France	-1	0	0	0	0
Greece	-1	n.r.	1	0.5	0.5
Iceland	n.r.	1	1	1	3
Ireland	-1	1	1	0	1
Israel	-1	0	1	1	1
Japan	-1	0	n.r.	0.5	0
Latvia	n.r.	1	0	0	1
Luxembourg	0	1	0	0	1
Mexico	0	n.r.	1	0.5	1.5
New Zealand	0	n.r.	1	1	2
Norway	0	1	1	1	3
Poland	n.r.	1	1	1	3
Singapore	-1	1	1	1	2
Slovak Republic	-1	1	0	0	0
Spain	0	0	1	0	1
Sweden	-1	1	1	1	2
Switzerland	0	1	0	0	1
United Kingdom (England)	0	1	0	1	2
United Kingdom (Northern Ireland)	-1	0	0	1	0
United Kingdom (Scotland)	-1	1	1	1	2
United States	0	1	1	0	2

Note: "Yes" is 1 point, a "Partial Yes" is 0.5 points and "No" is 0 points. n.a.: not applicable; n.r.: not reported.

1. See Oderkirk (forthcoming), Table 11. A score of -1 indicates that legal issues impeding dataset creation or data analysis were reported.
2. See Oderkirk (forthcoming), Table 13.
3. See Oderkirk (forthcoming), Table 11.
4. See Oderkirk (forthcoming, Table 14. A score of 0.5 indicates 1-2 key statistical or research programmes were reported.

Table 6.A2.2. **Technical and operational readiness to generate health information from EHRs**

	At least 70% of primary care physicians and hospitals are using EMR	National system includes information sharing among physicians and hospitals about treatment, medications, laboratory tests and images[2]	Minimum dataset has been defined[3]	Key data elements in all or most records are structured (coded to a terminology standard)[4]	Unique patient and provider identifiers in EHRs[5]	National organisation is responsible for clinical terminology and electronic messaging standards[6]	Legal requirement to adopt EHR systems that conform to clinical terminology and electronic messaging standards[7, 8]	Certification requires vendors to adopt standards and use structured data[7]	Financial incentives or penalties to adopt and maintain high-quality EHRs[7]	Total (max = 9)
Australia	0	1	1	0	1	1	0	0	1	5
Austria	1	1	0	1	1	1	1	n.r.	1	7
Canada	1	1	1	1	1	1	0	n.r.	1	7
Chile	0	0	0	1	0	1	0	1	1	4
Croatia	0	0	1	1	1	1	0.5	1	0	5.5
Czech Republic	1	0	1	n.r.	0.5	0.5	0	n.r.	0	3
Denmark	1	1	1	1	1	1	1	0	0	7
Estonia	1	0.5	1	1	1	1	1	n.r.	1	7.5
Finland	1	0.5	1	1	1	1	1	1	1	8.5
France	0	1	1	0	1	0	0.5	1	0	4.5
Greece	0	0.5	1	1	1	0	n.r.	n.r.	0	3.5
Iceland	1	0.5	1	1	1	1	0	n.r.	0	5.5
Ireland	0	0	1	n.r.	0.5	0	0.5	0	0	2
Israel	1	1	1	1	1	1	0	n.r.	1	7
Japan	0	0	1	1	0	1	0	n.r.	0	3
Latvia	1	0.5	1	1	1	0.5	0	n.r.	0	5
Luxembourg	n.r.	1	1	0	1	1	1	1	0	6
Mexico	0	0	0	1	1	0	0	1	0	3
New Zealand	1	1	1	1	1	1	0	0	0	6
Norway	1	0.5	1	1	1	0	n.r.	0	1	5.5

Table 6.A2.2. **Technical and operational readiness to generate health information from EHRs** *(cont.)*

	At least 70% of primary care physicians and hospitals are using EMR	National system includes information sharing among physicians and hospitals about treatment, medications, laboratory tests and images[2]	Minimum dataset has been defined[3]	Key data elements in all or most records are structured (coded to a terminology standard)[4]	Unique patient and provider identifiers in EHRs[5]	National organisation is responsible for clinical terminology and electronic messaging standards[6]	Legal requirement to adopt EHR systems that conform to clinical terminology and electronic messaging standards[7, 8]	Certification requires vendors to adopt standards and use structured data[7]	Financial incentives or penalties to adopt and maintain high-quality EHRs[7]	Total (max = 9)
Poland	0	1	1	0	1	1	1	n.r.	0	5
Singapore	1	1	1	1	1	1	0	1	1	8
Slovak Republic	1	0.5	1	1	1	1	1	1	0	7.5
Spain	1	1	1	0	0.5	1	0	n.r.	1	5.5
Sweden	1	1	1	1	1	1	0	0	0	6
Switzerland	0	1	1	0	1	1	0	n.r.	0	4
United Kingdom (England)	1	0.5	1	1	1	1	0	1	1	7.5
United Kingdom (Northern Ireland)	1	1	0	0	1	0	0	0	0	3
United Kingdom (Scotland)	1	0.5	1	1	0.5	1	0	1	1	7
United States	1	0	1	1	0.5	1	0	1	1	6.5

Note: "Yes" is 1 point, a "Partial Yes" is 0.5 points and "No" is 0 points. n.a.: not applicable; n.r.: not reported.
1. See Oderkirk (forthcoming), Table 2.
2. See Oderkirk (forthcoming), Table 3. A score of 0.5 indicates that some aspects of data sharing among physicians and hospitals were reported.
3. See Oderkirk (forthcoming), Table 5.
4. See Oderkirk (forthcoming), Table 6. A score of 1 indicates that at least 3 of 5 key elements are structured in all or most records.
5. See Oderkirk (forthcoming), Table 8. A score of 0.5 indicates that there is a unique ID for only one group (patients or providers).
6. See Oderkirk (forthcoming), Table 9. A score of 0.5 indicates that there is a national organisation responsible for either clinical terminology or electronic messaging standards (not both).
7. See Oderkirk (forthcoming) Table 10.
8. A score of 0.5 indicates that there is a legal requirement for electronic messaging standards only.

Table 6.A2.3. Projects where data from EHR systems are used to regularly monitor and report on health care quality at the health care system level

	Project	
Canada	Title	Continuing Care and Residential Care Reporting Systems
	Purpose	To capture demographic, clinical, functional and resource utilisation information on individuals receiving continuing care services in hospitals or long-term care homes in Canada and use this information to support secondary uses such as decision making regarding funding and resource allocation (for example).
	Description	The clinical data standard for the CCRS was developed by interRAI, an international research network, and modified with permission by CIHI for Canadian use. The interRAI Resident Assessment Instrument Minimum Data Set (RAI-MDS 2.0)© is used to identify the preferences, needs and strengths of continuing care hospital patients or long-term care home residents and provides a snapshot of their services. The information, gathered electronically at the point of care, provides real-time decision support for front-line care planning and monitoring, as well as for health system uses such as facility management, resource allocation and funding. Pan-Canadian reports are regularly published using point of care information, with evidence that this information has been used by decision makers within their respective jurisdiction/organisation.
	Publications	Depression Among Seniors in Residential Care *https://secure.cihi.ca/estore/productFamily.htm?pf=PFC1432&locale=en&lang=EN&mediatype=0.* Caring for Seniors with Alzheimer's Disease and Other Forms of Dementia *https://secure.cihi.ca/estore/productFamily.htm?locale=en&pf=PFC1534&lang=en&media=0.* Resident Safety: Characteristics Associated with Falling in Ontario Complex Continuing Care *https://secure.cihi.ca/estore/productFamily.htm?pf=PFC1032&locale=en&lang=EN&mediatype=0.*
	Title	Acute and Ambulatory Care Information Services Demonstration Projects
	Purpose	The purpose of the AACIS data supply demonstration projects is to identify opportunities to improve or streamline the flow/reporting of data to CIHI by leveraging eHealth or digital health solutions such as electronic health records. Improvements of particular interest include reducing the burden of manual data collection, increasing data timeliness, expanding data coverage and evolving data relevancy.
	Description	The benefits anticipated from this project include: • Understanding extent to which an Electronic Health Record (EHR) system contains data elements required for Discharge Abstract Database (DAD) and National Ambulatory Reporting System (NACRS) • Quantifying the benefits that can be realised by health care organisations, jurisdictions, CIHI and the health care system by leveraging electronic data sources for health system reporting, planning and management purposes
Denmark	Title	Health Data Programme
	Purpose	To make health data from national databases and registries available for secondary use
	Description	A national programme aiming at making data available in a secure manner across sectors and for relevant purposes
	Publications	Information about publications provided upon request
	Title	Danish Clinical Registries (RKKP)
	Purpose	Improve the use of registries for clinical, research and managerial purposes
	Description	67 joint regional databases used for analysing clinical data from various sources
	Publications	Homepage of RKKP in Danish *www.rkkp.dk/in-english/.* English RKKP homepage *www.rkkp.dk/in-english/.* Internet link to the 67 databases *www.sundhed.dk/sundhedsfaglig/kvalitet/kliniske-kvalitetsdatabaser/.*
Finland	Title	AvoHilmo
	Purpose	Primary Care Dataset for monitoring and research
	Description	Extracting data from EHR systems to the primary health care register on daily bases
	Publications	Information about publications provided upon request
	Title	HILMO upgrade
	Purpose	Hospital Dataset for monitoring and research
	Description	Developing the hospital discharge register to better provide the data directly from EHRs
Iceland	Description	Continuous quality management of patient safety and quality of care by the Directorate of Health
	Publications	Annual reports. Information about publications provided upon request.
	Description	Continuous monitoring of quality of care to the elderly (RAI)
	Publications	Annual reports. Information about publications provided upon request.

Table 6.A2.3. **Projects where data from EHR systems are used to regularly monitor and report on health care quality at the health care system level** *(cont.)*

	Project	
Japan	Title	Monitoring of cancer incidence in Japan
	Purpose	To estimate national cancer incidence on the basis of data from regional cancer registries.
	Description	Internet link provided to a summary in English. *http://ganjoho.jp/data/reg_stat/statistics/brochure/mcij2011_report.pdf.*
	Title	Cancer statistics in japan
	Purpose	To collect information about cancer statistics.
	Description	Information about publications provided upon request. Internet link provided to a summary in English. *http://ganjoho.jp/data/reg_stat/statistics/brochure/2015/cancer_statistics_2015.pdf.*
New Zealand	Title	National Patient Flow
	Purpose	Gather information on the outcome of referrals into secondary care and the time to access treatment to understand demand.
	Description	A national system to collect health care information tracking patient movement and events from first referral to treatment.
Poland	Purpose	Data collection and analysis
	Description	Electronic Platform of Collection, analysis and dissemination of digital resources for medical events
Spain	Title	BDCAP
	Description	A database where the data have been extracted from EHRs in the domain of Primary Care. The system is operated by Regions and is co-ordinated at the National level.
	Title	RAE-CMBD
	Description	A database where information is extracted from EHRs and paper records manually regarding hospital specialties. The database is operated by the Regions and is co-ordinated at the national level by the Ministry of Health.
	Title	BIFAP
	Description	A system where information is extracted from EHRs regarding prescription medications, based on notifications on a voluntary basis from health care providers. The database is managed by the Spanish Agency of Drugs and Medical Products.
	Title	Pharmacovigilance system:
	Description	This system automates the extraction of data from EHRs at the regional level. The data is aggregated at the national level.
Sweden	Title	IT-tool for healthcare-associated infections
	Purpose	To prevent healthcare-associated infections
	Description	When antibiotics are prescribed the cause is recorded in the EHR for follow up and inclusion in Quality registries used for monitoring and improvement.
	Publications	Information about publications provided upon request. Internet link provided to a summary in English. *http://skl.se/halsasjukvard/patientsakerhet/vardrelateradeinfektioner.746.html.*
	Title	Quality Registries in Sweden
	Purpose	To monitor quality in health care and to encourage and refine best practice guidelines for clinical care
	Description	A system of National Quality Registries has been established in the Swedish health and medical services in the last decades. There are about 100 registries that receive central funding in Sweden.
	Publications	Information about publications provided upon request. Internet link provided to a summary in English. *www.kvalitetsregister.se/englishpages/aboutqualityregistries.2422.html.*
United Kingdom (England)	Title	National Tariff System
	Purpose	Reimbursement
	Description	Capture of data from acute providers to support statistics and reimbursement
	Title	CQRS (Calculating Quality and reporting service)
	Purpose	Monitoring quality of primary care
	Description	Extraction of data from primary care systems to support monitoring (e.g. against Quality and Outcomes Frameworks)
United Kingdom (Scotland)	Title	NHS NSS Discovery
	Purpose	Quality improvement
	Description	NSS Discovery is an information system that provides approved users with access to a range of comparative information to support performance and quality improvement.

Table 6.A2.3. **Projects where data from EHR systems are used to regularly monitor and report on health care quality at the health care system level** *(cont.)*

	Project	
United States	Title	National Health Care Surveys
	Purpose	The Centers for Disease Control and Prevention's National Center for Health Statistics (NCHS) is asking for EHR data for the National Health Care Surveys from Eligible Professionals (EP), Eligible Hospitals (EH), and Critical Access Hospitals (CAH) to fulfill the Meaningful Use Electronic Health Records (EHR) Incentive Programs Public Health Objective, Measure 3, submission of data for specialised registry reporting.
	Description	NCHS will register all types of providers that have first registered with the Centers for Medicare & Medicaid (CMS) and received a CMS Registration ID. Once registration is complete, the National Center for Health Statistics will determine whether the registrant is part of the survey sample. If so, the National Center for Health Statistics will contact the organisational contact to set up data submission with the expectation to submit according to survey requirements. For example, General Practitioners participating in the National Ambulatory Medical Care Survey will be requested to send data on all office based encounters according to survey requirements. Currently, we will register providers planning to attest for either Stage 1 or Stage 2 of Meaningful Use. Beginning in 2017, we will also register providers planning to attest for Stage 3.
	Title	National Hospital Care Survey
	Purpose	The National Hospital Care Survey is an annual survey conducted by the Centers for Disease Control and Prevention's National Center for Health Statistics (NCHS) in order to gather critical information from hospitals on important issues facing the US health care system.
	Description	NCHS Data first determines hospital eligibility to participate, which is followed by an annual interview on the hospital's characteristics. Lastly, hospitals are asked to send in an electronic data component, where eligible hospitals are asked to submit electronic health record (EHR) or Uniform Bill (UB)-04 administrative claims data for all inpatient discharges and Emergency Department and Outpatient Department visits.

ORGANISATION FOR ECONOMIC CO-OPERATION AND DEVELOPMENT

The OECD is a unique forum where governments work together to address the economic, social and environmental challenges of globalisation. The OECD is also at the forefront of efforts to understand and to help governments respond to new developments and concerns, such as corporate governance, the information economy and the challenges of an ageing population. The Organisation provides a setting where governments can compare policy experiences, seek answers to common problems, identify good practice and work to co-ordinate domestic and international policies.

The OECD member countries are: Australia, Austria, Belgium, Canada, Chile, the Czech Republic, Denmark, Estonia, Finland, France, Germany, Greece, Hungary, Iceland, Ireland, Israel, Italy, Japan, Korea, Latvia, Luxembourg, Mexico, the Netherlands, New Zealand, Norway, Poland, Portugal, the Slovak Republic, Slovenia, Spain, Sweden, Switzerland, Turkey, the United Kingdom and the United States. The European Union takes part in the work of the OECD.

OECD Publishing disseminates widely the results of the Organisation's statistics gathering and research on economic, social and environmental issues, as well as the conventions, guidelines and standards agreed by its members.

OECD PUBLISHING, 2, rue André-Pascal, 75775 PARIS CEDEX 16
(81 2016 25 1 P) ISBN 978-92-64-26642-1 – 2017